Personality and Motivational Differences in Persons With Mental Retardation

Personality and Motivational Differences in Persons With Mental Retardation

Edited by

Harvey N. Switzky
Northern Illinois University

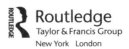

Routledge
Taylor & Francis Group
New York   London

Cover design is an image of the Roman god Janus,
the god of beginnings.

First published by
Lawrence Erlbaum Associates,
10 Industrial Avenue
Mahwah, NJ 07430
Reprinted 2010 by Routledge

Routledge
Taylor & Francis Group
270 Madison Avenue
New York, NY 10016

Routledge
Taylor & Francis Group
2 Park Square
Milton Park, Abingdon
Oxon OX14 4RN

Cover design by Kathryn Houghtaling Lacey

Library of Congress Cataloging-in-Publication Data

Personality and motivational differences in persons with mental
    retardation / Harvey N. Switzky, editor.
            p.   cm.
        Includes bibliographical references and index.
ISBN 0-8058-2569-X (cloth : alk. paper)
ISBN 0-8058-2570-3 (pbk. : alk. paper)
1. Mentally handicapped — Psychology. 2. personality development.
    3. Personality and motivation.   I. Switzky, Harvey N.
RC570.2 .P468   2001
616.82'88 — dc21   2001023009
                                                              CIP

Contents

Contributors

Elizabeth M. Dykens, Ph.D.
University of California, Los Angeles
Neuropsychiatric Institute and Hospital
Division of Child and Adolescent Psychiatry
760 Westwood Plaza
Los Angeles, CA 90024-1759

Linda Hickson, Ph.D.
Ishita Khema
Teachers College
Columbia University
Box 223
525 West 120th St.
New York, NY 10027-6696

Robert Hodapp, Ph.D
University of California, University Los Angeles
Graduate School of Education & Information Studies
Moore Hall
Box 951521
Los Angeles, CA 90095-1521

Steven Reiss, Ph.D
Nisonger Center UAP
Ohio State University
1581 Dodd Drive
Columbus, OH 43210-1296

Harvey N. Switzky, Ph.D. (Editor)
Department of Educational Psychology and Foundations
Northern Illinois University
DeKalb, Il 60115

Lisa Turner, Ph.D
Department of Psychology
LSCB 320
University of South Alabama
Mobil, AL 36688

James Van Haneghan, Ph.D
Department of Behavioral Studies and Education Technology
College of Education, ILB 104
University of South Alabama
Mobil, AL 36688

Michael Wehmeyer, Ph.D
Beach Center on Families and Disabilities
University of Kansas Teachers College
Lawrence, KS 66045

Edward Zigler, Ph.D.
Department of Psychology
P.O. Box 208205
Yale University
New Haven, CT. 06520-8205

Preface

The importance of the contribution of internal self-regulatory motivational and personality variables related to the outcome performance of persons with mental retardation has been sadly overlooked by scholars, teachers and practitioners within the area of mental retardation. In my opinion, internal personality and self-regulatory motivational system processes in learners with mental retardation have been ignored because of the historical reliance of the field on both Skinnerian behavioral models with their emphases on external stimuli as modulators of outcome performance, and on the rise of cognitive models that did stress that internal "thinking processes" mediated behaviour but left out the influence of mediational personality and self-regulatory motivational processes on outcome performance as well as the physical and social contexts in which learning and performance occurs (Belmont & Butterfield, 1971; Berkson, 1993; Bialer, & Sternlicht, 1977; Cobb & Bowers, 1999; Schroeder, 1990; Robinson, Patton, Pollaway, & Sargent, 1989). Concerns with developmental and internal self-regulatory motivational and personality processes per se were seen through a glass darkly, and viewed more as confounding variables needing to be controlled so as to allow practitioners and researchers to more clearly focus on the more important behavioral and cognitive processes underlying outcome performance (Switzky, 1999; Zigler, 1999. See also Zigler, this book). Without considering mediational personality and self-regulatory motivational processes along with contextual factors in determining outcome performance levels, both behavioral and cognitive models are inadequate for providing the foundation to increase the problem solving performance of persons with mental retardation (Borkowski, Day, Saenz, Dietmeyer, Estrada, & Groteluschen, 1992; Greeno, Collins, & Resnick, 1996; J. Heckhausen & Dweck, 1998; Switzky 1997, 1999; Zigler & Bennett-Gates, 1999).

Examining the literature of the last 40 years, there is considerable mention of the importance of motivational variables and their importance in facilitating the learning and performance of persons with mental retardation (Cromwell, 1963; Earl, 1961; Haywood, H.C., 1968; MacMillan, D.L., 1969; Siegel, 1979; Zigler, 1966). What is surprising is the lack of influence of this work on the field of mental retardation as a whole. This certainly was due to the narrow perspective of the dominant Skinnerian and cognitive information processing models which overshadowed all other paradigms to such an extent that motivational and personality researchers huddled together in self defense because they were viewed as heretical iconoclasts of the field (Switzky, 1999, E. Zigler, personal communication, August 7, 1995). Hence very little work on personality and motivation was disseminated to those who were concerned with improving the lives of mentally retarded persons.

Currently, interest in internal self-regulatory motivational and personality variables within a contextual and developmental framework has increased considerably and hence this book. One can only speculate about the reasons for this shift in paradigm and changes in the zeitgeist regarding mental retardation since the importance of motivational and personality have been recognized for many years even predating Skinnerian and cognitive models (Burack, Hodapp, & Zigler, 1998; Switzky, in press). The purpose of this book is to present both older and evolving newer models and applications involving personality and motivational operators to the field in order to demonstrate the power of motivational variables in understanding the behavior of persons with mental retardation with the purpose of enhancing the quality of life in persons with mental retardation and other developmental disabilities.

The book is organized into two parts: Part I which reviews the work of the few researchers who have investigated personality and motivational self-system processes, the Peabody-Vanderbilt and the Yale groups (Switzky, 1997). Part II presents a sampling of the new directions that have occurred within the last few years including theories of self-determination, theories of social intelligence and social decision making, the importance of biological factors influencing personality and motivational systems including psychopathological manifestations, the development of new omnibus theories of information processing linking cognition and motivation and performance based on the work of continental European theorists, specially Kuhl, and a new theory of motivation, Sensitivity Theory.

I would like to thank my mentor Carl Haywood for all his wisdom that he has imparted to me over the last 30 years. My fondest wish is that this book will stimulate generations of newer researchers to delve further into unraveling the intricacies of personality and motivational self-system processes in persons with mental retardation.

—Harvey N. Switzky

REFERENCES

Belmont, J. M., & Butterfield, E. C. (1971). Learning strategies as as determinants of memory deficiencies. *Cognitive Psychology, 2,* 411–420.

Berkson, G. (1993). Children with handicaps: A review of behavioral literature. Hillsdale, NJ: Lawrence Erlbaum Associates.

Bialer, I., & Sternlicht, M. (1977). (Eds.). *The psychology of mental retardation: Issues and approaches.* New York: Psychological Dimensions.

Borkowski, J. G., Day, J. D., Saenz, D., Dietmeyer, D., Estrada, T. M., & Groteluschen, A. (1992). Expanding the boundaries of cognitive interventions. In B. Y. L. Wong (Ed.), *Contemporary intervention research in learning disabilities* (pp. 1–21). New York: Springer Verlag.

Burack, J.A., Hodapp, R.M., & Zigler, E. (1998) (Eds.), *Handbook of mental retardation and development.* New York: Cambridge University Press.

Cobb, P., & Bowers, J. S. (1999). Cognitive and situated learning perspectives in theory and practice. *Educational Researcher, 28*(2), 4–15.

Cromwell, R. L. (1963). A social learning approach to mental retardation. In N.R. Ellis (Ed.). *Handbook of mental deficiency, psychological theory and research.* (pp. 41–91).

Earl, C.J.C. (1961). *Subnormal personalities: Their clinical investigation and assessment.* London: Bailliere, Tindall & Cox.

Greeno, J.G., Collins, A. M., & Resnick, L.B. (1996). Cognition and learning. In D. Berliner & R. Calfee (Eds.), *Handbook of educational psychology* (pp. 15–46). New York: MacMillan.

Haywood, H.C. (1968). Psychometric motivation and the efficiency of learning and performance in the mentally retarded. In B. W. Richards (Ed.), *Proceedings of the First Congress of the International Association for the Scientific Study of Mental Deficiency.* (pp. 276–283). Reigate, Surrey, England: Michael Jackson.

Heckhausen, J., & Dweck, C.S. (1998) (Eds.), *Motivation and self-regulation across the lifespan.* New York: Cambridge University Press.

MacMillan, D.L. (1969). Motivational differences: Cultural-familial retardates vs. normal subjects on expectancy for failure. *American Journal of Mental Deficiency, 74,* 254–258.

Robinson, G.A., Patton, J.R., Pollaway, E.A., & Sargent, L. R. (1989). (Eds.), *Best practices in mild mental disabilities.* Arlington, VA: Council for Exceptional Children.

Schroeder, S.R. (1990) (Ed.), *Ecobehavioral analysis and developmental disabilities.* New York: Springer-Verlag.

Siegel, P.S. (1979). Incentive motivation and the mentally retarded person. In N.R. Ellis (Ed.), *Handbook of mental deficiency, psychological theory and research* (second edition, pp. 1–61). Hillsdale, NJ: Lawrence Erlbaum.

Switzky, H.N. (1997). Individual differences in personality and motivational systems in persons with mental retardation. In W.E. MacLean, Jr. (Ed.), *Ellis' handbook of mental deficiency, psychological theory and research,* (third edition, pp. 343–377). Mahwah, NJ: Lawrence Erlbaum.

Switzky, H.N. (1999). Intrinsic motivation and motivational self-system processes in persons with mental retardation: A theory of motivational orientation. In E. Zigler & D. Bennett-Gates (Eds.), *Personality development in individuals with mental retardation.* (pp. 70–106). New York: Cambridge University Press.

Switzky, H.N. (in press). The cognitive-motivational perspective on mental retardation. In H. N. Switzky & S. Greenspan (Eds.), *What is mental retardation? Ideas for an evolving disability definition.* Washington, DC: AAMR

Zigler, E. (1966). Research on the personality structure in the retardate. In N.R. Ellis (Ed.), *International review of research in mental retardation* (vol. 1, pp. 77–108). New York: Academic Press.

Zigler, E. (1999). The individual with mental retardation as a whole person. In E. Zigler & D. Bennett-Gates (Eds.), *Personality development in individuals with mental retardation.* (pp. 1–16). New York: Cambridge University Press.

Zigler, E., & Bennett-Gates, D. (1999). *Personality development in individuals with mental retardation.* New York: Cambridge University Press.

Part I

Commentary:
Perspective and Retrospective

1

Looking Back 40 Years and Still Seeing the Person With Mental Retardation as a Whole Person

Edward Zigler

Yale University

In these pages I share some thoughts about the lessons I learned during 40 years of work in the field of mental retardation. While my principal focus is on the direction the science has taken, a primary lesson is that science is not an isolated enterprise. Over the years, I observed the vicissitudes of American history as they affected the discipline. Looking back, I see that many of the issues and purported solutions emphasized at any particular time represent the swinging of the historical pendulum. The path and speed of the pendulum are directed not only by knowledge derived from the latest scientific research, but also by political, economic, and social forces that have little to do with mental retardation but have a profound impact on professional approaches to it.

From a modern vantage point, the pendulum was launched during the mid-19th century when physicians such as Samuel Howe and Edouard Seguin attempted to treat people with mental retardation with dignity and compassion. Their efforts led to the rise of the residential institution, designed to provide retarded children and adults with education, humane treatment, and understanding in a place where they were valued and could succeed. The gesture that they should be treated "normally" progressed to the thought that they could become "normal." These hopes were dashed when, despite society's best efforts, individuals with mental retardation did not become smarter and succeed independently outside of the institutional cocoon. The treatment of retarded people then entered its dark age. Institutions became human warehouses where residents were hidden, neglected, and forgotten.

Parents of retarded children did not forget, however, and they fought for decent care. Their major victory was the passage of the Education for All Handicapped Children Act of 1975 (the predecessor of the Individuals with Disabilities Education Act or IDEA). The Act guaranteed children with intellectual and other handicaps a "free appropriate education" in the "least restrictive environment" and gave their parents clout and rights to assure that their special needs were met. Today, advocates are fighting for—and winning—the rights of individuals with handicaps to be fully included in the mainstream of society, exactly where they started at the beginning of this condensed history..

The science of mental retardation did not lead these changes but merely tagged along. Its growth as a science was, if anything, stymied by the moral and ideological battles surrounding the passage of the IDEA. No one wanted to be on the "wrong" side of the argument, which was based on human and constitutional rights. Recall that the IDEA was shaped by groups of "angry parents" and public officials sympathetic to minorities and other disadvantaged citizens they believed were wronged by segregation, prejudice, and denial of equal opportunities (Trent, 1994). The advocates' position drew on civil rights and constitutional guarantees, and they defended it in the courts and halls of Congress. Scientists were not invited into the process. In fact, "the validity of the methods and findings of behavioral science [was outwardly] rejected from the standpoint of an intellectual movement" (Jacobson & Mulick, 1996a, p. 3).

As the battle for public education for retarded children gained publicity and popular support, many scientists climbed on the bandwagon. Their endorsements gave the movement a degree of scientific credibility that it did not really deserve. A telling illustration is the push for normalization and deinstitutionalization that quickly gained momentum in the 1970s. Professionals supported these slogans although they had no evidence that these practices were of any benefit. Their enthusiasm drowned out their few colleagues who argued that research was needed to determine if these changes would do more good than harm and that institutions should remain in place until the findings were in (Zigler, 1978). As a result, institutions all but disappeared, but there is no proof that successors such as group homes are any better and there is some suggestion that they are just as bad or worse (Zigler, Hodapp, & Edison, 1990). Although not the same population, studies show that the deinstitutionalization of mentally ill individuals has had far-reaching, deleterious effects (Fuchs & Fuchs, 1995).

How did policies and practice in mental retardation drift so far from their foundations in knowledge (Paul & Rosselli-Kostoryz, 1997)? First, so called "best" practices have been determined by slogans and the loudest voices rather than by sound developmental principles; second, the current focus is on input, on where and what services are delivered, rather than on output, on how much progress individuals with disabilities actually make under the new system (MacMillan, Semmel, & Gerber, 1995). The science of mental retardation could be of great help in this area—at least it could have been before the discipline slipped toward "deprofessionalization," and the "elucidation of cognitive, affective, and behavioral functioning of people with MR [was] largely discarded" (Jacobson & Mulick, 1996a, p. 3).

I entered the fray shortly before research became irrelevant. There actually was a good deal of research being conducted, much of it focused on the intellectual deficits of mental retardation. How I moved from there to studying the personality dynamics in retarded functioning is the story of this chapter. Before I map the path my research took, I will discuss the positions I have taken over the years on some topics that remain contentious.

IQ VERSUS
SOCIAL ADAPTATION

Given the history of changing definitions in the area of mental retardation, definitions are a good place to start. While there is general agreement that the essential defining feature of mental retardation is lower intelligence than that displayed by the modal member of an appropriate reference group, there is disagreement over the meaning of intelligence that has only intensified in recent years.

One view is that intelligence refers to the quality of an individual's behavior assessed against some criterion of social adaptation. The polar argument is that a clear distinction must be drawn between underlying intelligence and manifest behaviors that are typically labeled "*intelligent.*" Inherent in this position is the belief that behaviors indicative of social adaptation do not inevitably reflect normal intellectual functioning any more than the relative absence of such behaviors in the psychiatric patient or criminal inevitably reflects intellectual subnormality. Researchers who espouse this view, including myself (Zigler, 1987), argue that the concept of social adaptation is much too vague and that the behaviors often placed within its rubric frequently stem from nonintellective influences. Supporting our position is the fact that measures of intelligence are very reliable and have high predictive validity, whereas adaptive behavior does not even have definitional and operational consensus and is far from having adequate standardized measurement (MacMillan, Gresham, & Siperstein, 1995; Simeonsson & Short, 1996).

However, in seeking a more satisfying definition of intelligence, this group, too, has reached no agreement. The fact is that definition making is an arbitrary exercise. This point is easily substantiated by looking at the similarities and differences in the definitions of mental retardation advanced by the American Association on Mental Retardation (1992), the American Psychiatric Association (1994), and Division 33 of the American Psychological Association (Jacobson & Mulick, 1996b), as well as reactions to them (e.g., Belmont & Borkowski, 1994; MacMillan, Gresham, & Siperstein, 1993). Obviously, even the professionals cannot agree on a "true" definition of the phenomenon. This proves to me that it is fruitless to argue whether a definition is true or false. The more appropriate point of contention is whether one definition is more useful than another with respect to organizing researchers' thinking and giving direction to empirical and treatment efforts.

With these criteria in mind, I, along with others, have argued that intelligence is a hypothetical construct having as its ultimate referents the cognitive processes of the individual, for example, thought, memory, concept formation, and reasoning. Approached in this way, the problem of defining intelligence becomes one with the problem of determining the nature of cognition and its development. The attention to development here owes much to classic works by Werner, Piaget and Inhelder, and Vygotsky, who all sought to understand mental retardation within the context of normal intellectual development (Hodapp, Burack, & Zigler, 1998). A review of the history of psychometrics some time later led Tuddenham (1962) to suggest that an adequate theory of intelligence must provide an explanation of the curve of change in cognitive ability throughout the life span.

The delineation of cognition and its development as the essential focus of intelligence, and thus of mental retardation, has a certain appeal since it relates so readily to at least one noncontroversial phenomenon that forever differentiates the retarded individual from one of average intellect. Two adults of quite disparate IQs (for example, one of 70 and one of 100) may be employed in the same occupation, participate in the same community and recreational activities, and each be happily married and raising families. In terms of social adaptation indices, these two individuals appear similar. However, when attention is shifted to the development and present manifestation of their formal cognitive characteristics, it is not difficult to distinguish between them. They function quite differently on a wide variety of cognitive tasks and on a wide array of psychometric measures that also assess, albeit far from perfectly, basic cognitive processes. The individual of IQ 100 is clearly superior to the individual of IQ 70 in meeting the cognitive demands posed by these tasks. Thus it can be stated with certainty that, at the peak of their intellectual development, the cognitive functioning of the adult with average intelligence is at a higher level than that of the adult with mental retardation.

If cognitive differences are approached from a developmental point of view, we can observe that a retarded child progresses through the same stages of cognitive development as a peer who is not retarded, but at a slower rate. The performance of a child with mental retardation will thus resemble that of a younger, non-retarded child who is at the same developmental level more than that of a nonretarded agemate whose cognitive system has matured at a faster rate. How well each child has adapted to his or her environment really does not matter in this comparison. we are looking at the sum total of cognitive processes each child has available or has mastered that are being looked at. This cognitive collection of course mediates inputs from the environment and responses that the child makes in efforts to adapt. But the quality and nature of their information-processing systems will continue to differentiate the retarded and nonretarded children as they grow , while their relative success at adaptation may not. Therefore, although many thinkers disagree with me, I believe that it is only through reference to differences in the rate of development and final level of formal cognitive functioning that the distinction between intellectually retarded and nonretarded people can be reliably drawn.

COGNITIVE VERSUS
MOTIVATIONAL DETERMINANTS OF BEHAVIOR

Now that I have presented a way to anchor an approach to mental retardation on a common ground—the nature and quality of cognitive processes—it must be noted that overemphasizing this basically sound position has resulted, at best, in incomplete and, at worst, totally erroneous explanations for the behavior of retarded persons. What happened is that workers generally concentrated on cognitive limitations and ignored other factors that could influence a retarded person's actions. What was often forgotten is that the behavior of retarded people, like that of all human beings, reflects a lot more than formal cognitive processes.

When I began my career, there was a clear tendency in the scientific literature to attribute *all* of the atypical behavior of retarded groups to their cognitive deficiency. Some of the more sophisticated theoretical efforts attempted to connect behaviors commonly observed in retarded individuals to specific hypothesized defects in the cognitive system. For example, ideas were put forth that retarded people suffer from a relative impermeability of the boundaries between regions in the cognitive structure, primary and secondary rigidity caused by subcortical and cortical malformations, inadequate neural satiation related to brain modifiability or cortical conductivity, impaired attention directing mechanisms, a relative brevity in the persistence of stimulus trace, or a dissociation between the verbal and motor systems.

I have long taken an adversarial stance toward the need to invoke such concepts when explaining differences in behavior between nonretarded and mildly retarded groups (e.g., Zigler, 1967). However, I have also defended these theoretical formulations as valuable in that they began to lead researchers away from a global approach toward a more fine-grained analysis of the cognitive processes of both retarded and nonretarded individuals. Thus, my contentions aside, the concepts on this list represent some of the most important programmatic theoretical efforts in the history of mental retardation research.

These concepts also comprise one side of the developmental versus difference controversy over the nature of mental retardation (Zigler, 1969; Zigler & Balla, 1982; Zigler & Hodapp, 1986). Difference theorists contend that all mental retardation stems from underlying organic dysfunctions that result in specific deficits in cognitive functioning and atypical cognitive development. Developmental theorists believe that this description applies only to individuals whose retardation is caused by organic impairments. Individuals with cultural-familial retardation are seen as those in the lower portion of the normal distribution of intelligence. They therefore follow the same overall pattern of development as nonimpaired individuals, but they progress at a slower rate and ultimately attain a lower asymptote of cognitive functioning. These predictions are referred to as the similar structure and the similar sequence hypotheses, respectively. To date, the majority of the research favors the developmental model (Bennett-Gates & Zigler, 1998).

It is not my intention to pick the winner of this long-standing controversy. I list some of the difference positions only to show how much theoretical and empirical energy was devoted to understanding the cognitive shortcomings of retarded persons. As the list of hypothesized cognitive deficiencies grew over the years, it became common to explain any differences in behavior between nonretarded and retarded individuals with a selection of one defect or another that appeared relevant. While the "defectol-ogists" thought they were on the right track, this fixation pre-vented researchers from dealing with the real complexities of the phenomena of mental retardation.

While no exception can be taken to circumscribed cognitive hypotheses concerning mental retardation, I must assert again that any cognitive theory of the behavior of retarded people is insufficient because few behaviors are purely cognitive in origin. While the analogy is far from perfect, consider that, as a group, children of lower socioeconomic status (SES) have lower IQs than middle-SES children. However, when differences in their behavior are found, IQ is but one of many factors considered in explaining them. Researchers look closely at the children's social environ-ments, educational histories, the child-rearing practices used in their homes, and the attitudes, motives, goals, and experiences that they bring to the assessment situation. In contrast, when dealing with children with mental retardation,researchers seem to assume that their cognitive deficiency is such a pervasive determinant of their total functioning as to make them impervi-ous to influences known to affect the behavior of everyone else.

This assumption is obvious in the research paradigm favored in the early decades of empirical work in mental retardation. Many studies employed comparisons of institutionalized, familial retarded children, many of whom were from the lowest SES, with middle-SES children who resided at home. These groups differed not only in respect to the quality of their cognitive functioning as defined by IQ, but also in respect to their total life histories and their current social–psychological interactions. Although individ-uals with mental retardation are generally no longer institutional-ized, they are still subjected to relatively more social deprivation and rejection than are those of normal intellect. Modern scientists are ready—even anxious—to invoke these experiences in explain-ing the behavior of children from lower-income families. Yet, in the case of retarded individuals, researchers still rely so heavily on the cognitive deficiencies of retarded individuals that they tend to ignore environmental events that are known to be central in the genesis of personality in individuals of normal intellect.

In defense of researchers who employed this paradigm, it could be argued that one need not be very sensitive to motiva-tional or personality differences between groups compared on tasks thought to be essentially cognitive in nature. In my opinion, such an argument is erroneous. Although it is true that the effects of particular motivational and emotional factors will vary as a function of the particular task employed, performance on no task can be considered the inexorable product of cognitive functioning, totally uninfluenced by other systems. Evidence in support of this point can be found in numerous studies that employed cognitive measures but found differences in performance to be associated with social class in IQ-matched individuals of normal intellect and related to institutional status in IQ-matched individuals of retarded intellect. Such findings lead me to reject the often implicitly held view that the cognitive deficiencies of the retarded individual are so ubiquitous in their effects that researchers may safely ignore personality variables which also distinguish our retarded subjects from their nonretarded comparison group. This strikes me as little more than a reaffirmation of a sound experimental dictum: A difference in performance on a dependent variable cannot safely be attributed to a known difference in subject characteristics (e.g., IQ) if the populations also differ on other factors which could reasonably affect, or have been demonstrated to affect, performance on the dependent measure.

The overly cognitive deterministic approach to the behavior of people with mental retardation stems from more than the implicit or explicit assumptions criticized here. It is also the result of the relative absence of sound empirical work dealing with personality factors in the behavior of retarded individuals. Had such a body of work developed over the years, it could have moderated the narrow cognitive orientation that for a time slowed progress in the understanding of mental retardation.

PERSONALITY MYTHS

Not only has relatively little work been done on the development and structure of personality in retarded individuals, but many of the views advanced have been inadequate and, in some instances, patently ridiculous. For example, in the early part of this century, a common opinion was that individuals of retarded intellect were essentially immoral, degenerate, and depraved. This point of view is apparent (and surprising, considering the source) in a statement made in 1912 by one of our nation's pioneer figures in mental retardation, Walter Fernald:

> The feebleminded are a parasitic, predatory class, never capable of self-support or of managing their own affairs. . . . Feebleminded women are almost invariably immoral and . . . usually become carriers of venereal disease or give birth to children who are as defective as themselves. . . . Every feebleminded person, especially the high-grade imbecile, is a potential criminal, needing only the proper environment and opportunity for the development and expression of his criminal tendencies. (In Zigler & Harter, 1969, p. 1066)

Unfortunately, the next half-century did not witness much abatement in the cliché-ridden and stereotypic thinking on the personality of retarded people. Several writers (Wolfensberger & Menolascino, 1968; Zigler, 1966) noted how some carried this deficit approach to the extreme, arguing that retarded persons represent a subspecies of less than human organisms. Not until the battle that led to passage of the IDEA did the realization spread that retarded individuals are fully human.

One cannot help but wonder why such prejudicial views about the personality of retarded people were perpetuated for so long. Some of this error can be traced to a common, but not necessary, outcome of the taxonomic practice of categorizing and labeling. It is fairly easy to differentiate people with respect to the rate of their cognitive development and the ultimate level of cognition achieved. The ability to differentiate quickly lends itself to categorizing and labeling individuals along some dimension of intellectual adequacy. The grossest example of this is the typical textbook presentation of the distribution of intelligence: A line is arbitrarily drawn through the distribution so that it intersects the abscissa at the point representing an IQ of 70, with everyone below this point categorized as mentally retarded.

If one is not careful, this straightforward and certainly defensible practice can subtly and deleteriously influence one's opinions of those on either side of the line. If one fails to appreciate both the arbitrary nature of the 70 IQ cutoff point and the fact that people are being divided on nothing more than the grossest overall measure of cognitive functioning, it is a short step to believing that those who are below this point are subnormal. Since the conceptual distance between "subnormal" and "abnormal," the latter with its age-old connotation of disease and defect, is minimal, it is tempting to regard those on the retarded side of the fence as a unitary group defective in all spheres of functioning and forever separated, by their very nature, from all persons possessing higher IQs.

This type of thinking is apparent in the general difference approach to the behavior of people with mental retardation. For years, researchers directed a large amount of scientific effort toward discovering how retarded individuals are different from more intelligent members of society, and very little attention was paid to how they are similar. I believe that, while the difference orientation might have had a certain viability in the early stages of investigations of cognitive differences between retarded and nonretarded groups, its value shrinks drastically when it comes to the issue of personality differences. Indeed, the difference orientation in the personality sphere is indefensible when it generates stereotypes such as those portrayed by Fernald.

The great heterogeneity in personality that one can grossly observe in any group of retarded individuals makes it unlikely that a particular set of personality traits is an invariable feature of low intelligence. In this group are people who are shy and gregarious, timid and outgoing, serious and frivolous. Retardation cannot explain these differences. It seems more parsimonious to me to view the development of personality in retarded individuals as no different in nature than the development of personality in individuals of normal intellect.

PERSONALITY DEVELOPMENT

Once we accept such a view, we can turn our attention away from personality traits thought to manifest themselves as a consequence of intellectual retardation and toward those particular experiences in the socialization process which give rise to the emotional and motivational features that constitute the personality structure. When researchers shift their orientation in this way, they may discover that the personality of a retarded individual will be like that of a nonretarded individual in those instances where the two have had similar socialization histories. One might also expect differences to the extent that their socialization histories differ. This is not to deny the influence of innate differences in temperament and personality style that contribute to individuality. These innate elements alone speak against some personality pattern supposedly unique to mental retardation and shared by everyone whose intellectual features led them to be labeled as retarded. By appreciating the contributions of both nature and nurture, researchers can begin to look for the source of variations in personality functioning between groups of retarded and nonretarded individuals, as well as intragroup variation—a search that will be far more productive than one confined to stereotypes and IQ scores.

If the process of personality development is the same regardless of IQ level, how do we explain the common finding of stylistic differences between groups of retarded children and middle-SES children of normal intellect. This finding does not contradict my thesis at all if one remembers that many children with mental retardation have had very depriving and atypical social histories. However, one must keep in mind that their backgrounds, and the extent to which they are atypical, may vary from one retarded child to the next. Two sets of parents who are themselves retarded may provide quite different rearing environments for their children. At one extreme, we may find a retarded child who is ultimately removed from the home, not because of low intelligence, but because the home represents an especially poor environment. At the other extreme, a retarded set of parents may provide their children with a relatively normal home even though it might differ in certain important respects—values, goals, attitudes, and opportunities for learning—from a home in which the family is of average or superior intelligence.

In the first example, the child not only experiences a quite different socialization history while still living at home, but also differs from the child in the second situation to the extent that residential placement has its own effects on personality. Add a third child who is not retarded and lives with parents of average intelligence and economic means. The difference in life experiences between child one and child three is enormous. Yet, much of our knowledge about personality features in mental retardation was derived from just such a comparison. One cannot help but wonder how many of the differences discovered reflected the effects of institutionalization, the factors that led to the child's institutionalization, or some complex interaction between these factors, rather than some purely cognitive aspect of mental retardation.

To add even more complexity, the socialization histories of many cultural-familial retarded persons differ markedly from the histories of retarded individuals who are organically impaired. Those with organic etiologies do not show the same gross differences from the nonretarded population in the frequency of good versus poor family environments. They do differ, however, from both the cultural-familial retarded and nonretarded groups in their pattern of cognitive development. Because of genes, biochemistry, or environmental insult, their cognitive apparatus is damaged and/or its functioning impaired. Their intellectual performance, therefore, has operating features that deviate from the norm. Years ago, I proposed a two-group approach to mental retardation in which cultural-familial retardation is conceptualized as the lower part of the normal distribution of intelligence (Zigler, 1967). Thus the same rules that govern normal development would still apply. Retarded individuals with organic etiologies have their own distribution located to the left of the normal curve, with a small amount of overlap. Their cognitive development follows different rules imposed by the particular type of damage their neural systems suffered.

Amazing advances in medical research have now pinpointed many types of damage and their results in behavior and development (see Hodapp, Burack, & Zigler, 1990; Pennington & Bennetto, 1998). However, these leaps in science have not uncovered any new explanations for cultural-familial retardation, supporting my belief that these individuals received a genetic draw that places them at the lower end of the normal IQ distribution— which, by definition, must have a low end as well as a high end. Furthermore, genes are not linked to personality as closely as they are to intelligence, although scientists are beginning to identify certain behavioral phenotypes in specific types of organic retardation (Dykens, 1999).

In the face of this complexity, it is not necessary to consider the problem unassailable, nor to assert that each retarded child is so unique that it is impossible to isolate the ontogenesis of those factors that are important in determining level of functioning. I believe we should conceptualize retarded persons as essentially rational human beings, responding to environmental events in much the same way as individuals of normal intellect. Then (unless science eventually proves otherwise), we can allow our knowledge of normal personality development to give direction to our efforts.

This does not mean that the importance of lowered intelligence per se can be ignored, since personality traits and behavior patterns do not develop in a vacuum. However, many features of personality can arise from environmental factors that have little or nothing to do with intellectual endowment. For example, the effects of residential placement may be constant, regardless of the person's intelligence level. In other instances, one must think in terms of an interaction; that is, given a lowered intellectual ability, a person will have certain experiences and develop certain behavior patterns different from those of a person with higher intelligence. An obvious example is the greater amount of failure that retarded individuals typically experience. Again, though, what must be emphasized is that the behavior pattern developed as a result of this history may not differ in kind or ontogenesis from that developed by individuals of normal intellect who, by some environmental circumstance, also experience an inordinate amount of failure. Similarly, one can expect the behavior of retarded persons who are treated to a more typical history of success to be more typical, independent of their intellectual level.

This last statement, alluding to changes in behavior through the manipulation of the experiences that affect motivation, prompts me to raise a note of caution. Some knowledgeable workers (Milgram, 1969; Zeaman, 1968) attributed to me a motivational theory of mental retardation. This is an error. I have never asserted that motivation is responsible for the deficiency in retarded functioning. I consider the essential difference between retarded and nonretarded individuals to be cognitive. No amount of change in the motivational structure of retarded persons will make them intellectually normal, when normalcy is defined in terms of those formal cognitive processes discussed at the outset of this chapter. However, one can speak of improving the performance of a retarded individual on a task, through the manipulation of motivational factors, to the extent that performance on that task is influenced by more than the cognitive demands it poses.

This point is especially crucial when one considers the everyday social competence of the retarded individual. Even a complete overhaul of the motivational structure will not make it possible for him or her to become a rocket scientist. However, rather circumscribed changes in motivation may make the difference between successful and unsuccessful employment at an occupation that has cognitive demands within the limits of that person's cognitive ability. My point is that a concern with motivational factors holds no promise of a dramatic cure for mental retardation, defined in terms of its essential cognitive foundation. A motivational approach does hold the promise of informing workers how to help people with mental retardation to utilize their intellectual capacity optimally.

Although not terribly dramatic, this goal is at least realistic. It is also of the utmost social importance in light of the now well-documented evidence that the everyday adjustment of the majority of retarded people residing in our communities is more a function of personality than it is of cognitive ability. Such evidence bolsters a recurring theme in my thinking: As important as the formal cognitive processes are, their roles have been overestimated, especially with respect to the everyday demands of many jobs and social situations.

THE RISE AND FALL OF STUDIES
OF PERSONALITY

Over the years, my colleagues and I attempted to delineate a number of motivational variables not necessarily unique to retarded persons, but ones commonly observed in their behavior as a group. We gathered evidence to demonstrate that the performance of retarded persons, which many attributed to cognitive shortcomings, is often the product of particular motives. We have also been interested in discovering the particular experiences that give rise to particular motives, attitudes, and styles of problem solving and how variation in these experiences leads to variation in the personality features of individuals of both retarded and normal intellect. This interest does not mean that we invariably championed the importance of motivational over cognitive variables, since it is clear that both, independently and in interaction, influence performance on any given task. Our studies made us aware that, while it is conceptually feasible to draw a distinction between cognitive and motivational operants in behavior, this division is difficult if not totally artificial in practice.

Our contributions to the understanding of personality functioning in mental retardation began at a time when care and treatment practices were radically different than they are today. Many of the participants in our (and others') research resided in institutions where they experienced much more social deprivation than later generations of retarded individuals, most of whom reside in the community, yet many of the personality features we identified were not peculiar to institutional residents but were also observed to some extent in our noninstitutional groups. Traits such as low expectancy of success, fear of failure, need for social reinforcement, outerdirectedness, and overdependency were often found to affect our retarded subjects regardless of where they lived. This is not really surprising because people of low intelligence undoubtedly fail more, rely more on adults to help them, and experience social rejection more than people with greater intellectual endowment. This is as true today as it was when institutions were common. In fact, now that children with mental retardation are exposed more to nonretarded peers in mainstreamed or fully inclusive classrooms, their shortcomings may be more obvious and the effects on motivation more pronounced. This is an empirical question that unfortunately has not been given the serious attention that it—and the children with mental retardation affected—deserve.

Nor does the demise of the residential institution erase the relevance of social deprivation to the behavior of retarded individuals. Even though the ability to identify specific causes of mental retardation has become highly sophisticated over the years, about half of the retarded population is still classified as having a "subcultural" or cultural-familial etiology (Simonoff, Bolton, & Rutter, 1998; Zigler & Hodapp, 1986). This type of retardation is most common in the lower SES, which can be a more socially depriving environment than that available in wealthier surroundings. Thus, social deprivation can still be a driving factor in the performance and personality development of many individuals with mental retardation.

Most unfortunately, the serious study of personality features in mental retardation has dwindled in recent decades. An exception is the increased attention to psychiatric disorders and dual diagnosis in the clinical literature (Dykens, 1998). Perhaps the importance of this type of work was overshadowed by the exciting advances that have occurred in biogenetic and biochemical fields. A review of the mental retardation literature since 1975 revealed that the number of studies published each year (about 1,000) remained relatively constant (King, State, Shah, Davanzo, & Dykens, 1997). The focus, however, shifted. In the past decade, proportionately more work was conducted in the areas of diagnosis, classification, epidemiology, and genetics than in psychology, etiology, or rehabilitation. I have no complaints with the interest in nonpsychological features of mental retardation. My complaint is that, like the narrow interest in low IQ in earlier years, the rest of the retarded person is being ignored. Yet that person still has a personality—a complex array of motivational and emotional features that permeate his or her everyday functioning. And unlike the categorical issues or genetic properties, these are features we can work with to help that functioning be more adaptive. The rest of this chapter describes the theoretical and empirical origins of the approach to mental retardation that I have pursued.

THE LEWIN-KOUNIN
FORMULATION

My work began in the late 1950s when my graduate school advisor, Harold Stevenson, and I became interested in the Lewin-Kounin rigidity formulation. Back then, this theory had a strong influence on how mental retardation was conceptualized as well as on treatment and training practices (see Zigler, 1962).

The essence of the Lewin-Kounin theory is that, due to the nature of the development of retarded individuals, they are inherently more rigid than are chronologically younger, nonretarded people who are at the same mental age level. This view derived initially from Lewin's general behavior theory. He saw the individual as a dynamic system and explained individual differences as arising from differences in the structure of the total system, the material and state of the system, or its meaningful content. The first two factors played the most important role in Lewin's theory of mental retardation. He viewed the retarded child as cognitively less differentiated, that is, having fewer regions in the cognitive structure, than an intellectually average child of the same chronological age. Thus, with respect to the number of cognitive regions, the retarded child resembles a nonretarded younger child. However, in terms of the material and state of the system, Lewin (1936) argued that these children are still not cognitively similar. He conceived "the major dynamic difference" between a retarded and a nonretarded child of the same degree of differentiation to be "a greater stiffness, a smaller capacity for dynamic rearrangement in the psychical systems of the former."

Lewin presented a considerable amount of observational and anecdotal material, as well as the findings of one experiment, to support his theoretical position. His findings, however, were ambiguous at best. It was left for Kounin to provide stronger empirical support for the hypothesis that retarded individuals are more rigid than nonretarded individuals.

Kounin (1941a, 1941b, 1948) advanced the view that rigidity is a positive, monotonic function of chronological age. By "rigidity," Kounin, like Lewin, was referring to "that property of a functional boundary which prevents communication between neighboring regions" and not to phenotypic rigid behaviors, as such. Thus, with increasing chronological age, the individual becomes more differentiated, that is, has more cognitive regions, which results in a lower incidence of rigid behaviors; at the same time, the boundaries between regions become less permeable.

Kounin offered evidence from five experiments in which he employed older and younger retarded individuals and nonretarded comparisons. (It is important to note that only the retarded participants resided in institutions.) Degree of differentiation was controlled by equating the groups on mental age. The children were presented with a variety of similar tasks. For example, they were first instructed to draw cats until satiated and then to draw bugs until satiated, or first told to lower a lever and then to raise it to release marbles.

As predicted from the Lewin-Kounin hypothesis, the nonretarded group showed the greatest amount of transfer effects from task to task, the younger retarded group a lesser amount, and the older retarded group the least amount of transfer. That is, following satiation on the first task, both retarded groups performed longer on the second task than did their nonretarded peers. Kounin also found that the retarded individuals spent considerably more total time on the tedious tasks, a finding not derivable from the Lewin-Kounin formulation. This he attributed to the "rigid state" of people with mental retardation, which spells itself out behaviorally in persistence on boring tasks. Another unpredicted finding was that the older retarded group had a negative "cosatiation" score; that is, the group spent less time on the first task than on subsequent, highly similar tasks. I will say more about this rather intriguing finding later.

On the lever-pressing task, the greatest number of errors (lowering rather than raising the lever on task two) was made by the nonretarded group, the least number by the older retarded group, and the younger retarded children fell in between. Note that on this task the lesser "rigidity," as defined by Lewin and Kounin, of the nonretarded group resulted in a higher incidence of behavioral responses often characterized as rigid, that is, perseverative responses. In the retarded participants, there was a lack of influence of one region on another. This resulted in fewer errors on task two because they were "psychologically" placed into a new region by instructions ("push down; now push up"). In those instances where they must move from one region to another on their own, the Lewin-Kounin formulation predicts more difficulty and thus more errors.

This prediction was confirmed in Kounin's concept-switching task, consisting of a deck of cards that could be sorted on the basis of one (form) or another (color) principle. Participants were first asked to sort the cards and then asked to sort them some other way. Here the nonretarded group had the least difficulty, and the older retarded group the most difficulty, in shifting from one sorting principle to another. Thus, when they must move through a cognitive boundary on their own, older retarded individuals make more perseverative responses.

The Lewin-Kounin theory is a conceptually demanding one in that it sometimes predicts a higher, and sometimes a lower, incidence of "rigid" behaviors in retarded compared to nonretarded individuals. However, the fact that it generates specific predictions as to when one or the other state of affairs will obtain is a tribute to this theory. Kounin's work seemed to offer impressive experimental support for the formulation as well.

Stevenson and I (1957) conducted a study to test the validity of the Lewin-Kounin theory. We investigated the ability of retarded and nonretarded children to acquire one response and then to switch to a new response in a discrimination-learning situation. Moving from Kounin's postulate that the boundaries between cognitive regions are more rigid in mental retardation, we hypothesized that the solution of a reversal problem would require movement to a new region and thus would be more difficult for retarded children. We chose as our measure the incidence of previously correct responses during the solution of the second problem, reasoning that such a perseverative response following the switch is the most direct evidence that the child has remained in a prior region.

We employed younger and older institutionalized retarded children and a nonretarded group, all equated on mental age. We found a striking equivalence in performance among groups. They did not differ on the number of trials required to learn the initial discrimination problem, on the number of correct choices on the reversal problem, or on the direct measure of rigidity employed (the frequency with which they made the response on the reversal problem which had been correct on the initial problem).

Stevenson and I entertained the possibility that this switching problem was too easy to allow group differences to be observed. We therefore conducted a second experiment using a more difficult problem. This time we rejected the Lewin-Kounin formulation, testing instead the hypothesis that rigidity is a general behavior mechanism related to the complexity of the task at hand. We predicted that the frequency of rigid responses (perseverations) would be greater for both the nonretarded and the retarded groups on the more difficult reversal problem, but that there would be no differences between the groups. All predictions were confirmed, forming evidence against the Lewin-Kounin formulation.

SOCIAL DEPRIVATION AND MOTIVATION FOR SOCIAL REINFORCEMENT

In pondering the disagreement of our findings with those of Kounin, Stevenson and I directed our thinking to the differences in tasks employed across the two sets of experiments and, probably more important, to the characteristics of the participants that could have influenced their performance. Beyond IQ, the most obvious characteristic was that the retarded groups lived in institutions where they probably did not have many positive social contacts. As for the differences in tasks, in our studies the participants had minimal interaction with the experimenter, while on Kounin's tasks they received instructions from an adult. We began to wonder whether Kounin's retarded groups played longer on his tasks not because they were rigid, but because they wanted to prolong the social contact. Our participants, on the other hand, had little opportunity to interact with the experimenter and thus no reason to persevere. We thus evolved the hypothesis that institutionalized retarded children are relatively deprived of adult contact and approval, so they have a higher motivation to procure these desirables than do nonretarded children.

In our first test of this motivational hypothesis (Zigler, Hodgden, & Stevenson, 1958), we constructed three simple motor tasks. Like Kounin's instruction-initiated tasks, each had two parts and provided satiation, cosatiation, and error scores. The study deviated from Kounin's procedure in that two conditions of reinforcement were used. In one, the experimenter maintained a nonsupportive role; in the other, the experimenter made positive comments and, in general, reinforced the child's performance. We found that the retarded participants spent more time on the games in both conditions. They played the longest when they received support, whereas mental-age-matched, nonretarded children were unaffected.

The sensitivity of the retarded group to social reinforcement lent credibility to the social deprivation hypothesis. However, our findings did not invalidate the Lewin-Kounin rigidity formulation. In fact, some of our results were reminiscent of Kounin's. Regardless of reinforcement condition, our retarded participants performed an inordinately long time on the relatively boring, monotonous tasks we employed. In addition, as Kounin found with his older retarded group, our retarded sample in the support condition played the second part of the task longer than they did the first part, even though both parts were extremely similar. (I must confess that this strange increase from part one to part two remained a mystery to me for several years. I think I began understanding this phenomenon, which will be discussed in the next section, when I gave up trying to interpret it in terms of theories with which I was conversant and relied instead on a closer and more clinical observation of the child's behavior in the experimental setting.)

The Zigler, Hodgden, and Stevenson findings hardly constituted a deathblow to the Lewin-Kounin rigidity formulation. At most, these findings indicated that the production of phenotypically rigid behaviors is also influenced by motivational effects, a view not very much at variance with Lewin and Kounin's own stance on motivation. At this point, what appeared to be in order was a more convincing test of our view that the seemingly rigid behaviors of retarded individuals are a result of social deprivation rather than cognitive rigidity.

Green and I (1962) therefore designed a study in which we included both institutionalized and noninstitutionalized retarded groups as well as nonretarded children. All three groups were equated on mental age, and the two retarded groups were also equated on chronological age. The Lewin-Kounin formulation generates the prediction that the performance of the two retarded groups would be similar and that both would differ from the children of average intellect. The social deprivation hypothesis predicts that the performance of the two noninstitutionalized groups would be similar and that both would differ from the institutionalized retarded children. The latter hypothesis was supported. The institutionalized participants showed the relatively long satiation times, a preservative behavior often interpreted as evidence of rigidity. I then conducted another study in which I included a group of institutionalized children of average intellect (Zigler, 1963a). I found that regardless of intelligence level, institutionalized children played the socially reinforced, satiation-type task longer than did noninstitutionalized children. This convinced me that social deprivation, not rigidity inherent in mental retardation, could explain Kounin's and many of our own findings.

Before we could adequately test this hypothesis, we needed a measure that reflects socialization deficits. The cluster of events that constitute social deprivation had never been adequately delimited, so I devised a procedure for raters to evaluate children's preinstitutional social histories (Zigler, 1961). Based on these ratings, I selected retarded children who were either high or low in social deprivation. The children were given a socially reinforced, two-part satiation game similar to those used earlier. I found that the more socially deprived children spent a greater amount of time on the game, more frequently made the maximum number of responses allowed, and spent more time playing part two than part one of the game.

The Lewin-Kounin theory could not explain differences in rigid behaviors between groups of retarded children equated on both chronological and mental age. My findings instead supported the view that the "rigidity" observed in the earlier studies reflected motivation to maintain interaction with an adult and to secure social approval through compliance and persistence. These results also provided evidence that this motivation is related to the amount of preinstitutional social deprivation retarded children experience.

To build on this work, we had to tackle the thorny issues of the nature and measurement of social deprivation. This was an arena of psychology that had a murky conceptual foundation and a sizable literature of inconsistent and contradictory findings. To this day I have found few constructs in psychology that are more frequently employed, yet more inadequately defined, than social deprivation. As Gewirtz (1957) once put it, the concept of social deprivation has been loosely applied to certain events in early childhood which, in turn, are considered antecedent to certain social behaviors. The problem, of course, is that there is little agreement as to either the early events or the subsequent behaviors.

To operationalize the social deprivation construct for use with retarded children, I initially entertained the possibility of using length of institutionalization. However, I soon realized that institutionalization is not, in itself, a psychological variable. At best, it refers to some vague social status of the individual. To relate this setting to social deprivation, one must designate specific social interactions in the institution that give rise to particular behaviors. Given these qualms, another possibility came to mind: Many institutionalized children tend to come from relatively depriving homes, so it might be their preinstitutional experiences that should be evaluated. Within this framework, institutionalization would be analyzed for its particular psychological features and for its effects as they interact with the effects of the earlier psychological environment.

These considerations led us to construct a standard, objective measure of preinstitutional social deprivation (Zigler, Butterfield, & Goff, 1966). Initially, we asked two experienced psychologists to read the social histories of 60 consecutively admitted, familial retarded children and to independently rate them on a social deprivation scale. The scale consisted of nothing more than a line subdivided into six areas ranging from *"very protected"* to *"very deprived."* The judges were not instructed as to what these terms meant beyond being told that they related to the amount and quality of interactions that the children had had with important adults in their lives. The judges were also asked to list the specific factors in the case histories that influenced their ratings.

In spite of the vagueness of the social deprivation construct, we found respectable interjudge reliability. There was clearly some commonality in the early histories of the retarded children to which seasoned psychologists responded in deducing the amount of social deprivation experienced. To determine what these common factors might be, we examined the events the raters had listed as important in their judgments. They most frequently cited factors such as the child had been removed from the home, parents' divorce or poor mental health, and child abuse. From this list we assembled a collection of items thought to be the experiential referents of social deprivation.

We continued to refine the measure over several years until we developed a scale that could be reliably rated, even by people untrained in psychology. The scale also included a single subjective estimate of social deprivation which the rater assessed prior to scoring the objective items. The subjective scale was retained to capture nuances of deprivation that might not be reflected in the objective items. Factor analyses found the scale to yield four discernible components, reflecting the preinstitutional continuity of the child's residences, the parents' attitude toward institutionalization, their marital harmony, and the intellectual and economic richness of the family.

This social deprivation scale was first used in a study by Zigler, Balla, and Butterfield (1968). Our goal was to clarify my earlier findings (Zigler, 1961) of a positive relation between degree of preinstitutional social deprivation and motivation for social reinforcement (measured by how long the child persisted in playing a monotonous but socially reinforced game). By using the scale, we hoped to discover the particular aspects of preinstitutional deprivation that resulted in the heightened desire for reinforcement. We also tried to correct a weakness in my earlier study, which employed children who had already been institutionalized for an average of 2 years. This made it difficult to tell if their strong social motivation was due to their preinstitutional histories or to the deprivation inherent in institutionalization. We thus tested the children shortly after their admission. We also included children of both familial and organic etiologies.

Our findings supported the general hypothesis that social deprivation results in a heightened motivation for social reinforcement. A positive relation was found between preinstitutional deprivation and the effectiveness of social reinforcers dispensed by an adult. This relation held for the nonfamilial as well as the familial retarded groups. Particular aspects of the preinstitutional history were found to be critical, namely, the harmony and richness of the child's family and the parents' attitude toward institutionalization.

This motivational interpretation rests on the assumption that institutionalized retarded individuals have been deprived of adult social reinforcement, so they are highly motivated to obtain this particular class of reinforcers. Evidence supporting this view came from a study by Harter and myself (1968). We found that an adult experimenter was a more effective social reinforcer than a peer experimenter for retarded children who lived in institutions but not for those who lived at home. It thus appeared that the institutionalized retarded child's motivation to obtain social reinforcement is relatively specific to attention and praise dispensed by an adult, rather than a more generalized desire for reinforcement dispensed by any social agent.

Balla (1967) contributed an important missing link in the chain of evidence we were attempting to forge. He conducted observations in the homes of retarded and nonretarded children and in several institutions which housed children of both intelligence levels. He found direct support for the assumption of an adult social reinforcement deficit. With respect to the quantity and quality of adult social interactions, the institutionalized groups were similar to one another and the home groups were similar to one another, regardless of intelligence level. However, when looking at the comparison most often made in the literature, institutionalized retarded children were found to interact with adults significantly less often than nonretarded children who lived at home. It is therefore not surprising that when these retarded children are placed in a situation where social interaction is readily available, they choose to linger.

Although I have been couching this discussion in terms of an alternate explanation for apparently rigid behavior, heightened motivation for social reinforcement has also been used as an indicator of an important developmental phenomenon, namely, dependency. Thus, with a slight shift in terminology, we might conclude that our findings indicate a general consequence of social deprivation is overdependency—a trait that has a profound impact on the lives of retarded individuals. Zigler and Harter (1969) concluded that, given some minimal intellectual level, the shift from dependency to independence is the most important factor enabling retarded persons to become self-sustaining members of society. Social deprivation can impede this developmental shift by leading deprived individuals to try to satisfy certain affectional needs before they can cope with independent activities.

Evidence on this point came from a study by Harter (1967). She found that institutionalized retarded individuals took longer to solve a concept-formation problem in a social condition, where they were face-to-face with a supportive experimenter, than when the experimenter was silent and out of view. Their motivation to interact with the adult competed with their attention to the learning task, so learning suffered. This interpretation was supported by Balla's (1967) observation of institutionalized retarded children in a school setting. He found that they used the school not as a place to learn but as a place to connect with adults, apparently compensating for the lack of such relationships in the other parts of their life space.

Our findings suggest that because severely deprived retarded individuals are highly motivated to maximize interpersonal contact, they are relatively unconcerned with the performance expected of them. Of course, the two activities are not always incompatible, but in many instances they are. The absence of institutionalization today does not absent the social deprivation that can lead familial retarded individuals to care more about social interactions than the task at hand in school or on the job.

SOCIAL DEPRIVATION AND THE NEGATIVE REACTION TENDENCY

Once we began to view mental retardation beyond its cognitive component alone, we became more aware of the complexity of retarded individuals. This approach led us to a phenomenon seemingly at variance with their increased desire for social reinforcement (a phenomenon I labeled the "*positive-reaction tendency*"). One does not have to look hard to notice that retarded children often have a reluctance and wariness to interact with adults. This orientation (which I labeled the "*negative-reaction tendency*") helped me understand certain group differences reported by Kounin.

Recall that Kounin employed a cosatiation task as one measure of rigidity. In this type of task, participants are allowed to perform until they wish to stop. They then play a very similar game until again satiated. The cosatiation score is the measure of the degree to which performance on the first task influences performance on the second task. The theoretical positions of Lewin and Kounin, as well as Stevenson and Zigler, predict that the absolute playing time of retarded individuals on task two, after satiation on task one, would be greater than that of nonretarded individuals. However, neither of these positions could explain the recurring finding that, as a group, retarded children perform longer on the second task. Nonretarded children, on the other hand, invariably spend more time on the first part.

I hypothesized that institutionalized children learn during task one that the experimenter is not like other strange adults they have met who initiated painful experiences (physical examinations, shots, etc.) with supportive comments. This reappraisal of the experimental situation results in a reduction of the negative-reaction tendency. When they switch to task two, they meet it with a positive-reaction tendency and play for a long time while they enjoy the social reinforcement. Nonretarded children have a relatively low negative-reaction tendency when they begin. On part one their positive-reaction tendency is reduced, through fatigue and satiation effects, so they have no reason to persist on part two.

This thinking led me to wonder if the cosatiation score mirrors motivational factors rather than inherent rigidity. Shallenberger and I (1961) tested this proposal by presenting three games before the two-part task. The games were given under two conditions of reinforcement. Under positive reinforcement, all of the participants' responses met with success, and they were further rewarded with verbal and nonverbal support from the experimenter. We assumed that this condition would reduce the negative-reaction tendency the child brought to the setting. In a negative reinforcement condition, all responses met with failure, and the experimenter gave further negative feedback by noting this lack of success. We assumed that this condition would increase the negative-reaction tendency.

These assumptions were tested with mental-age-matched groups of retarded and nonretarded children. We found that regardless of intellectual level, children in the negative condition spent more time on part two than on part one of the criterion task than did those in the positive condition. These findings indicated that cosatiation effects do not reflect rigidity but the relative strength of the positive- and negative-reaction tendencies. These tendencies seem to be the product of experience and, apparently, are open to modification.

Instead of the time scores we used, Weaver (1966) employed a more direct measure of the child's approach and avoidance tendencies. His task, developed in our laboratory, required the child to place felt pieces onto a long felt board, at one end of which sat an adult. In one condition, the adult positively reinforced the child; in another, negative comments were made. The reaction tendencies were assessed by how far from the adult the child placed the shapes. Weaver found that, over the series of trials, noninstitutionalized children in the positive condition moved toward the experimenter, whereas children in the negative condition moved away. A subsequent study (Klaber, Butterfield, & Gould, 1969) indicated that this and our standard time measure were significantly correlated.

A logical conclusion to this line of research is that a wariness of adults and of the tasks they present leads to a general attenuation in the retarded child's effectiveness. Failure on tasks initiated by adults is, therefore, not to be attributed entirely to low intelligence. Rather, the atypically high negative-reaction tendency of many retarded individuals may cause behaviors (for example, avoidance), that hamper their performance on tasks that they have the intellectual capacity to master.

THE REINFORCER HIERARCHY

Another concept my colleagues and I advanced to explain differences in performance between retarded and nonretarded individuals of the same mental age is that of the reinforcer hierarchy. This term pertains to the ordering of reinforcers in the individual's motivation system from most to least effective. The seed of this line of thinking germinated when I puzzled over Kounin's finding that retarded children had greater difficulty than their nonretarded peers on his concept-switching task. This was the task on which they had to sort cards on the basis of one feature and then another. In trying to understand why the retarded group performed so poorly, I realized that the only reinforcer available to participants for correctly switching concepts was whatever satisfaction inheres in being correct. Being correct is probably more reinforcing for a nonretarded than for a retarded child, who may place greater value on interacting with the adult.

A related idea came from a line of research indicating that middle-SES children are more motivated to be correct for its own sake than are lower-SES children. Specifically, middle-SES children were found to do better on a discrimination-learning task when an intangible rather than a tangible reinforcer was employed, while lower-SES children did better when the reinforcer was a tangible one. Kounin employed institutionalized familial retarded children, who are drawn predominantly from the low SES. They may not have been motivated by the intangible reinforcement. Thus, the differences obtained by Kounin may have resulted in part from comparing lower-SES retarded with middle-SES nonretarded children—groups who differed in the value they placed on the available reward.

This view was tested by Zigler and deLabry (1962) in an experiment utilizing Kounin's concept-switching task with groups of familial retarded and lower- and middle-SES nonretarded children. In one condition, Kounin's original reinforcer (that inherent in a correct response) was employed. In a second condition, the reinforcer was tangible (a small toy). We found that the retarded and lower-SES nonretarded children took fewer trials to switch in the tangible condition, while the middle-SES children did slightly better in the intangible condition. Reminiscent of Kounin's results was the finding of significant differences among the three groups who received intangible reinforcers. However, no differences were found among the three groups that received their preferred reinforcement (retarded tangible, lower-SES tangible, and middle-SES intangible).

I argued that shifts in the position of particular reinforcers in the individual's reinforcer hierarchy are related to advancing cognitive-developmental stages (Zigler, 1963b). However, these changes cannot account for differences in the value of certain reinforcers between retarded and nonretarded children who are matched on mental age, and thus grossly on cognitive-developmental level. I began to wonder if these differences could be attributed to their social histories instead. For instance, among retarded students the likelihood of failure is high, so teaching methods often center on doing one's best rather than being right. This deemphasis of right for right's sake alone could lower the motive to be correct in the child's motive hierarchy. Another possibility is that the enhanced effectiveness of tangible reinforcers for institutionalized retarded and lower-SES children may stem from the relative deprivation of material rewards, such as toys and candy, in their environments.

Up to this point, our work on the reinforcer hierarchy focused on how particular reinforcers external to the child, but dispensed by some social agent, take on their effectiveness in the child's motivational system. Later, we shifted our attention to the more general phenomenon of the intrinsic reinforcement that inheres in being correct, regardless of whether or not an external agent dispenses a reinforcer. This line of thinking derived from White's (1959) ideas about the nature of the effectance motive in the human behavior system. Whether or not one accepts his view that the need for effectance or mastery is a basic need that parallels other primary drives, the effectance concept does provide a rubric for a variety of human behaviors from infancy through senility.

Harter and I (1974) collaborated on a study to operationally purify the effectance motive construct and to examine this motivation in retarded and nonretarded children. We began by constructing a battery of tasks to measure the motivation to master, to explore, to conceptualize tasks as challenging problem-solving situations, to be curious, and to solve a task for the sake of being correct. Our efforts were partially guided by our intuitive attempts to design a set of tasks that reflect behaviors we observed to be important in the development of children of average intellect, but seemingly absent or less predominant among retarded populations. The typical pattern of our findings was that nonretarded children showed the greatest desire to master a problem for the sake of mastery, to choose the most challenging task, and to demonstrate the greatest curiosity and exploratory behavior. Noninstitutionalized retarded children showed less of this type of behavior; institutionalized retarded children, in most cases, demonstrated the least mastery motivation.

We hypothesized that cognitive mastery could drop in the motive hierarchy as a result of experiences that either extinguish this motive or elevate other motives more important to the individual's needs. In the case of retarded children whose efforts to achieve cognitive mastery so frequently meet with failure, such a motive could easily become associated with anxiety. As a result, they become more motivated to escape the anxiety associated with the effort than to gratify the mastery motive. Such a process may underlie the common finding that retarded children are more motivated to avoid failure than to achieve success. (This trait is the topic of the next section.) Retarded children who reside in institutions may have not only a depressed mastery motive but a strong motive to receive adult reinforcement. Here again, we find support for the idea that inter- and intragroup performance differences among retarded and nonretarded children may arise from diverse social histories.

EXPECTANCY OF SUCCESS

A frequently noted trait of individuals with mental retardation is their high expectancy of failure. This propensity is thought to be learned after frequent confrontations with tasks with which they are intellectually ill-equipped to deal. That failure experiences and expectancies affect a wide variety of behaviors was first documented in children of average intellect. However, early research employing success-failure manipulations with retarded individuals was somewhat inconsistent. Some studies found that retarded children performed better following success and poorer following failure compared to their nonretarded peers. Others found the opposite or that both types of children responded in the same way.

One problem in these studies was that the experimental conditions typically involved very simple, circumscribed experiences of success or failure. They did not constitute an analogue of the pervasive history of failure assumed for the retarded participants. Such prolonged failure could produce a *"failure set"* (Zeaman & House, 1960) and a willingness to settle for a relatively low degree of success. To test this hypothesis, Stevenson and I (1958) employed a three-choice discrimination task in which one stimulus was reinforced some of the time and the other two stimuli were never reinforced. Although we later discovered that performance on this task is also influenced by a number of other factors, our rationale was that maximizing behavior (persistent choice of the partially reinforced stimulus) should be more characteristic of retarded children because they have come to expect and settle for lower amounts of success. As predicted, we found retarded children to maximize more than children of average intelligence.

Of course, these findings could also be interpreted as consonant with the Lewin-Kounin rigidity formulation. That is, maximization (consistently responding to one stimulus) could be conceptualized as perseverative behavior, which might be expected of retarded children because of their inherent rigidity. A procedure for differentially testing the Stevenson-Zigler motivational and Lewin-Kounin rigidity positions suggested itself. If a low expectancy of success stemming from a high incidence of failure causes retarded individuals to maximize behavior, then this same type of behavior should be found in children of average intellect who also experienced relatively high amounts of failure. Such a history is not uncommon among lower-SES children. The motivational position, therefore, predicts similarity in performance by retarded and lower-SES children on a partially reinforced, three-choice problem. The position that rigidity is inversely related to IQ leads to the expectation that their performance will be dissimilar, with the lower-SES children performing more like their middle-SES peers of the same IQ.

Gruen and I (1968) tested this hypothesis with groups of middle- and lower-SES nonretarded and noninstitutionalized familial retarded children of comparable mental ages. Before the learning problem, one-third of the children in each group were administered pretraining tasks in which they experienced a high degree of success; one-third experienced a low level of success; and one-third did not receive any pretraining. The expectation here was that the low success condition would lower the child's general expectancy of success and thus result in more maximizing behavior on the learning task. Preliminary success, on the other hand, was expected to lead to more patterning. This is a common strategy of children of this mental age and entails a left, middle, right (or vice versa) response pattern. This strategy indicates an attempt to find a "solution" that results in 100% reinforcement (which is actually unattainable on this task).

Our findings allowed us to conclude that motivational factors, not cognitive rigidity, determine behavior on the probability task. Nonretarded, lower-SES children had the most maximizing (correct choices) and the least patterning responses, while middle-SES children had the least maximizing and most patterning responses. Retarded children fell between these two groups on both measures. No effects as a result of prior conditions of success and failure were found for the lower-SES and retarded children. However, for middle-SES children, the preliminary success condition resulted in even less maximization and more patterning than did the other two conditions. For this group, early success apparently led them to believe they could also succeed on this task.

Our data analyses permitted certain conclusions about the processes that mediate performance on the discrimination problem. During the early trials, all children rely rather heavily on the pattern response, a strategy dictated by their cognitive (mental age) level. The child's willingness to give up this cognitively congruent strategy for a maximization strategy (which, although not meeting the goal of 100% success, does provide the best possible payoff) has some relation to his or her expectancy of success. In middle-SES children, this expectancy is relatively high and, therefore, they are unwilling to settle for that degree of success provided by the maximization response. In search of greater rewards, they can do little more than continue with the patterning response which, at this mental age level, is a relatively complex strategy. On the other hand, the retarded and lower-SES children have a lower expectancy of success and are, therefore, more willing to give up patterning in favor of maximization.

The tendency for the lower-SES children we tested to accept a relatively low degree of success might be explained by the fact that they attended classes with middle-SES, probably higher-achieving children. It is possible that the lower-SES child in the middle-SES oriented schoolroom experiences more failure than retarded children who attend special classes conducted especially · for them. These lower-SES children come to distrust their own cognitive strategies and are more ready to abandon them.

These findings should not be interpreted to mean that social class or intellectual level determine the child's expectancy of success. Rather, it is the particular incidence of success or failure experienced by the individual child. This notion was supported by Kier, Styfco, and myself (1977), who asked teachers to rate groups of lower- and middle-SES, nonretarded students as being successful or unsuccessful in school. We found that, independent of SES, children ranked as unsuccessful by their teachers were the most willing to settle for a low degree of success and thus adopt a maximization strategy on our probability task. The point is that any child's behavior is more predictable when it is approached from a psychological point of view rather than from an IQ or demographic frame of reference.

OUTERDIRECTEDNESS

Another line of investigation in our work, revealed that, in addition to a lowered expectancy of success, the high incidence of failure experienced by retarded individuals generates a style of problem solving characterized by outerdirectedness. That is, retarded persons come to distrust their own solutions to problems and therefore seek guides to action in the immediate environment. In an early study (Zigler et al., 1958), we found that institutionalized retarded children tended to terminate their performance on experimental games following a suggestion from an adult that they might do so. Nonretarded children tended to ignore these suggestions, stopping instead of their own volition. We originally interpreted this finding to mean that social deprivation results in an enhanced motivation for social reinforcers and, hence, in greater compliance in an effort to obtain them. (Here one can see a clear instance of how a commitment to a particular viewpoint leads one to avoid interpretations of data other than those to which he or she is committed.)

However, Green and I (1962) found that noninstitutionalized retarded children had the highest tendency to terminate their performance upon a cue from the experimenter. This finding is incongruent with the social deprivation position, which led us to expect that retarded and nonretarded children who live at home would be similar in their sensitivity to adult cues. The fact that they were not led us to suggest that sensitivity to external cues is most appropriately viewed as a general component of problem solving, having its antecedents in the child's history of success or failure.

Of the three groups who participated in our study, the nonretarded children are assumed to have had the highest incidence of success emanating from self-initiated solutions to problems. As a result, they should be the most willing to employ their own thought processes in problem-solving situations. Antithetically, the self-initiated solutions of retarded children are assumed to result in a high incidence of failure, making them lack confidence in their ability to solve problems. They should therefore be more sensitive to external cues, particularly those provided by social agents, in the belief that these cues will be more reliable than their own cognitive efforts. But because institutionalized retarded children live in an environment adjusted to their intellectual shortcomings, they probably experience less failure than retarded children who live in the community. This latter group continues to face the complexities and demands of an environment that is beyond their intellectual capacities and should, as we found, manifest the greatest sensitivity to external cues.

This position was tested by Turnure and myself (1964). In a first experiment, we examined the imitation behavior of retarded and nonretarded children of the same mental age on two tasks. One task involved the imitation of an adult and the other a peer. First, the children played some games under either a success or a failure condition. The specific hypotheses tested were that retarded children are generally more imitative and that all children are more imitative following failure than following success experiences. These hypotheses were confirmed on both imitation tasks. Our findings suggested that the outerdirectedness of the retarded child results in behavior characterized by an oversensitivity to external models. While this can result in a lack of spontaneity and creativity, it can also be a productive use of role models.

Turnure and I conducted a second experiment (1964) to demonstrate that outerdirectedness may be either detrimental or beneficial, depending on the nature of the situation. Nonretarded and noninstitutionalized retarded children of the same mental age were instructed to assemble an item, reminiscent of the object-assembly items on the WISC, as quickly as they could. While the child worked, the experimenter put together a second item. The hypothesis was that the outerdirectedness of retarded children leads them to attend to what the adult is doing rather than concentrating on their own task, thus interfering with performance. When the child had completed the puzzle, the experimenter took apart the puzzle he himself had been working on and gave it to the child to assemble. Here, the cues that the retarded

child had picked up as a result of outerdirectedness should facilitate performance. The predictions were confirmed. The nonretarded children were superior on the first task, whereas the
retarded children were superior on the second task. Further con-
firmation of the outerdirectedness hypothesis was obtained by a
direct measure of how often the children glanced at the experimenter. As expected, the retarded children glanced significantly
more often.

Sanders, Zigler, and Butterfield (1968) addressed whether the
outerdirectedness of retarded children, found on simple imitation
tasks, is also manifested in a discrimination-learning situation. If
so, this style of problem solving would be relatively pervasive and
should be considered when evaluating the general behavior of
retarded persons. Groups of retarded and nonretarded children of
the same mental age were presented with a size discrimination
task that involved a cue which the child could use in choosing
among stimuli. Three conditions were employed: one in which
the cue led to success (positive condition), one in which the cue
led to failure (negative condition), and one in which no cue was
presented. The expectation was that the cue would be more
enhancing in the positive and more debilitating in the negative
condition for the retarded than for the nonretarded children.
Although some rather complex findings were obtained in the positive condition, which lent weight to the outerdirectedness
hypothesis, this hypothesis received its strongest support under
the negative condition. The retarded children made more errors
than the nonretarded children in response to the erroneous cue.
Thus children of retarded intellect relied heavily on the negative
cue even though it led to errors, while children of average intellect
did not.

Achenbach and I (1968) reformulated this hypothesis in
terms of a distinction between two learning strategies. One, which
we called the cue-learning strategy, was characterized by a
reliance on concrete situational cues with little attempt to educe
relations among problem elements. The contrasting problem-
learning strategy was an active attempt to educe abstract relations
among problem elements in order to find the solution.

Although our procedure varied somewhat in a series of experiments, essentially we utilized a three-choice size discrimination

task in which a light came on in association with the correct stimulus. On the first few trials, the light came on almost immediately. As time progressed, the interval between the onsets of the trial and of the light became longer. During the task, participants were occasionally prodded to make their choice of stimuli as quickly as possible. This procedure was intended to create a somewhat ambiguous situation in which children could either continue waiting for the light to direct their choice or begin responding to the abstract relation (relative size) among the problem elements. Correct responses before the light onset were utilized as the measure of the successful employment of the problem-learning strategy.

In our first experiment, we found that noninstitutionalized retarded children relied on the cue longer than did an institutionalized group, while nonretarded children were the first to abandon this strategy. In a second experiment, participants were presented the learning task immediately after preconditions of success or failure. We also attempted to assess whether waiting for the light cue inhibited learning of the size relation or whether it was just a conservative response strategy whereby the child decided to wait for the light even though he or she knew which stimulus was correct. We replicated the findings of our first experiment and also demonstrated that reliance on the cue by the retarded children involved an inhibition of learning rather than caution in responding.

Contrary to our expectations, our failure and success manipulations did not influence any group's reliance on cues. However, we obtained serendipitous support for our view that these experiences influence outerdirectedness. We discovered a class of 16 retarded children whose teacher employed methods that could affect precisely those variables we thought to mediate outerdirectedness. Observation of his classroom revealed that he showered new pupils with success and reinforced what he called "figuring things out for yourself," rewarding independent thought more highly than correct responses. We looked at the performance of these classmates on our learning task and discovered not only that they relied on cues significantly less than our other retarded participants, but that they relied on them less (albeit not significantly so) than did the children of average intellect.

Again, one can see that it is not retardation per se that produces a behavior, but the child's particular experiences.

Our studies in this area led us to theorize that how outerdirected a child will be depends on two factors: level of cognition attained (for example, mental age) and the degree of success experienced through employing whatever cognitive resources he or she has available. Concerning the first factor, the lower the mental age, the more outerdirected the child, because this is more conducive to successful problem solving than dependency upon immature cognitive abilities. With cognitive growth and development, the child should become more innerdirected. This is due both to expanded cognitive ability and to the fact that with increasing age there is a gradual reduction in cues provided the child by adults (further reducing the effectiveness of an outerdirected style). Thus the shift from outer- to innerdirectedness in typical child development is a gradual process that culminates in autonomy as an adult.

This general developmental factor does not explain our findings that retarded children are more outerdirected than nonretarded children even when matched on mental age. Apparently, the crucial variable here is the amount of success children experience when employing their cognitive abilities. It appears that certain age expectancies are firmly built into child-rearing practices and that society reacts to a child more on the basis of chronological age than mental age. In nonretarded children these ages are fairly equivalent, so they are usually presented problems that are in keeping with their cognitive resources. With increasing maturity, they experience increasing success in utilizing these resources. Retarded children, on the other hand, are continuously confronted with problems appropriate to their chronological age but inappropriate to their mental age. These problems are too difficult, so they do not experience the success that would lead them to discard an outerdirected style. This style comes to have a negative effect on their performance in the classroom (Bybee & Zigler, 1998).

Our findings can be conceptually extended to retarded children affected by the current practices of mainstreaming and inclusion. It may very well be that noninstitutionalized retarded children, benevolently placed in an environment that is too demanding for them, are more outerdirected than institutionalized or segregated retarded children, who experience an environment more geared to their intellectual shortcomings. Our findings are in keeping with ideas presented long ago that residential care is more likely to foster the retarded child's self-confidence than is the non-sheltered school in the community setting. For example, Rosen, Diggory, and Werlinsky (1966) found that institutionalized retarded children set higher goals, predicted better performance for themselves, and actually performed at a higher level. Edgerton and Sabagh (1962) also pointed out certain positive features of the sheltered setting for the higher IQ retarded child. Their argument echoed that of Johnson and Kirk (1950), who favored separate classes for retarded children in public schools, since they tend to be isolated and rejected in regular classes.

These opinions and hypotheses came before implementation of the IDEA and the practice of educating most retarded children in community schools. The effect of this practice on the performance and motivational drivers of these students has been sparsely studied. It is as if the existence of the law and the ideology surrounding it negated the need for scientific evaluation. Should empiricists ever resurrect their interest in what motivates retarded children to learn (or not learn), they might be surprised to discover that the groundwork for their efforts was laid long ago.

THE EZ-PERSONALITY QUESTIONNAIRE

To be fair, part of the reason the relation between personality-motivational factors and performance in retarded individuals was not examined more thoroughly has to do with measurement difficulties. There simply was no standardized instrument to assess the personality traits common in individuals with mental retardation. Our group at Yale used individual experimental tasks to gauge separately each of the motivational factors discussed above. Although the face validity of the tasks has been demonstrated, it is clear that they are not pure measures of the constructs they are thought to operationalize. Nor is it be feasible to administer all of them to derive personality profiles for scientific or clinical use.

In recent years we have been working to develop an instrument to measure personality functioning in individuals with mental retardation—the EZ-Yale Personality Questionnaire, or EZPQ (Zigler, Bennett-Gates, & Hodapp, 1999). The 37-item, seven-scale instrument has been found to have good internal reliability, temporal stability, and concurrent validity with the samples employed. The measure is also quite successful in distinguishing between individuals with and without mental retardation.

The scales identified in the factor analyses of EZPQ scores both confirm and refine the original five hypothesized constructs of outerdirectedness, expectancy of success, effectance motivation, positive reaction tendency, and negative reaction tendency. The two additional constructs we found, obedience and curiosity/creativity, represent refinements in the conceptualization of outerdirectedness and effectance motivation, respectively. In addition to the separate scores, total scores from the EZPQ accurately predicted whether an individual is functioning in the range of retarded or nonretarded intelligence.

The next steps in the development of the EZPQ involve broadening the standardization sample and delineating the measure's utility for researchers, educators, and therapists. Thus far our samples have been limited to retarded individuals without an identified organic etiology. The factor structure of the EZPQ should be examined using samples of individuals with biological bases for their impairments. Because some of the constructs tapped by the measure have shown a developmental progression (e.g., outerdirectedness), age norms should be established

The advantage of being able to assess functioning on several dimensions of personality, the ease of administration, and the psychometric properties of the EZPQ should facilitate not only research but also treatment practices. In applied settings, the EZPQ can eventually be used to screen for maladaptive behaviors so that clinicians and educators can plan interventions. The measure can also be used pre- and postintervention to assess attainment of behavioral objectives. Once refined, it is hoped the EZPQ will yield a better understanding of the relation between personality and both adaptive and cognitive functioning in individuals with mental retardation and that it will be a useful guide in treatment regimens.

A NOTE
ON INSTITUTIONALIZATION

Much of the empirical work on the performance of retarded children was conducted during a time when institutionalization was common. Many theories were therefore derived almost solely from institutionalized populations. I hope that I have made clear by now that it is a serious error to assume that the behavior of retarded persons reflects their intellectual retardation, uninfluenced by the effects of where they live and attend school.

In the 1960s and 1970s, some rather dramatic exposés of horrible conditions in institutions led lay people and professionals to condemn all institutions as having some negative, monolithic effect on every single resident. Contradicting this view are some of my and my colleagues' findings that the protected environment of the institution can result in retarded children being less outerdirected, and thus more spontaneous in utilizing their cognitive resources, than is the case with their noninstitutionalized counterparts. Yet even this more substantive argument must be made with caution.

Before one can assert that institutionalization will have one effect and its opposite, inclusion, will have another, one must be prepared to argue that important social-psychological phenomena are constant within each setting. It is difficult for me to see how such an argument can be defended when so little systematic work has been done in this area. Few investigators have gone beyond a concern with the characteristics of gross setting and begun the painstaking search for the particular features and practices of these settings that might differentially encourage the development of children who differ among themselves in respect to psychological traits and social histories.

In our work on institutionalization, my colleagues and I entertained two assumptions that retain their relevance in today's climate. The first is that institutions (or special or inclusive classes) differ among themselves in the effects they have on children who come to them for care. The second is that the same institution (or special or inclusive class) may affect children differently depending upon the child's personality dynamics, which may have been determined long before the child arrived in the setting.

An old study by Butterfield and myself (1965) is illuminating with respect to how particular practices in institutions give rise to particular behaviors. We examined differences in motivation for social reinforcement among retarded children in two equally large residential schools. Our samples were matched on a wide range of variables, thus allowing us to attribute stylistic differences to where they lived.

In institution A, efforts were made to provide a noninstitutional, home-like environment. School classes and social events were all coeducational. Meals were prepared in the living units, where the children ate in small groups. Emphasis was placed on individual responsibility rather than on external control by the staff. No buildings were locked, and children moved freely about the grounds. In institution B, classrooms and most social events were segregated by gender. Meals were prepared and children ate in a large central dining room with virtually no individual attention. All buildings were locked, and a large staff of security officers patrolled the grounds. The social climate at institution A strikes one as being much more conducive to constructive, supportive interactions between the children and their caregivers than the social climate at institution B.

As predicted from our work on social deprivation, we found that the children from the more—well, institution-like—institution had a higher motivation to obtain social reinforcement. We also found institutional differences in performance on the concept-switching task employed by Kounin to assess cognitive rigidity.

Because no one begins life anew when he or she changes residence, my colleagues and I also looked at the interaction between the effects of institutionalization and the child's social history. As a follow-up to a study I did on motivation for social reinforcement (Zigler, 1961), we retested children who were still in the original institution 3 years later (Zigler & Williams, 1963). We found that their desire for social reinforcement increased over time. However, most striking was the finding that children who came from relatively good homes evidenced a much greater increase in their motivation for social reinforcers between the two testings than did children from more socially deprived homes.

These same children were again given our perseveration measure 5 and 8 years after my original testing (Zigler, Butterfield, & Capobianco, 1970). This time we found a general decrease in motivation for social reinforcement. This is not surprising since, by this time, the children were well into adolescence and should not have been as motivated to receive praise on a simple task involving little more than dropping marbles into a hole. However, we found that the effects of early deprivation still lingered even after the children had been institutionalized this long. Children from highly deprived backgrounds showed a greater decrease in their motivation for social reinforcement than children from less depriving backgrounds. This finding again shows that institutionalization is not a uniform experience. Furthermore, while the effects of early social deprivation appear amenable to subsequent environmental events, these events do not act upon children in a uniform manner.

Nor, I submit, does the gross event of mainstreaming or fully including a retarded child in school or in the community. Just as the effects of institutions were found to be mediated by the child's unique personality and set of experiences, so too would do we expect the effects of some type of public setting to vary among children who arrive there. And just as we found differences between institutions A and B, there are also going to be differences between inclusive classrooms A and B. The type of setting simply does not tell much about the socioemotional environment provided there.

Researchers can make a grand contribution to the field of special education by picking up where earlier research on personality variables in mental retardation left off. By studying the person-environment interaction, we can come to understand the positive and—dare I say—negative aspects of various degrees of inclusion on children whose social histories may have skewed their motivational approaches. To encourage this work, I offer the experiences of my colleagues and I when we made the politically incorrect discovery that not all institutions for retarded people were bad in themselves or for the residents. While we were not reprehended or ostracized, what happened may actually have been worse. In the wake of the anti-institution movement, we were ignored.

PERSONALITY FACTORS
AND EVERYDAY ADJUSTMENT

The research agenda I began some 40 years ago centered on the systematic evaluation of experiential, motivational, and personality factors in the behavior of retarded persons. I believed then, and I still believe, that an understanding of these noncognitive domains can provide a better understanding of the socialization process in individuals with mental retardation. I emphasize socialization for a simple but potent reason: While most environmental manipulations designed to improve cognitive functioning in retarded people have been relatively unsuccessful (Spitz, 1986; Zigler, 1988), there is proof that some motivational and personality factors relevant to social adjustment or maladjustment can be modified. Thus, the area of motivation is where workers can do the most good in helping retarded persons to be effective in their everyday lives.

As is arguably the case for people of average intelligence, there is not a strong relation between cognitive status of retarded individuals and their successful adaptation in the community. This conclusion was long ago formed in Windle's (1962) review of over 100 studies dealing with the adjustment of retarded residents discharged from institutions. Windle found that the vast majority of studies reported no relation between intellectual level and outcome. Among even earlier workers in this country, such as Fernald and Potter, many felt that the differences in social adequacy among mildly retarded individuals were a matter of personality rather than intelligence.

Today, most persons with mental retardation reside in the mainstream society, so social adaptation has become the goal of education and treatment practices. In fact, "adaptive behavior" is now part of most official definitions of mental retardation. Yet the specific personality factors relating to adjustment have still not been adequately studied. The research program I undertook was only a small step in this direction. My colleagues and I tried to isolate motivational factors underlying the behavior of individuals with mental retardation and to discover the particular experiences which give rise to them. While we made some progress, we never got to the point where we could study the psychological processes and motive states in combination rather than in isolation. This left us far from achieving the stage where we could propose changes in treatment practices that could promote healthy personality and hence healthy adaptation.

This brings me to the topic of applied research, which, when I started out, was an unthinkable use of the talents of basic researchers such as myself. Yet even then I found myself pondering the words of Davies (1959) when he stated, "The constructive efforts of (community) agencies are especially directed toward those elements of personality which have been shown not to be fixed, which are susceptible to improvement, and which are more decisive factors in socialization than intelligence alone" (p. 216). After reading his discussion of these rehabilitative efforts, it seemed to me that much of this work was being carried out without much scientific evidence to support it. Regrettably, the situation is little changed today. Retarded children are in public schools and retarded adults are in the neighborhood and workplace, and we still do not know enough about their personality dynamics to help in their adjustment. Although interpersonal and social skills are vital to that adjustment, these personality traits have been deemphasized in favor of "increasing emphasis on the achievements of valued lifestyle outcomes" (Jacobson & Mulick, 1996b, p. 213). It is a small wonder that, in the absence of sound information, national policy decisions about the care and education of people with mental retardation are based on little more than vague generalizations, stereotypes, and political ideologies.

The psychological science of mental retardation, I am afraid, has itself become an ideology, detached from its roots in science as the quest for knowledge. This is not the case with other aspects of empirical work in the field, especially biochemical and genetic studies, which have produced some impressive results. Using modern empirical techniques and analytic methods, social scientists too can build a knowledge base and use it to enhance treatment practices and to enlighten social policies. To embark on this empirical voyage, once again the retarded individual must be viewed as a whole person—one with a past and a present that are brought to whatever setting or intervention is provided and combine with it to determine his or her future.

REFERENCES

Achenbach, T., & Zigler, E. (1968). Cue-learning, associative responding, and school performance in children. *Developmental Psychology, 1,* 717–725.

American Association on Mental Retardation. (1992). *Mental retardation: Definition, classification, and systems of supports* (9th ed.). Washington, DC: Author.

American Psychiatric Association. (1994). *Diagnostic and statistical manual of mental disorders* (4th ed.). Washington, DC: Author.

Balla, D. (1967). *The verbal action of the environment on institutionalized retardates and normal children of two social classes.* Unpublished doctoral dissertation, Yale University, New Haven.

Belmont, J. M., & Borkowski, J. G. (1994). Prudence, indeed, will dictate . . . [Review of the book *Mental retardation: Definition, classification, and systems of support* (9th ed.)]. *Contemporary Psychology, 39,* 495–496.

Bennett-Gates, D., & Zigler, E. (1998). Resolving the developmental-difference debate: An evaluation of the triarchic and systems theory models. In J. A. Burack, R. M. Hodapp, & E. Zigler (Eds.), *Handbook of mental retardation and development* (pp. 115–131). New York: Cambridge University Press.

Butterfield, E. C., & Zigler, E. (1965). The effects of differing institutional climates on the effectiveness of social reinforcement in the mentally retarded. *American Journal of Mental Deficiency, 70,* 48–56.

Bybee, J., & Zigler, E. (1998). Outerdirectedness in individuals with and without mental retardation. In J. A. Burack, R. M. Hodapp, & E. Zigler (Eds.), *Handbook of mental retardation and development* (pp. 434–461). New York: Cambridge University Press.

Davies, S. P. (1959). *The mentally retarded in society.* New York: Columbia University Press.

Dykens, E. M. (1998). Maladaptive behavior and dual diagnosis in persons with genetic syndromes. In J. A. Burack, R. M. Hodapp, & E. Zigler (Eds.), *Handbook of mental retardation and development* (pp. 542–562). New York: Cambridge University Press.

Dykens, E. M. (1999). Personality-motivation: New ties to psychopathology, etiology, and intervention. In E. Zigler & D. Bennett-Gates (Eds.), *Personality development in individuals with mental retardation* (pp. 249–270). New York: Cambridge University Press.

Edgerton, R. B., & Sabagh, G. (1962). From mortification to aggrandizement: Changing self-conception in the careers of the mentally retarded. *Psychiatry, 25,* 263–272.

Fuchs, D. & Fuchs, L. S. (1995). Inclusive schools movement and the radicalization of special education reform. In J. M. Kauffman & D. P. Hallahan (Eds.), *Illusion of full inclusion* (pp. 213–242). Austin, TX: Pro-Ed.

Gewirtz, J. (1957). *Social deprivation and dependency: A learning analysis.* Paper presented at the meeting of the American Psychological Association, New York, NY.

Green, C., & Zigler, E. (1962). Social deprivation and the performance of feebleminded and normal children on a satiation type task. *Child Development, 33,* 499–508.

Gruen, G. E., & Zigler, E. (1968). Expectancy of success and the probability learning of middle-class, lower-class, and retarded children. *Journal of Abnormal Psychology, 73,* 343–352.

Harter, S. (1967). Mental age, IQ, and motivational factors in the discrimination learning set performance of normal and retarded children. *Journal of Experimental Psychology, 5,* 123–141.

Harter, S., & Zigler, E. (1968). Effectiveness of adult and peer reinforcement on the performance of institutionalized and noninstitutionalized retardates. *Journal of Abnormal Psychology, 73,* 144–149.

Harter, S., & Zigler, E. (1974). The assessment of effectance motivation in normal and retarded children. *Developmental Psychology, 10,* 169–180.

Hodapp, R. M., Burack, J. A., & Zigler, E. (Eds.). (1990). *Issues in the developmental approach to mental retardation.* New York: Cambridge University Press.

Hodapp, R. M., Burack, J. A., & Zigler, E. (1998). Developmental approaches to mental retardation: A short introduction. In J. A. Burack, R. M. Hodapp, & E. Zigler (Eds.), *Handbook of mental retardation and development* (pp. 3–19). New York: Cambridge University Press.

Jacobson, J. W., & Mulick, J. A. (1996a). Introduction. In J. W. Jacobson & J. A. Mulick (Eds.), *Manual of diagnosis and professional practice in mental retardation* (pp. 1–8). Washington, DC: American Psychological Association.

Jacobson, J. W., & Mulick, J. A. (Eds.). (1996b). *Manual of diagnosis and professional practice in mental retardation.* Washington, DC: American Psychological Association.

Johnson, G. O., & Kirk, S. A. (1950). Are mentally handicapped children segregated in the regular grades? *Exceptional Children, 17,* 65–68.

Kier, R. J., Styfco, S. J., & Zigler, E. (1977). Success expectancies and the probability learning of children of low and middle socioeconomic status. *Developmental Psychology, 13,* 444–449.

King, B. H., State, M. W., Shah, B., Davanzo, P., & Dykens, E. (1997). Mental retardation: A review of the past 10 years. Part I. *Child and Adolescent Psychiatry, 36,* 1656–1663.

Klaber, M. M., Butterfield, E. C., & Gould, L. J. (1969). Responsiveness to social reinforcement among institutionalized retarded children. *American Journal of Mental Deficiency, 73,* 890–895.

Kounin, J. (1941a). Experimental studies of rigidity: I. The measurement of rigidity in normal and feebleminded persons. *Character and Personality, 9,* 251–272.

Kounin, J. (1941b). Experimental studies of rigidity: II. The explanatory power of the concept of rigidity as applied to feeblemindedness. *Character and Personality, 9,* 273–282.

Kounin, J. (1948). The meaning of rigidity: A reply to Heinz Werner. *Psychological Review, 55,* 157–166.

Lewin, K. (1936). *A dynamic theory of personality.* New York: McGraw-Hill.

MacMillan, D. L., Gresham, F. M., & Siperstein, G. N. (1993). Conceptual and psychometric concerns about the 1992 AAMR definition of mental retardation. *American Journal on Mental Retardation, 98,* 325–335.

MacMillan, D. L., Gresham, F. M., & Siperstein, G. N. (1995). Heightened concerns over the 1992 AAMR definition: Advocacy versus precision. *American Journal on Mental Retardation, 100,* 87–95.

MacMillan, D. L., Semmel, M. I., & Gerber, M. M. (1995). The social context: Then and now. In J. M. Kauffman & D. P. Hallahan (Eds.), *Illusion of full inclusion* (pp. 19–38). Austin, TX: Pro-Ed.

Milgram, N. A. (1969). The rationale and irrational in Zigler's motivational approach to mental retardation. *American Journal of Mental Deficiency, 73,* 527–532.

Paul, J. L., & Rosselli-Kostoryz, H. (1997). The future of special education. In J. L. Paul, M. Churton, H. Rosselli-Kostoryz, W. C. Morse, K.

Marfo, C. Lavely, & D. Thomas (Eds.), *Foundations of special education* (pp. 229–235). Pacific Grove, CA: Brooks/Cole.

Pennington, B. F., & Bennetto, L. (1998). Toward a neuropsychology of mental retardation. In J. A. Burack, R. M. Hodapp, & E. Zigler (Eds.), *Handbook of mental retardation and development* (pp. 80–114). New York: Cambridge University Press.

Rosen, M., Diggory, J. C., & Werlinsky, B. (1966). Goal setting and expectancy of success in institutionalized and noninstitutionalized mental subnormals. *American Journal of Mental Deficiency, 71,* 249–255.

Sanders, B., Zigler, E., & Butterfield, E. C. (1968). Outer-directedness in the discrimination learning of normal and mentally retarded children. *Journal of Abnormal Psychology, 73,* 368–375.

Shallenberger, P., & Zigler, E. (1961). Rigidity, negative reaction tendencies, and cosatiation effects in normal and feebleminded children. *Journal of Abnormal and Social Psychology, 63,* 20–26.

Simeonsson, R. J., & Short, R. J. (1996). Adaptive development, survival roles, and quality of life. In J. W. Jacobson & J. A. Mulick (Eds.), *Manual of diagnosis and professional practice in mental retardation* (pp. 137–146). Washington, DC: American Psychological Association.

Simonoff, E., Bolton, P., & Rutter, M. (1998). Genetic perspectives on mental retardation. In J. A. Burack, R. M. Hodapp, & E. Zigler (Eds.), *Handbook of mental retardation and development* (pp. 41–79). New York: Cambridge University Press.

Spitz, H. H. (1986). *The raising of intelligence: A selected history of attempts to raise retarded intelligence.* Hillsdale, NJ: Lawrence Erlbaum Associates.

Stevenson, H. W., & Zigler, E. (1957). Discrimination learning and rigidity in normal and feebleminded individuals. *Journal of Personality, 25,* 699–711.

Stevenson, H. W., & Zigler, E. (1958). Probability learning in children. *Journal of Experimental Psychology, 56,* 185–192.

Trent, J. W., Jr. (1994). *Inventing the feeble mind: A history of mental retardation in the United States.* Berkeley, CA: University of California Press.

Tuddenham, R. D. (1962). The nature and measure of intelligence. In L. Postman (Ed.), *Psychology in the making* (pp. 469–525). New York: Knopf.

Turnure, J. E., & Zigler, E. (1964). Outer-directedness in the problem-solving of normal and retarded children. *Journal of Abnormal Psychology, 69,* 427–436.

Weaver, J. (1966). *The effects of motivation-hygiene orientation and interpersonal reaction tendencies in intellectually subnormal children.* Unpublished doctoral dissertation, George Peabody College for Teachers.

White, R. (1959). Motivation reconsidered: The concept of competence. *Psychological Review, 66,* 297–333.

Windle, C. (1962). Prognosis of mental subnormals. *American Journal of Mental Deficiency, 66* (Monogr. Suppl. 5).

Wolfensberger, W., & Menolascino, F. (1968). Basic considerations in evaluating ability of drugs to stimulate cognitive development in retardates. *American Journal of Mental Deficiency, 73,* 414–423.

Zeaman, D. (1968). Review of N. R. Ellis, *International review of research in mental retardation: Vol. 1. Contemporary Psychology, 13,* 142–143.

Zeaman, D., & House, B. J. (1960). Approach and avoidance in the discrimination learning of retardates. In D. Zeaman et al., *Learning and transfer in mental defectives* (Progress Report No. 2, pp. 32–70). NIMH, USPHS, Res. Grant M-1099 to University of Connecticut.

Zigler, E. (1961). Social deprivation and rigidity in the performance of feebleminded children. *Journal of Abnormal and Social Psychology, 62,* 413–421.

Zigler, E. (1962). Rigidity in the feebleminded. In E. P. Trapp & P. Himelstein (Eds.), *Readings on the exceptional child* (pp. 141–162). New York: Appleton-Century-Crofts.

Zigler, E. (1963a). Rigidity and social reinforcement effects in the performance of institutionalized and noninstitutionalized normal and retarded children. *Journal of Personality, 31,* 258–269.

Zigler, E. (1963b). Social reinforcement, environment and the child. *American Journal of Orthopsychiatry, 33,* 614–623.

Zigler, E. (1966). Research on personality structure in the retardate. In N. R. Ellis (Ed.), *International review of research in mental retardation* (Vol. 1, pp. 77–108). New York: Academic Press.

Zigler, E. (1967). Familial mental retardation: A continuing dilemma. *Science, 155,* 292–298.

Zigler, E. (1969). Developmental versus difference theories of mental retardation and the problem of motivation. *American Journal of Mental Deficiency, 73,* 536–556.

Zigler, E. (1978). National crisis in mental retardation research. American *Journal of Mental Deficiency, 83,* 1–8.

Zigler, E. (1987). The definition and classification of mental retardation. *Upsala Journal of Medical Science, Supplement,* 1–10.

Zigler, E. (1988). The IQ pendulum. [Review of the book *The raising of intelligence: A selected history of attempts to raise retarded intelligence.*] *Readings, 3,* 4–9.

Zigler, E., & Balla, D. (1982). Motivational and personality factors in the performance of the retarded. In E. Zigler & D. Balla (Eds.), *Mental retardation: The developmental-difference controversy* (pp. 9–26). Hillsdale, NJ: Lawrence Erlbaum Associates.

Zigler, E., Balla, D., & Butterfield, E. C. (1968). A longitudinal investigation of the relationship between preinstitutional social deprivation and social motivation in institutionalized retardates. *Journal of Personality and Social Psychology, 10,* 437–445.

Zigler, E., Bennett-Gates, D., & Hodapp, R. (1999). Assessing personality traits of individuals with mental retardation. In E. Zigler & D. Bennet-Gates (Eds.), Personality development in individuals with mental retardation (pp. 206–225). New York: Cambridge University Press.

Zigler, E., Butterfield, E. C., & Capobianco, F. (1970). Institutionalization and the effectiveness of social reinforcement: A five- and eight-year follow-up study. *Developmental Psychology, 3,* 255–263.

Zigler, E., Butterfield, E. C., & Goff, G. A. (1966). A measure of preinstitutional social deprivation for institutionalized retardates. *American Journal of Mental Deficiency, 70,* 873–885.

Zigler, E., & deLabry, J. (1962). Concept-switching in middle-class, lower-class, and retarded children. *Journal of Abnormal and Social Psychology, 65,* 267–273.

Zigler, E., & Harter, S. (1969). Socialization of the mentally retarded. In D. A. Goslin & D. C. Glass (Eds.), *Handbook of socialization theory and research* (pp. 1065–1102). New York: Rand McNally.

Zigler, E., & Hodapp, R. M. (1986). *Understanding mental retardation.* New York: Cambridge University.

Zigler, E., Hodgden, L., & Stevenson, H. W. (1958). The effect of support on the performance of normal and feebleminded children. *Journal of Personality, 26,* 106–122.

Zigler, E., Hodapp, R. M., & Edison, M. R. (1990). From theory to practice in the case and education of mentally retarded individuals. *American Journal on Mental Retardation, 95,* 1–12.

Zigler, E., & Williams, J. (1963). Institutionalization and the effectiveness of social reinforcement: A three-year follow-up study. *Journal of Abnormal and Social Psychology, 66,* 197–205.

2

Personality and Motivational Self-System Processes in Persons With Mental Retardation: Old Memories and New Perspectives

Harvey N. Switzky

Northern Illinois University

INTRODUCTION

The psychological and educational literature over the past 40 years regarding the personality and motivational characteristics of individuals with mental retardation has swelled. Ironically very little of the knowledge contained in that literature has been communicated to researchers, practitioners, educators, families, and others who are concerned with improving the quality of life of persons with mental retardation. Personality and motivational self-system processes are the energizing forces that drive all other psychological, learning, and self-regulatory processes underpinning the performance of persons with mental retardation. Personality and motivational self-system processes influence what information gets stored in the long-term memory system, how that information is organized, and what information is retrieved to enable persons with mental retardation to perform in an adaptive and functional manner. This chapter allows both practitioners and researchers to become better acquainted with the theory of motivational orientation and motivational self-system processes in persons with mental retardation so that they may be energized by the knowledge and to redirect their theories and practices to improve the quality of life of persons with mental retardation.

The chapter has three sections. Section 1 presents a brief historical review and critical examination of the various conceptual models and theories regarding personality and motivational self-system processes in persons with mental retardation which have evolved over the last 40 years. (See also Hickson and Khemka, chap. 4, this volume). Section 2 presents a brief description of a theory of intrinsic and extrinsic motivation (motivational orientation) as developed by a group of researchers that I call the Peabody-Vanderbilt Group (Switzky, 1996, 1997, 1999), of which I was a member, and the evidence which supports their model. Section 3 presents some practical implications of the theory of motivational orientation applicable to the daily lives of persons with mental retardation.

I. MOTIVATIONAL AND SELF-SYSTEM PROCESSES IN PERSONS WITH MENTAL RETARDATION: A BRIEF HISTORY

Forty years ago, conceptions of personality and motivational process in persons with mental retardation were for the most part only ephemerally related to ideas deriving from the psychological models of that period, and few conceptions derived from systematic and sustained analysis of the behavior of persons with mental retardation. Mental retardation researchers were concerned primarily with the role of cognitive processes and the differences in performance between persons with mental retardation compared to persons without mental retardation on a variety of learning tasks in order to identify the deficits which were believed to characterize persons with mental retardation. Developmental, contextual, and personality–motivational processes per se, were not of great interest and were conceived more as threats to internal validity needing to be controlled to allow researchers to more clearly focus on the immensely more important cognitive and learning processes (Haywood & Switzky, 1986; Hobbs, 1963; Hodapp, Burack, & Zigler, 1990; Lipman, 1963; Switzky, 1997, 1999).

Recently, there has been a massive explosion of knowledge concerning persons with mental retardation from more of a holistic, developmental, contextual, motivational, and cognitive perspective (Burack, Hodapp, & Zigler, 1998; Haywood & Switzky, 1986; Merighi, Edison, & Zigler, 1990; Switzky, 1997, 1999, in press; Zigler & Bennett-Gates, 1999; Zigler & Hodapp, 1991), hence the reason for this volume. This new perspective recognizes that the performance of persons with mental retardation reflects the complex interplay of personality and motivational processes with cognitive processes within a developmental and contextual perspective (Borkowski, Carr, Rellinger, & Pressley, 1990; Deci, Hodges, Pierson & Tomassone, 1992; Ford, 1992; 1995; Harter, 1999; Haywood & Switzky, 1992; Hodapp et al. 1990; Pintrich, Anderman, & Klobucar, 1994; Ryan & Deci, 2000; Switzky, 1997, 1999, in press; Switzky & Haywood, 1984; Switzky & Heal, 1990). This point of view not only reflects a new conception of mental retardation, but also reflects mainstream psychological thought concerning the development of human beings as active problem solvers (Bandura, 1997; Deci & Ryan, 1991; Dweck, 1999; Gollwitzer & Bargh, 1996; Heckhausen & Dweck, 1998; Lambert & McCombs, 1998; Lepper, 1996; Lepper & Hodell, 1989; McCombs & Whisler, 1997; Ryan, 1995, 1998; Ryan, Deci, & Grolnick, 1995; Skinner, 1995; Sternberg & Berg, 1992; Stipek, 1998; Zimmerman, 2000). The author views these trends as reflecting the accelerating integration between a psychology of mental retardation and a developmental and contextual psychology of human growth for all human beings (Boekaerts, Pintrich, & Zeidner, 2000; Borkowski et al. 1990; Feuerstein, Klein, & Tannenbaum, 1991; Haywood & Tzuriel, 1992; Hodapp et al.; Pintrich, 2000; Pintrich & Schrauben, 1992; Switzky, 1997, 1999; Weiner, 1994).

Major historical attempts to conceptualize the behavior of persons with mental retardation in terms of personality and motivational constructs to explain the initiation, direction, intensity, and persistence of goal-directed behavior generally followed the prevailing zeitgeist of psychological thought at the time. However, they were derived primarily from the behavior of persons without mental retardation and often needed to be forced, extended, and revised in order to incorporate and explain "motivated" behavior in persons with mental retardation. Sometimes these attempts led to dead ends, while other attempts were quite systematic and fruitful for both psychological theory building and research resulting in a better understanding of the behavior of persons with mental retardation (Haywood & Switzky, 1986, Switzky, 1997).

I review the following theoretical models in Section 1: (a) *the rigidity hypothesis* (Balla & Zigler, 1979; Balla, Butterfield, & Zigler, 1974; Bybee & Zigler, 1992; Harter & Zigler, 1968; Kounin, 1941a, 1941b; Lewin, 1936; Lustman & Zigler, 1982; Zigler, 1961; Zigler, chap. 1, this volume; Zigler & Bennett-Gates, 1999; Zigler, Butterfield, & Goff, 1966); (b) *social learning theories* (Atkinson, 1964; Balla & Zigler, 1979; Bialer, 1961; Covington, 1987; Cromwell, 1963, 1967; Gruen & Zigler, 1968; Harter & Zigler, 1972; Haywood & Switzky, 1986; Hoffman & Weiner, 1978; Horai & Guarnaccia, 1975; Luthar & Zigler, 1988; MacMillan, 1975; McManis & Bell, 1968; McManis, Bell, & Pike, 1969; Miller, 1961; Moss, 1958; Rotter, 1954; Schwartz & Jens, 1969; Stevenson & Zigler, 1958; Switzky, 1997; Weiner, 1986; Zigler & Bennett-Gates, 1999); (c) *self-concept theories* (Balla & Zigler, 1979; Collins & Burger, 1970; Evans, 1998; Glick, 1999; Glick & Zigler, 1985; Haywood & Switzky, 1986; Haywood, Switzky, & Wright, 1973; Leahy, Balla, & Zigler, 1982; Piers & Harris, 1964; Ringness, 1961; Switzky & Hanks, 1973; Zigler, Balla, & Watson, 1972); (d) *anxiety theories* (Balla & Zigler, 1979; Cantor, 1963; Castaneda, McCandless, & Palermo, 1956; Cochran & Cleland, 1963; Lipman, 1960; Lipman & Griffith, 1960; Zigler, 1966a); and (e) *effectance motivation and intrinsic motivation theories* (Harter, 1999, 1983; Harter & Pike, 1984; Harter & Zigler, 1974; Haywood, 1968a, 1968b, 1971, 1992; Haywood & Switzky, 1985, 1986; Hodapp et al. 1990; Switzky, 1997, 1999; Switzky & Haywood, 1974, 1984; Switzky & Heal, 1990; Switzky, Haywood, & Isett, 1974; Switzky, Ludwig, & Haywood, 1979; White, 1959; Zigler, 1966b; Zigler & Balla, 1981, 1982; Zigler & Bennett-Gates, 1999; Zigler & Hodapp, 1991).

A. The Rigidity Hypothesis

The rigidity hypothesis was one of the earliest formulations regarding the cognitive and personality structure of persons with mild mental retardation. It was derived from the work of Lewin (1936) and Kounin (1941a, 1941b) who viewed the structure of cognition as developmentally dynamic and consisting of inner regions of needs, skills, and habits of behavior. As the individual developed there was an increase in the number and the complexity of these inner regions, a process called *differentiation,* which corresponded with the mental age of the individual. The boundaries of each inner region were viewed as also varying in *permeability,* which allowed information to communicate and flow throughout the whole cognitive structure. As an individual matured it was believed that the boundaries between inner regions became less permeable, a quality referred to as *rigidity.* To account for the deficient performance of persons with psychosocial mental retardation compared to persons without mental retardation even when matched on mental age (which controlled for the amount and degree of differentiation of cognition) on different laboratory learning tasks, Lewin and Kounin proposed that the cognitive structure of persons with mental retardation was fundamentally different from that of persons without mental retardation. The boundaries between the inner regions of persons with mental retardation were believed to be less permeable and more rigid, accounting for the greater perseveration, concreteness, and sterotypic performance, all personality traits observed in the samples of individuals with mental retardation persons.

The Lewin-Kounin studies provided a springboard for the most systematic, successful, and sustained series of studies over the past 40 years. They emphasize that the behavior of persons with mental retardation is not primarily due to a fundamentally different and defective cognitive structure but to overlooked motivational and environmental interactions common in persons with and without mental retardation.

The behavior observed in psychosocial persons with mental retardation was hypothesized by Zigler and his colleagues from Yale University (the Yale group) to be due to: (a) their history of repeated failure in attempting to cope with their life experiences; (b) their chronic social deprivation caused by a lack of continuity of care by parents or caretakers, an excessive desire by parents to separate from or institutionalize their child, impoverished economic circumstances, or a family history of marital discord, mental illness, abuse, or neglect, and the experience of living in regimented, harsh, and joyless institutional settings; (c) their history of chronic disapproval by parents, siblings, and other important social agents in their social world; and (d) their cognitive deficiencies and inefficient learning.

As the result of the operation of these environmental variables, the Yale group characterized the personality and motivational characteristics in persons with mental retardation. The Yale group's system combines and derives from themes emanating from social learning models and theories of effectance and intrinsic motivation, as well as self-concept and anxiety theories, and are characterized in terms of the following constructs.

1. *Positive reaction tendencies and overdependency* are the tendencies in persons with mental retardation to be overly dependent and highly motivated to sustain social interactions resulting in social reinforcement from supportive adults to a greater extent than those observed in of the same mental age without mental retardation.

2. *Negative reaction tendencies and wariness* are the tendencies in persons with mental retardation to be initially reluctant, fearful, cautious, and mistrustful (i.e., wary) in social interactions with strange adults in their environment. As a result of their histories of social deprivation, persons with mental retardation appear to be motivated by strong ambivalent feelings to interact with supportive adults (positive reaction tendencies) as well as a reluctance and caution to do so (negative reaction tendencies and wariness). These initial tendencies toward wariness may be replaced by positive reaction tendencies toward adults as a result of a history of interaction where the adult is perceived as less threatening and harmful.

3. *Expectancies of success and failure* are the degree to which an individual expects to succeed or fail when presented with a new task. Generally persons with mental retardation have a higher expectancy to fail on a task compared to persons without mental retardation.

4. *Outerdirectedness* is a learning style of problem solving in persons with mental retardation characterized by a distrust of one's own inner-derived solutions to difficult problems which is characterized by an overreliance on imitating external mediators and generally seeking external stimulus cues as

guides to finding solutions compared to persons of the same mental age without mental retardation.

5.   *Effectance motivation and intrinsic versus extrinsic motiva-* *tion* is associated with the pleasure and sustained perform-ance individuals derive from using their own cognitive resources for their own sake and independence from environ-mentally derived external reinforcement (i.e., task-intrinsic motivation), usually in the domains of exploration, play, curiosity, and mastery of the environment. Individuals lack-ing in effectance motivation are characterized by being heav-ily dependent on receiving environmentally derived external-reinforcement feedback in order to perform a task (i.e., task-extrinsic motivation). Compared to persons without mental retardation of the same mental age, persons with mental retardation generally have less effectance motivation and more of an extrinsic motivational orientation leading to different patterns of incentives and reinforcement hierar-chies. (See the related research of the Peabody-Vanderbilt group described in Section 2.)

6.   *Self-concept* as viewed by the Yale group is viewed develop-mentally as a set of self-images: (a) the real self-image (i.e., the person's current self-concept); (b) the ideal self-image (i.e., the way the person would ideally like to be); and (c) the self-image disparity (i.e., the difference between the real self-image and the ideal self-image). According to developmental theory (Glick, 1999; Glick & Zigler, 1985), the difference between the person's real self-image and ideal self-image increases with higher levels of development. This is assumed to occur because higher levels of development lead to increasing cognitive differentiation, which results in a greater likelihood for disparity between an individual's conceptual-ization of the real self and the ideal self. Additionally, because an individual's capacity to experience guilt increases develop-mentally as the individual incorporates social demands, mores, and values, the individual must measure up to many more internalized demands, and these greater self-demands and the guilt that accompanies them should be reflected in a greater disparity between real and ideal self-images. The expectation is that when children with and without mental

retardation are matched on both mental age and chronological age, children with mental retardation will have lower ideal self-images and lower self-image disparities than children without mental retardation because of their extensive history of failure experiences and low expectancy of success. These ideas are very similar to Markus' theory of possible selves (Markus & Nurius, 1986), which was recently applied by Borkowski et al. (1992) as motivational operators which energize metacognitive self-system processes in children without mental retardation. For the most part, these expectancies regarding the self-concept of children with mental retardation were confirmed in research studies (Leahy, Balla, & Zigler, 1982; Zigler, Balla, & Watson, 1972; see also the section on self-concept theories).

7. *Anxiety* levels of persons with mental retardation are higher than in their chronological age and mental age peers without mental retardation. These high anxiety levels, which are a result of their history of social deprivation and repeated failure in attempting to cope with their life experiences, may depress even more their ability to solve problems in school, at work, and in the community (see also the section on anxiety).

The work of the Yale group over the past 40 years has demonstrated the interaction of experiential, motivational, and personality processes in persons with mental retardation as it affects all aspects of their daily life experiences. Their work has emphasized the operation of motivational processes and has provided some counterbalance to the field's historic research preoccupation with the role of cognitive processes in accounting for the behavior of persons with mental retardation.

B. Social Learning Theories

Social learning theories were initially developed to explain the acquisition of socially relevant behaviors mediated by the operation of a set of internal cognitive processes rather than through the operation of isolated stimulus-response externally reinforced behavioral contingencies. Rotter (1954), an early social learning theorist, emphasized the individual's cognitive expectancies (beliefs) concerning the occurrence of reinforcing events (the contingencies of reward or reinforcement) in the individual's social world as well as the perceived value of these reinforcing events in determining the individual's behavior. Expectancies were determined not only by beliefs about the occurrence of reinforcing events in a particular situation but also by generalized expectancies concerning the occurrence of reinforcing events in other similar situations. Rotter referred to an individual's generalized expectancies regarding the occurrence of reinforcing events as their *locus of control*. Locus of control is the extent to which an individual believed that one's own behavior (e.g., hard work) or a relatively permanent personal characteristic (e.g., physical strength) can be instrumental in determining what happened to one's self (*internal locus of control*), as opposed to the extent to which an individual believed that what happened to one's self was random (e.g., luck, chance, fate) or under the control of external persons (e.g., biased others), examples of an *external locus of control*.

Another construct deriving from Rotter was the notion of success-striving versus failure-avoiding motivational expectancies in individuals. According to Rotter, an individual with a high generalized expectancy for success, the *success-striving* individual, is primed to respond primarily to cues in the social environment which lead to continued success. An individual with a low generalized expectancy for success, *the failure-avoiding individual*, is primed to respond primarily to cues in the social environment which lead to the prevention of additional failure. Such an individual stops trying to be successful as a general motivational orientation and instead is primarily concerned with the prevention of additional failure.

Rotter's (1954) version of social learning theory greatly influenced the work of Cromwell (1963, 1967) and his colleagues (Bialer, 1961; Miller, 1961; Moss, 1958) in their application and extension of social learning theory to the personality and motivational processes of persons with mental retardation. In general (Cromwell, 1963; Haywood & Switzky, 1986, Zigler & Bennett-Gates, 1999), persons with mental retardation were found to be more characterized by (a) an external locus of control and failure-avoiding motivational expectancies than persons without mental retardation; that is, persons with mental retardation had stronger tendencies to be failure-avoiders than success-strivers; (b) entering a novel situation with a performance level depressed below that expected in terms of their psychometric mental age and intelligence; (c) fewer tendencies to increase effort following a mild failure experience; and (d) fewer tendencies to be moved by failure experiences. An internal locus of control developed as a joint function of both mental and chronological age and was positively correlated with task persistence and learning efficiency. In a series of studies, MacMillan and his colleagues (MacMillan & Keogh, 1971) showed that children with mental retardation were more dominated by feelings of failure than children without mental retardation. In these studies, the children were prevented from finishing several tasks and then asked why the tasks were not completed. Children with mental retardation consistently blamed themselves for the lack of task completion compared to the children without mental retardation who blamed their failure on external causes.

Atkinson (1964), another early social learning theorist, derived an expectancy value model of behavior based on an individual's unconscious expectancies for success (the motive for success or need to achieve) or for failure (the motive to avoid failure) in accomplishing the task, and also on an individual's conscious beliefs about that particular situation (i.e., the perceived probability of success associated with the expectations to feel proud, the incentive value of success, and the perceived probability of failure associated with the expectations to feel shame, the incentive value of failure). The tendency to approach a task was determined by an unconscious personality factor (the motive for success or need to achieve) and two conscious situational factors (expectations for success and pride). The tendency to avoid a task was determined by an unconscious personality factor (the motive to avoid failure) and two conscious situational factors (expectations for failure and shame). The resultant tendency to approach or avoid a task was a function of the tendency to approach minus the strength of the tendency to avoid the task. The tendency to approach a task was a multiplicative function of the motive for success the perceived probability of success the incentive value of success. The tendency to avoid a task was a multiplicative function of the motive to avoid failure the perceived probability of failure the incentive value of failure.

Theories of achievement motivation derived from Atkinson's model are based on the idea that the need for achievement is derived from a conflict between striving for success and a need to avoid failure. Individuals showed extreme individual differences in the ways they resolved this conflict (Covington, 1987): Some approach success despite the risk of failure, while others act defensively to avoid failure with its implications for low ability. Success-oriented persons with strong needs to achieve prefer achievement tasks where the probability of success is equal to the probability of failure, thus ensuring themselves of sufficient successes to sustain further effort without too easy a victory. Failure-prone persons with strong needs to avoid failure prefer achievement tasks that are either too easy or too difficult, thus increasing the probability of success in the former case and establishing excuses in advance for failure in the latter case.

Atkinson's (1964) version of social learning theory also influenced researchers in mental retardation (McManis & Bell, 1968; McManis, Bell, & Pike, 1969; Schwarz & Jens, 1969). However, much of this work led to inconsistent results and was never followed up by other researchers in mental retardation. Atkinson's ideas concerning an individual's performance as being dependent on personality factors, expectations concerning success and failure, and emotional states profoundly affected later motivational theorists who extended his work (Ames & Ames, 1984, 1985, 1989; Borkowski et al., 1992; Covington, 1987; Deci & Ryan, 1985, 1991, 1995; Dweck, 1989, 1998, 1999; Ford, 1992, 1995; H. Heckhausen, 1967, 1983, 1991; Kuhl, 1987, 2000; Maehr & Pintrich, 1991; Nicholls, 1989; Pintrich, 2000; Ryan & Deci, 2000; Skinner, 1995; Zimmerman, 2000; Zimmerman & Schunk, 1989).

A more fruitful line of research based on the zeitgeist of early social learning models focused on the effects of success and failure expectancies on problem-solving behavior. Typically a probability learning paradigm was used which is a variant of a three-choice discrimination problem in which one stimulus is partially reinforced (usually 66% of the time) and the other two stimuli are never reinforced. Thus, the subject is faced with an insoluble problem; that is, they can never be correct 100% of the time. If an individual persistently chooses a partially reinforced stimulus, he or she is using a maximizing strategy of reinforcement success. It has been hypothesized that because of their low expectancies of success, children with mental retardation are more likely than children with higher expectancies of success to use a maximizing strategy. Children with higher expectations of success believe that the problem has a solution and that they can be successful all of the time, so they tend not to use a maximizing strategy. It has been shown that children with mental retardation are found to use more maximizing strategies than children without mental retardation (Gruen & Zigler, 1968; Stevenson & Zigler, 1958; Zigler, this volume; Zigler & Bennett-Gates, 1999).

Weiner (1986), building on the work of Rotter (1954) and Atkinson (1964), developed a cognitive model of need for achievement and the behavior of success-striving, success-oriented individuals and failure-avoiding, failure-prone individuals, based on the individuals' own interpretations of the causes to which they attributed their own success or failure experiences. Weiner expanded Rotter's single internal-external locus of control dimension into three separate dimensions: locus, stability, and control. The locus dimension referred to the source of the behavior, that is, whether the behavior was due to internal or external causes. The stability dimension referred to the relative permanence or impermanence of the cause of the behavior, that is, one's ability level was viewed as relatively permanent, whereas one's effort, luck, or mood were viewed as more labile. The control dimension referred to the perceived amount of control an individual has over the cause of the behavior; that is, although one can control the amount of effort expended on a task, one has no control regarding luck on a task. In general, failure-prone individuals attributed their failures to a lack of ability (a permanent quality) and ascribed their successes to impermanent external causes such as positive teacher bias, good luck, or an easy task, whereas success-oriented individuals ascribed their poor performances to lack of effort (an impermanent quality) (Covington, 1987).

Weiner's attributional theory (Weiner, 1986) has inspired some studies with persons with mental retardation. Horai and Guarnaccia (1975) gave a coding task under success feedback (subjects were informed that they had done well) and failure feedback (subjects were informed that they had done poorly and that others had done much better) experimental conditions. Horai and Guarnaccia (1975) interviewed their subjects (male adults with mild mental retardation from a community-based training center) with an exhaustive forced-choice procedure to determine their attributions of success or failure (ability, effort, task difficulty, or luck). It was expected, that because of their history of failure, persons with mental retardation would have cognitive attributions similar to those associated with a failure-prone cognitive orientation: they would make more attributions to lack of ability under failure feedback than attributions to ability under success feedback, and they would make more attributions to increased effort under success feedback than attributions to lack of effort under failure feedback.

Successful subjects were found more likely to credit their high ability for their performance than were failure subjects to credit their low ability for their failure. Failure subjects were more likely to blame their lack of effort than were successful subjects to say that they tried harder on the task. Failure subjects were more likely to attribute their failure to bad luck than were successful subjects to attribute their success on the task to good luck. There were no differences in attributions to task difficulty between the two groups. This study demonstrated that Weiner's attribution theory could be applied to adults with mental retardation and that the attributions of adults with mental retardation could be assessed. Furthermore, contrary to the expectation that all persons with mental retardation show homogeneous personality structures with regards to their reactions to success and failure experiences, that is, in this case they would use the attributions predicted for failure-prone individuals, the persons with mental retardation in this study functioned more like success-oriented individuals. This study showed that contrary to Cromwell's (1963) generalization that persons with mental retardation expect failure and have fewer tendencies to be moved by it than persons without mental retardation, persons with mental retardation show great individual differences in their responses to success and failure.

Hoffman and Weiner (1978) performed a partial replication of the Horai and Guarnaccia (1975) study on a group of TMR adults using a coding task to give success and failure experiences. This study used three causal attributions (ability, effort, and task difficulty). These adults with moderate retardation behaved to the success and failure feedback in a most realistic manner similar to the pattern observed in adults without mental retardation. The learning and performance of persons with mental retardation can be facilitated if adaptive attributions are combined with outcome information leading to a pattern of cognitive attributions ascribing high ability for success feedback and ascribing lack of effort for failure feedback. Both these studies show that the state of being mentally retarded does not inevitably lead to a failure-prone cognitive orientation and that one must be cognizant of the variety of individual differences existing in persons with mental retardation. Only a subset of persons with mental retardation have been found to make attributions that are counterproductive to achievement strivings (Zoeller, Mahoney, & Weiner, 1983).

Social learning theories have provided a fruitful model to understand the motivational systems of persons with mental retardation. Social learning approaches have evolved considerably over the past 40 years, influencing research with both and populations with and without mental retardation (Bandura, 1997; Boekaerts, Pintrich, & Zeidner, 2000; Dweck, 1999; J. Heckhausen & Dweck, 1998; Switzky, 1997, 1998; Zigler & Bennett-Gates, 1999).

C. Self-Concept Theories

Self-concept theories have increasingly dominated mainstream psychological research from the 1940s (Rogers, 1947; Snygg & Combs, 1949) to today (Boekaerts, Pintrich, & Zeidner, 2000; Harter, 1983, 1990, 1993, 1999; Leahy, 1985, Marsh & Holms, 1990; Marsh & Shavelson, 1985; Marsh & Hattie, 1996; Markus & Wurf, 1987; McCombs, 1988, 1989; McCombs & Marzano, 1990; McCombs & Whisler, 1989; Zimmerman & Schunk, 1989). Research on the self-concept of persons with mental retardation has been sparse and inconsistent because of the extreme difficulty of studying populations so limited in verbal behavior (Balla & Zigler, 1979; Glick, 1999; Haywood & Switzky, 1986).

It might be expected that because of their long history of failure and lack of success, stigmatization, rejection, and cognitive deficiencies persons with mental retardation would have lower self-concepts and extreme negative self-perceptions compared to persons without mental retardation (Balla & Zigler, 1979; Covington, 1987; Harter, 1999; Haywood & Switzky, 1986; Merighi et al., 1990). This expectation has been only partially supported (see also Zeidner, 1995).

Collins and Burger (1970) found no overall differences in self-concept between adolescents with and without mild mental retardation. Piers and Harris (1964) suggested that there might be a positive correlation between self-concept and measured intelligence. Their groups with mental retardation scored significantly lower on the Piers-Harris Children's Self-Concept Scale than either third or sixth grade children of normal intelligence. They also found that in their groups without mental retardation, subjects of higher psychometric intelligence and academic achievement had more positive self-concepts. Similarly, Gorlow, Butler, and Guthrie (1963) found that adolescents with mental retardation who scored lower on three self-concept scales also scored lower on the WAIS, the California Achievement Test, and a measure of arithmetic achievement.

Ringness (1961) found that children with mild mental retardation tended to overestimate their own success more than did average or intellectually superior children. The children with mental retardation rated themselves less favorably than did those in the intellectually superior group but not less favorably than did those in the average group. Self-concept measured as expectancy of success in children with mental retardation was found to be less realistic, in terms of actual achievement, than in the children without mental retardation. It was also found that the self-concept ratings of children with mental retardation were found to be less reliable than for average or intellectually superior children.

Haywood, Switzky, and Wright (1974) and Switzky and Hanks (1973) reported on a set of studies trying to relate vocational training success (as measured by supervisor's rating and production rates of subjects) to personality and intelligence measures in a group primarily consisting of 67 adults with mild mental retardation. (See Zewdie, 1995, for a similar study on African-American adults with moderate mental retardation). Each subject was given a battery of nine instruments: the Tennessee Self-Concept Scale, Clinical and Research Form (Fitts, 1965), a global self-concept measure; the Junior Eysenck Personality Inventory (Eysenck, 1965), a measure of extraversion—introversion and neuroticism—emotionality; the Piers-Harris Children's Self-Concept

Scale (Piers & Harris, 1969), a global self-concept measure; the Children's Personality Questionnaire (Porter, Cattell, & Ford, 1968), a global personality measure; the Children's Locus of Control (Bialer, 1961); Miller's Adult Locus of Evaluation (Miller, 1965), a measure of the individual's reliance on one's self (internal) or others (external) in evaluating one's own performance; the Raven Coloured Progressive Matrices (Raven, 1956) and the Raven Standard Progressive Matrices (Raven, 1960), measures of cognition; the Matching Familiar Figures (Kagan, 1964), a measure of impulsivity—reflectivity; and the Picture Motivation Scale (Kunca & Haywood, 1969), a measure of intrinsic or extrinsic motivational orientation. Together, the Piers-Harris Children's Self-Concept Scale, the Raven Progressive Matrices, the Matching Familiar Figures, and age accounted for 41% of the variance in supervisor's rating ($R = .64$, $p < .001$). For 27 subjects, both supervisor's ratings and production rates were available. Production rates correlated significantly with supervisor's rating ($r = .50$, $p < .01$). For the 27 subjects, the Piers-Harris Children's Self-Concept Scale, the Matching Familiar Figures, and the Picture Motivation Scale together accounted for 57% of the variance in supervisor ratings ($R = .76$, $p < .025$). For the subset of the 27 subjects, individuals who had lower reported self-concepts about their academic and intellectual ability were rated higher by their supervisors and were producing at a higher rate. Those who gave higher reports of their ability were rated lower and produced at a lower rate. The supervisors may have given higher ratings to those vocational trainees who showed a more realistic assessment of their abilities. Furthermore, production rates may have been higher for vocational trainees with more accurate self-concepts. The results of this study replicate Ringness' (1961) findings. This study seemed to indicate either an unrealistically high self-concept in poor achievers with mental retardation or a problem with the reliability of self-concept measures in individuals with mental retardation. The study also illustrates the very large individual differences regarding personality and motivational variables existing in the group of vocational trainees.

    Zigler and his colleagues in the Yale group (Glick, 1999; Glick & Zigler, 1985) developed a developmental theory of self-concept which has been applied successfully to persons with mild mental retardation and mental ages of nine years or older (Leahy et al.,

1982; Zigler et al., 1972) that may give self-concept research new vigor and thrust. Self-concept is viewed by the Yale group as a set of self-images: the real self-image, the ideal self-image, and the self-image disparity. As development (mental age, MA) increases the differences between the person's real self-image and ideal self-image becomes greater. This is assumed to occur because higher levels of development lead to increasing cognitive differentiation. This greater cognitive differentiation results in a greater likelihood for disparity between an individual's conceptualization of the real self and an individual's conceptualization of the ideal self. Additionally, because an individual's capacity to experience guilt increases developmentally as the individual incorporates social demands, mores, and values, the individual must measure up to many more internalized demands, and these greater self-demands and the guilt that accompanies them should be reflected in a greater disparity between real and ideal self-images (Bybee & Zigler, 1991; Bybee, Ennis & Zigler, 1990; Zigler & Glick, 1986).

Importantly, the Yale group has come up with a set of scales measuring the various aspects of self-concept that may have construct validity for a person with mild mental retardation (MA > 9 years) the Katz-Zigler adjective checklist of real, ideal, and negative future self-images (1967), the Self-Perception Profile for Children (Harter 1985), and spontaneous self-descriptions of real, ideal, and negative future self-images (Bybee, Glick, & Zigler, 1990). In essence, these developments may facilitate new research in the self-concepts of persons with mild mental retardation because of more valid instruments.

D. Anxiety Theories

Anxiety theories have also long dominated mainstream psychological research (Cantor, 1963; Covington, 1987; Hill, 1984; Hill & Wigfield, 1984; Sarason, Davidson, Lighthall, Waite, & Ruebusch, 1960; Spielberger, 1972), but have not been fruitfully applied in allowing researchers to understand the motivational systems operating in persons with mental retardation, perhaps because of the same reasons which have hampered the application of self-concept theories to persons with mental retardation (limited verbal ability and the lack of suitable research instruments having adequate reliability and construct validity in populations with mental retardation). Balla and Zigler (1979) believe that there are suitable instruments which can be applied to persons with mental retardation, that is, the Children's Manifest Anxiety Scale (CMAS) (Castaneda et al., 1956), even though it requires a fourth grade reading level, as well as the Test Anxiety Scale for Children (TASC) (Sarason et al., 1960).

It might be expected that, because of their history of failure, social deprivation, and cognitive deficiencies, persons with mental retardation may have higher levels of anxiety regarding their ability to cope with their life experiences compared to persons without mental retardation and that these levels of higher anxiety may depress even more their competence to solve problems in school, at work, and in the community. These expectations have for the most part been supported (see also Zeidner, 1995).

Lipman (1960) compared the CMAS scores of institutionalized females with mild mental retardation to their mental-age-matched peers without mental retardation and found evidence of higher levels of anxiety in the group with mental retardation. Lipman and Griffith (1960) attempted to determine the relationship between CMAS scores and a test of verbal abstraction in a group of institutionalized persons with mild mental retardation. There was a moderate negative correlation between CMAS scores and verbal abstracting performance and a strong positive correlation between psychometric intelligence and the total abstracting score. Anxiety depressed performance on the hard items but did not facilitate performance on the easy items, a kind of Yerkes-Dodson law (Yerkes & Dodson, 1908). Cochran and Cleland (1963) found greater levels of anxiety in an institutionalized sample with mental retardation than in either a chronological age or an academically matched sample of persons without mental retardation. Generally, persons with mental retardation have higher levels of anxiety than their mental and chronological age peers without mental retardation, with institutionalized individuals with mental retardation being more anxious than individuals with mental retardation living in the community (Balla & Zigler, 1979).

More recently, Glick (1999) and Glick, Bybee, and Zigler (1997) found evidence that the newer measures of self-concept (i.e., the Katz-Zigler Scale, 1967; the Self-Perception Profile for Children, Harter, 1985; and spontaneous descriptions of self-images, Bybee et al. 1990), when used on adolescents with mild mental retardation, show that low self-esteem is related to depression as measured by the Children's Depression Inventory (CDI) (Kovacs, 1983). The Pearson Correlation Coefficients among the CDI score and Harter Self-Perception measure scores varied from $r = .64-.47$, $p < .05$, and the CDI scores and the Real Self-Image scores derived from the Katz-Zigler scale were $r = .47$, $p < .01$. The less positive the real self-images were, the greater the amount of depression found demonstrating predictive validity of the measures used. Again, these developments may expand further research on depression in adolescents with mild mental retardation because of the availability of valid instruments.

E. Effectance Motivation and Intrinsic Motivation Theories

Effectance motivation and intrinsic motivation theories have greatly influenced our understanding of exploration, curiosity, mastery, and play behavior in persons with mental retardation and in persons without mental retardation (Harter & Zigler, 1974; Haywood, 1992; Haywood & Switzky, 1986, 1992; Switzky, 1997, 1999, in press; Switzky & Haywood, 1974, 1984, 1991, 1992; Switzky & Heal, 1990; Switzky et al. 1974, 1979; Zigler & Balla, 1982; Zigler & Bennett-Gates, 1999; Zigler & Hodapp, 1991). This area of research has been one of the most productive areas of experimentation in aiding researchers to understand personality and motivational processes in persons with mental retardation. Much of this work has been done by two research groups, the Yale group (Zigler, chap. 1, this volume; Zigler & Bennett-Gates, 1999) and the Peabody-Vanderbilt group (Haywood & Switzky, 1986; Switzky, 1997, 1999). Both groups were greatly influenced by White's (1959) formulation of effectance motivation or mastery motivation which theorized that everyone has an intrinsic need to feel competent in their interactions with their world. This competence is associated with the pleasure and sustained performance individuals derive from using their own cognitive resources for their own sake and being independent from environmentally derived external reinforcement, especially in the domains of exploration, play, curiosity, and mastery of the environment. White theorized that effectance motivation is relatively undifferentiated and global in young children and directed toward environmental features that capture their attention. Very young children may repeatedly engage in the same activity (e.g., banging on a drum) for the shear joy of the experience. As children become older their effectance motivation becomes more focused and they may direct their effectance motivation toward mastery of specific activities (e.g., sports, and specific school subjects). In adults, effectance motivation is directed toward job skills.

The Yale group conceptualized the motivational problems of persons with mental retardation as due in part to deficient effectance motivation and lack of concern for the intrinsic motivation that inheres in being correct regardless of whether or not an external agent dispenses the reinforcer for such correctness. This lack of effectance motivation is characterized by being heavily dependent on receiving environmentally-derived external reinforcement feedback in order to perform a task (i.e., task extrinsic motivation) and an overreliance on clues from the external environment to help guide behavioral performance (i.e., outerdirectedness), with a concomitant increase in extrinsically motivated behavior. Generally, because of their socially depriving life histories, their greater cognitive deficiencies, and related failure experiences, persons with mild mental retardation have less effectance motivation and more of an extrinsic motivational orientation leading to different patterns of incentives and reinforcement hierarchies compared to persons of the same mental age without mental retardation (Balla & Zigler, 1979; Hodapp et al., 1990, Merighi, et al., 1990; Zigler & Balla, 1981, 1982; Zigler & Bennett-Gates, 1999; Zigler & Hodapp, 1991).

Harter and her colleagues (Harter, 1978, 1981a, 1981b, 1982, 1983, 1987, 1992; Harter & Connell, 1984; Harter & Pike, 1984; Harter, Whitesell, & Kowalski, 1992; Renick & Harter, 1989; Silon & Harter, 1985) recently developed a program of developmental research in which White's (1959) theories of effectance and mastery motivation have been refined, extended, and operationalized.

Harter (1978, 1981a, 1983) presented a model of effectance motivation that could have implications for the development of extrinsic and intrinsic motivational orientations in persons with mental retardation. According to her basic model, the developmental pathways that lead to an intrinsic orientation are associated with positive reinforcement and approval by socialization agents for independent mastery attempts early in children's development. Additionally, socialization agents may model this approval and not reinforce children for dependency on adults. As a result, children internalize two critical self-systems: (a) a self-reward system, and (b) a system of standards or mastery goals that diminishes the children's dependency on external extrinsic social reinforcement. This leads to feelings of competence and feelings of being in control of one's successes and failures and increases children's effectance and intrinsic motivation. This increased sense of intrinsic pleasure enhances one's motivation to engage in subsequent mastery behavior. Thus, children's social environments support their inherent need for mastery over their worlds with the result that their behavior and incentive systems may be characterized as intrinsically motivated.

The developmental pathways that lead to an extrinsic orientation consist of negative outcomes such as lack of reward for or disapproval of independent mastery attempts, and modeling of such disapproval, as well as reinforcement for dependency by adults. Children in these environments increasingly manifest strong needs for external approval and dependence on externally-defined behavioral goals. This leads to feelings of low perceived competence and perceptions that external agents and events are controlling what is happening. These feelings of not being in control of one's successes and failures lead to feelings of anxiety in mastery situations and attenuate the motivation to be engaged in mastery behavior. Thus, such effectance motivation is blocked and reduced, resulting in an extrinsic motivational orientation. Children who have experienced early failure and disapproval by socialization agents become children whose behavior is extrinsically motivated. This latter pattern may be especially characteristic of children who are behaviorally incompetent and children with mental retardation (e.g., those who are behaviorally disordered, learning disabled, or have motoric or sensory handicaps), leading them to display greater behavioral deficits than would have been predicted on the basis of their initial incompetence, that is, the mental age deficit. This analysis is very similar to models derived and extended from the Peabody-Vanderbilt group (Haywood, 1992; Haywood & Burke, 1977; Haywood & Switzky, 1986, 1992; Haywood & Tzuriel, 1992; Schultz & Switzky, 1990,

1993; Switzky, 1997, 1999; Switzky & Haywood, 1984, 1991; Switzky & Heal, 1990; Switzky & Schultz, 1988), as well as models derived and extended from the Yale group (Hodapp et al., 1990; Weisz, 1979, 1981, 1990, 1999; Zigler & Bennett-Gates, 1999).

Weisz (1999) showed that children and adults with psychosocial retardation, because of their lifetime exposure to failure experiences, appear to be more susceptible to learned helplessness (Abramson, Seligman, & Teasdale, 1978) (i.e., a learned perception that one cannot control outcomes) than are children and adults without mental retardation. Persons with mental psychosocial retardation may show extreme performance deterioration in problem-solving ability in response to failure feedback. Persons with psychosocial mental retardation may have a high expectancy of failure: when confronted with failure experiences, they may just stop performing.

Harter developed several self-report instruments to measure components of her model of effectance motivation. The Scale of Intrinsic Versus Extrinsic Orientation in the Classroom (Harter, 1981b) is intended to measure motivational orientation in the classroom in children in Grades 2–9 without mental retardation. Factor analysis resulted in two factors, a motivational factor labeled curiosity/interest and a cognitive-informational factor labeled independent judgment versus reliance on teacher's judgment. Different developmental trends were shown for the motivational factor and the cognitive-informational factor. On the motivational factor, children began with high intrinsic scores in the third grade, which shifted to high extrinsic scores by the ninth grade. This shift toward increasing extrinsic orientation is difficult to interpret. It might reflect an adaptive reaction of students to the teaching styles and school socialization climate created by teachers in the school who use extrinsic reinforcers and performance feedback in a controlling fashion rather than in an informational manner, thereby supporting an extrinsic orientation learning style in the students. The informational classroom environment conveys relevant information to the student about the student's competence at a task, thus supporting self-autonomy and intrinsic motivation in the learner. The controlling classroom environment is designed to bring about a particular behavioral outcome in the student, thus supporting dependency and extrinsic motivation in the learner (Connell & Ryan, 1984; Decharms, 1968, 1976,

1984; Deci & Ryan, 1985; Deci, Nezlek, & Scheinman, 1981; Deci, Schwartz, Scheinman, & Ryan, 1981; Ryan & Deci, 2000; Ryan, Connell & Deci, 1985; Schultz & Switzky, 1990; Switzky, 1997; Switzky, & Schultz, 1988).

On the cognitive-informational factor, an opposite linear trend was observed. Third-grade children had high extrinsic scores, representing dependency on the teacher's judgment and external sources of evaluation, whereas ninth-grade children had high intrinsic scores representing reliance on their own judgment and self-evaluation of success and failure. These trends may represent the internalization of the mastery goals of the classroom as well as its performance criteria and the children's increasing knowledge of the rules of the school.

Harter (1992) has modified her scales to include a subscale to assess internalized motivation. The questionnaire contains 24 items to assess three motivational orientations (extrinsic, intrinsic, internalized). The students are asked to rate the truth value of a series of statements that reflect different goals and reasons for performing one's school work. An item assessing internalized motivation ("I do my schoolwork because I've learned for myself that it's important for me to do it") can be contrasted with an intrinsic reason ("I do my schoolwork because what we learn is really interesting") and an extrinsic reason ("I do my schoolwork because my teacher will be pleased with me if I do it").

Abhalter and Switzky (1992) use of Harter's Scale of Intrinsic Versus Extrinsic Orientation in the Classroom on a population of upper middle class children in the second through fifth grade only partially replicated Harter's (1981b) findings. On the motivational factor (curiosity/interest) children began with high intrinsic scores which sharply increased with grade level; that is, there was an increasing intrinsic orientation. On the cognitive-informational factor, a similar trend was observed: intrinsic scores increased with grade level. The Abhalter and Switzky (1992) finding supports the importance of the school climate variables operating. In the particular school system studied, it was observed that classroom teachers tended to function in more of an informational than a controlling manner.

Silon and Harter (1985) have used the Scale of Intrinsic Versus Extrinsic Orientation in the Classroom with a sample of 9- to 12-year-old children with mild mental retardation. Factor analysis resulted in two factors similar to those found in the sample of children without mental retardation: a motivational factor labeled motivation for hard work and a cognitive/informational factor labeled autonomous judgment. The most salient motivational theme for the sample of children with mental retardation was wanting to do either difficult or easy schoolwork rather than a more global intrinsic or extrinsic orientation. The concern of the children with mental retardation seemed to be more on what one wants to do in the classroom (hard vs. easy work) rather than on the reasons why one performs in the classroom (curiosity). Although there are differences in what is being measured by this scale with groups of and children with and without mental retardation, the children with mental retardation appear considerably more extrinsically oriented than do the children without mental retardation, replicating the findings of the Peabody-Vanderbilt group which has studied intrinsic and extrinsic motivational self-system processes for more than 30 years. The details of their research findings will be discussed in Section 2.

Harter (1982) developed another self-report scale, the Perceived Competence Scale for Children, in an attempt to measure domain-specific feelings of competence in children in Grades 3–9 without mental retardation. Four domains of perceived competence were hypothesized: cognitive competence, with an emphasis on academic performance; social competence, with an emphasis on peer relationships; physical competence, with an emphasis on sports and outdoor games; and a general sense of self-worth. Confirmatory factor analysis supported these four domains of competence.

Silon and Harter (1985) used the Perceived Competence Scale for Children on a sample of children ages 9 to 12 years with mild mental retardation. Factor analysis resulted in two factors similar to those found by Harter and Pike (1984) in children ages 4 to 7 years without mental retardation: a factor composed of the cognitive competence and physical competence subscales labeled general competence, and a factor composed of items from the social competence subscale labeled popularity. No general self-worth factor emerged. Children with mild mental retardation with mental ages less than 8 years appeared not to make distinctions about specific competence domains but rather simply made judgments about one's competence at activities in general, judging people to be competent or not competent, as do young children without mental retardation.

Research (Harter & Pike, 1984; Nicholls, 1984, 1990; Nicholls & Miller, 1984a, 1984b) has shown that self-perceptions of competence change developmentally. Children without mental retardation below the age of 8 years do not make judgments concerning their holistic worth as persons. They have not yet developed the concept of the self as a global entity that can be evaluated in terms of general worth. Preschool children through Grade 2 have a broadly defined concept of competence that includes social behavior, performance, and effort (Blumenfeld, Pintrich, Meece, & Wessels, 1982; Stipek, 1984; Yussen & Kane, 1985). As the children proceed developmentally they increasingly differentiate among their competence domains (Marsh, Barnes, Cairns, & Tidman, 1984; Nicholls, 1989).

Many of the hypothesized relationships among variables in Harter's model have been supported. As levels of intrinsic motivation increase in children, their perceptions of perceived competence and internal control increase also (Harter, 1981a; Harter, 1999; Harter & Connell, 1984). Children who perceive themselves as competent enjoy tasks more and display greater levels of intrinsic motivation than children who perceive themselves as incompetent (Boggiano, Main, & Katz, 1988; Gottfried, 1985, 1990). These children also obtain greater pleasure from succeeding on more difficult tasks compared with easier tasks (Harter, 1978, 1981a). Bandura (1986a) showed that models and reinforcement affect children's mastery attempts and internalization of self-reinforcement systems and mastery goal systems. Licht and Kistner (1986) and Schunk (1989b) showed that children with learning problems perceive themselves as incompetent, often fail in school, and have decreased levels of intrinsic motivation. Children at risk for academic failure are often held in low esteem by their peers and have parents who have low academic expectations; thus, motivation suffers when families do not reward mastery attempts and students do not associate with mastery-oriented peers (Bryan & Bryan, 1983). For further information regarding the Yale group's model of effectance and intrinsic motivation, see Zigler (chap. 1, this volume), and Zigler and Bennett-Gates (1999).

2. THE PEABODY-VANDERBILT
MODEL OF EFFECTANCE
AND INTRINSIC MOTIVATION

More than 30 years have passed since the Peabody-Vanderbilt group began its study of intrinsic motivation in a cognitive theory of motivational orientation (Haywood, 1992; Haywood & Burke, 1977; Haywood & Switzky, 1986, 1992; Schultz & Switzky, 1990; Switzky,1997,1999; Switzky & Haywood, 1974, 1984, 1991, 1992; Switzky & Schultz, 1988; Switzky et al., 1974, 1979) based on the idea that behavior for its own sake and using one's cognitive resources to the fullest are intrinsically gratifying and motivating for all persons. Our group has investigated individual differences in task-intrinsic and task-extrinsic motivation and how these differences affect behavior under various contextual conditions in persons with and without mental retardation.

The theory of motivational orientation is related to White's (1959) theory of effectance motivation and was influenced by Hunt's (1963, 1965, 1966, 1971) conception of motivation inherent in information processing and action, the two-factor theory of work motivation formulated by Herzberg (Herzberg, 1966; Herzberg & Hamlin, 1961, 1963; Herzberg, Mausner, & Snyderman, 1959), Bandura's social cognitive learning theories (Bandura, 1977, 1978, 1986a, 1997), and Feuerstein's theory of mediational learning experiences (MLE) (Feuerstein & Rand, 1974, Feuerstein, Rand, Hoffman, & Miller, 1980; Feuerstein, Klein, & Tannenbaum, 1991).

The constitutive definition of intrinsic motivation evolved as the theory of motivational orientation developed. As influenced by Hunt's system, intrinsic motivation refers to Hunt's (1963, 1971) conception of "motivation inherent in information processing and action". It is behavior in the absence of external stimulation or the possibility of external consequences, arising from the expectation of the joy of the information-processing activity itself. Individuals explore for the satisfaction of taking in and processing new information, even though encountering new information may result in an increase rather than a decrease in the total level of tension within one's psychological system (Haywood & Burke, 1977; Haywood & Switzky, 1992; Hunt, 1965, 1966, 1971). Hunt

(1963), in a very perceptive paper that foreshadowed many current issues, advanced eight questions that theories of motivation must answer:

1. *The instigation question* is concerned with what initiates behavior and what terminates behavior.
2. *The energization question* is concerned with what controls the vigor of an activity.
3. *The direction-hedonic question* is concerned with what controls the direction of behavior and what selects the cognitive activities individuals perform from among an array of available options.
4. *The cathexis question* is concerned with the choice of objects, places, and persons that individuals may form attachments with.
5. *The choice of response question* is concerned with what controls the particular response individuals finally make from among an array of responses.
6. *The choice of goals question* is concerned with what controls the particular end-goal individuals finally make from among an array of goals.
7. *The learning question* is concerned with identifying the factors that underlie and influence behavioral, conceptual change and performance for individuals.
8. *The persistence question* is concerned with why individuals persist in utilizing responses that fail to achieve their goals and why they persist in seeking goals they do not achieve.

Haywood (1992) answered Hunt's questions regarding a theory of intrinsic motivation as follows: Intrinsic motivation instigates activity, especially mental activity, because activity is more pleasant and more exciting than inactivity. Intrinsic motivation leads to more vigorous behavior than does extrinsic motivation, thus energizing behavior. Intrinsic motivation directs behavior toward the more psychologically exciting or interesting alternative paths. Intrinsic motivation aids in the formation of unique attachments or cathexes specifically leading individuals to return to intrinsically motivating tasks. Choice of response and goal may be the most powerful function of intrinsic motivation. Given an array of choices, intrinsically motivated individuals will select responses that are more difficult to perform and will move individuals toward distant goals compared to extrinsically motivated persons. Intrinsic motivation will increase learning efficiency and the persistence of performance for individuals in using responses that fail to achieve their goals and in pursuing goals that are not achieved, simply because it is the activity itself that is rewarding and not the mere attainment of external goals.

A second use of the term intrinsic motivation (Haywood & Switzky, 1986; Switzky, 1999) refers to task-extrinsic vs. task-intrinsic motivation, which is viewed as a learned personality trait by which individuals may be characterized in terms of the location of incentives that are effective in motivating their behavior. Individuals may be motivated by task-intrinsic incentives (e.g., responsibility, challenge, creativity, opportunities to learn, and task achievement) or by task-extrinsic incentives (e.g., ease, comfort, safety, security, health, and practicality aspects of the environment). Individuals who are motivated by task-intrinsic incentives are referred to as intrinsically motivated, whereas, individuals who are motivated by task-extrinsic incentives are referred to as extrinsically motivated. While all persons respond to each kind of incentive, it is the relative balance between the two sources of motivation, that is, the relative number of situations in which one is likely to be motivated by task-intrinsic versus task-extrinsic incentives, that constitutes a stable and measurable personality trait.

This trait theory of motivational orientation was derived from the two-factor theory of work motivation formulated by Herzberg's group (Herzberg, 1966; Herzberg et al., 1959). Herzberg's group was looking for sources of job satisfaction and dissatisfaction in industrial workers. The group asked workers to think of times when they had been quite satisfied with their jobs and times when they had been so dissatisfied that they had thoughts of changing jobs and then to identify the variables to which they attributed their dissatisfaction or satisfaction. In characterizing periods of dissatisfaction, the workers listed such variables as low pay; poor, unhealthy, hazardous, or uncomfortable work conditions; the context in which the job was performed; and lack of security—all conditions extrinsic to the job (to the task) itself, that is, task-extrinsic motivation. In characterizing periods of positive job satisfaction, instead of referring to the opposite poles of the dissatisfying task-extrinsic conditions the workers listed such task-intrinsic variables as the sheer psychological satisfaction of doing a task, opportunities to learn new things, to exercise creativity, to take responsibility, or to experience aesthetic aspects of the job (the task)—all conditions intrinsic to the job (to the task) itself, that is, task-intrinsic motivation. Herzberg's group conceived of these variables not as lying on a single bipolar dimension but as constituting two nonoverlapping dimensions that could vary simultaneously. Subsequent research revealed the power of the *motivator* (i.e., task-intrinsic factors in the theory of motivational orientation) variables over the *hygiene* (i.e., task-extrinsic factors in the theory of motivational orientation) in improving job satisfaction and job performance in a variety of industrial settings. A significant relationship to mental health was demonstrated by Herzberg and Hamlin (1961, 1963) who showed that intrinsic motivation appeared to be positively correlated with mental health and negatively correlated with mental illness.

The Peabody-Vanderbilt group (Haywood, 1992; Haywood & Burke, 1977; Haywood & Switzky, 1986, 1992; Haywood, Tzuriel & Vaught, 1992; Switzky, 1997, 1999; Switzky & Haywood, 1984; Tzuriel, 1991) conceive that the processes of thinking, learning, and problem-solving develop transactionally with task-intrinsic motivation and related attitudes about learning and thinking, self-concept variables, and habits of working, thinking, and learning. They suggest that there is a transactional relationship among fluid intelligence, cognitive development, and the development of motivational orientation.

All children, regardless of their level of fluid intelligence, are born with a general motive to explore and gain mastery over their worlds, that is, with both curiosity and competence motives (Switzky et al. 1974, 1979). What happens to these motives is a direct function of the consequences of their successive attempts to explore and to gain mastery over their world and their success or failure experiences to do so constitute forces that lead to acceleration or deceleration of these behaviors. Parents' responses to the exploratory and mastery behaviors of their children's performance provide feedback regarding the success or failure of the outcomes. Exploratory behaviors of relatively incompetent children (e.g., mentally retarded, learning disabled, behaviorally disordered, motoric or sensory-impaired), meeting often with failure, become increasingly less frequent, resulting in a lower inclination of these relatively incompetent children to expose themselves to novel stimuli, to derive information from their (increasingly less frequent and less intense) encounters with their environments, and to accumulate basic knowledge about their worlds to evaluate, to understand, and to elaborate subsequent new information to induce generalizations about the rules and structures of their worlds. The deficient cognitive development of these children leads toward the development of the personality trait of task-extrinsic motivation, that is, the tendency to attend to nontask and therefore nonfailure producing aspects of the environment in order to avoid dissatisfaction and failure rather than to seek satisfaction and success. In contrast, relatively competent children engage similarly in initial attempts to explore and gain mastery; however, these attempts are met by successful feedback by parents and other socializing agents, thereby strengthening exploratory and curiosity behaviors, resulting in a greater inclination of these relatively competent children to expose themselves to novel stimuli, to derive increasingly more information from their encounters with their environments, to accumulate more basic knowledge about their worlds in order to understand and to elaborate subsequent new information to induce generalizations about the rules and structures of their worlds, and to develop the personality-trait of task-intrinsic motivation, that is, the tendency to seek success and satisfaction by attending to task-intrinsic aspects of the environment such as creativity, increased responsibility, new learning, psychological excitement, and task-intrinsic aesthetics. This personality trait of task-intrinsic motivation is later expressed as a greater frequency of choices of activities in response to task-intrinsic incentives than in response to task-extrinsic incentives. On the other hand, the personality trait of task-extrinsic motivation is later expressed as a greater frequency of choices of activities in response to task-extrinsic incentives than in response to task-intrinsic incentives. The cognitive and motivational aspects of individuals thus develop in a transactional way. For less competent individuals, lack of external and social feedback of successful exploratory behavior by parents and other socializing agents results in fewer attempts at exploration and knowledge acquisition and the creation of an extrinsic-motivational orientation that creates the conditions of even less exploration and knowledge acquisition and a further slowing of cognitive development and an increasing extrinsic-motivational orientation which is known as the poor-get-poorer phenomenon (Haywood, 1992; Haywood & Switzky, 1992; Haywood et al., 1992). The poor-get-poorer phenomenon is related to the earlier concept of the mental age deficit (Haywood & Switzky, 1986; Haywood et al., 1992). The mental age deficit refers to the phenomenon that even if persons with mental retardation are matched on mental age with younger persons without mental retardation, the persons with mental retardation do less well on a variety of measures of learning and behavioral effectiveness (Lipman, 1963; Stevenson & Zigler, 1958; Zigler, chap. 1, this volume, Zigler & Bennett-Gates, 1999). For more competent individuals, the presence of external and social feedback of successful exploratory behavior by parents and other socializing agents results in accelerating increasing attempts at exploration and knowledge acquisition and the creation of an intrinsic-motivational orientation that creates the conditions of even more exploration and knowledge acquisition and an increasing intrinsic-motivational orientation (the rich-get-richer" phenomenon; Haywood, 1992; Haywood & Switzky, 1992; Haywood et al., 1992).

The primary instrument used by the Peabody-Vanderbilt group to measure motivational orientation in persons with and without mental retardation was the Picture Choice Motivation Scale (Kunca & Haywood, 1969). In this scale, each item is a pair of pictures of people engaged in various activities, vocations, or endeavors determined to be qualitatively either extrinsic or intrinsic. For each of the 20 pictures illustrating an intrinsically motivated (e.g., opportunity to learn, challenge, intense psychological satisfaction, responsibility) or an extrinsically motivated (e.g., opportunity for safety, ease, comfort, security) activity, the individual is asked which one would be preferred. The final score used to classify the individual is the number of intrinsically motivated choices out of the 20 pairs. The Picture Motivation Scale is useful with persons from a mental age of 3 years up to adolescence and has yielded reliability coefficients generally in the 0.80–0.90 range

(Kunca & Haywood, 1969; Miller, Haywood, & Gimon, 1975; Switzky & Haywood, 1992). Several studies have shown that the picture scale yields a roughly normal distribution of scores down to about the mental age of 3 years and that this distribution tends to become skewed (i.e., higher frequencies of intrinsic responses) with increasing chronological and mental age and psychometric intelligence up to middle adolescence (Call, 1968; Haywood, 1968a, 1968b; Haywood & Switzky, 1986; Switzky & Haywood, 1992). Generally, having an intrinsically motivated orientation is an increasing function of chronological age, mental age, psychometric intelligence, and social class. Usually persons with mental retardation as a group are more extrinsically motivated compared with persons of similar age without mental retardation. However, some persons with mental retardation are intrinsically motivated. (See Switzky & Heal, 1990, for an extensive discussion of the construct validity of the Picture Motivation Scale.) The theory of motivational orientation predicts the following:

1. Having an intrinsically motivated orientation is helpful to learners both with and without mental retardation in terms of learning more effectively. However, having an intrinsically motivated orientation is more important for learners with mental retardation in increasing performance and learning. On the whole, these predictions have been confirmed. Intrinsically motivated learners work harder, longer, and more effectively on a task compared to extrinsically motivated learners (Dobbs, 1967; Haywood, 1968a, 1968b; Haywood & Switzky, 1986; Haywood & Wachs, 1966; Schultz & Switzky, 1993; Wooldridge, 1966; Zewdie, 1995).

2. There is an interaction between motivational orientation and incentives such that one must match incentive systems to the unique motivational orientations of individuals, that is, the performance of intrinsically motivated individuals will be optimally reinforced by task-intrinsic incentives, whereas the performance of extrinsically motivated individuals will be optimally reinforced by task-extrinsic incentives. These predictions have been strongly confirmed (Gambro & Switzky, 1988, 1991; Haywood & Switzky, 1975, 1985, 1986, 1992; Haywood & Weaver, 1967; Haywood, Tzuriel, & Vaught, 1992;

Schultz & Switzky, 1990, 1993; Switzky, 1985; Switzky & Haywood, 1974, 1984, 1991, 1992; Switzky & Heal, 1990; Switzky & Schultz, 1988).

3.   Intrinsically motivated persons may be characterized by the operation of self-monitored reinforcement systems that make them less dependent on external reinforcement conditions, whereas extrinsically motivated persons may be characterized by an extreme dependence on the external reinforcement environment. Intrinsically motivated persons are more sensitive to task-intrinsic incentives, have high performance standards of internal self-reward, and are more likely to self-reinforce their own behavior, while extrinsically motivated persons are intensively outerdirected (in Zigler's sense), have very low performance standards of internal self-reward, and are extremely sensitive to the external reinforcement environment. These predictions have been strongly confirmed (Gambro & Switzky, 1988, 1991; Haywood & Switzky, 1975, 1985, 1986, 1992; Switzky & Haywood, 1974, 1991, 1992).

The next section presents in detail the research evidence that supports the theory of motivational orientation.

A. Intrinsically Motivated Learners Learn More Effectively

Intrinsically motivated learners may be characterized as overachievers and extrinsically motivated learners as underachievers on tests of school achievement, where the effects increase as the psychometric intelligence levels of the students decrease. This means that IM learners perform more effectively on tasks than would be predicted by knowledge of their psychometric intelligence alone and that extrinsically motivated learners perform less effectively than would be predicted by knowledge of their psychometric intelligence alone.

In a set of studies (Haywood 1968a, 1968b; Switzky & Heal, 1990) relating motivational orientation to academic achievement levels on the reading, arithmetic, and spelling subtests of the Metropolitan Achievement Test for a sample of 10-year-old students across three levels of intelligence (educable mentally retarded,

IQs 65–80; intellectually average, IQs 95–109; and intellectually superior, IQs 120 and above) the following findings were made.

a. Overachievers were found to be relatively more intrinsically motivated and underachievers relatively more extrinsically motivated in all three academic areas. Overachievers tended to be motivated to a greater extent by factors inherent in the performance of academic tasks, while underachievers tended to be motivated more by factors extrinsic to the task itself.

b. The difference in motivational orientation between over-achievers and underachievers was largest for the group of students who are educably mentally retarded and smallest for the group of students who are intellectually superior. The effects of motivational orientation increased as the intellectual ability levels of the students decreased, so that a disproportionate number of lower ability students were assessed to be extrinsically motivated.

c. When the groups of students were matched on age, sex, and IQ, it was found that in all three curricular-achievement areas, intrinsically motivated students were performing at a higher level than extrinsically motivated students. However, the effects varied with level of intelligence. Individual differences in motivational orientation were associated with 0% of the variance (using eta-squared) in achievement scores of the intellectually superior students, but such differences were associated with 10% of the variance (using eta-squared) of the intellectually average students and up to 30% of the variance using (eta-squared) of the students who are educably mentally retarded. On the average, the intrinsically motivated students in the average-IQ and the groups who are educably mentally retarded had achievement test scores about one full school-year higher than those of the extrinsically motivated students in the same IQ group. The achievement test scores of the intrinsically motivated students who are educably mentally retarded were not significantly different from those of the extrinsically motivated students with average-IQ. Thus, there was compelling evidence that intrinsic motivation is associated with higher school achievement and that the effects of the individual differences in motivational orientation appeared to be greater as psychometric intelligence decreased. While these students were not given the test of intrinsic motivation until they were 10-years-old, retrospective examination of their school achievement scores showed that the achievement score differences were already present by the first grade. Thus, a relatively intrinsically motivated orientation can compensate by increasing curricular-achievement performance levels in students of lower intelligence. A relatively extrinsically motivated orientation will decrease curricular achievement performance levels in students even below that predicted by their mental age levels.

Schultz and Switzky (1993) examined how intrinsic motivation affected reading comprehension and mathematics achievement on the Basic Achievement Skills Individual Screener (BASIS; Sonnenschein, 1983) in a group of urban minority elementary and junior high school students with behavior disorders in the second through seventh grades with an average age of 11 years as compared to their peers without behavior disorders. The purpose of the study was to demonstrate how differences in motivational orientation contributed to the academic performance deficits often observed in children with behavior problems by using a design analogous to that used by Haywood (1968a, 1968b) where groups of students were matched on age, sex, and IQ, thereby potentiating the effects of motivational orientation on academic achievement scores. Previous studies (Schultz & Switzky, 1990, Switzky & Heal, 1990; Switzky & Schultz, 1988) suggested that the lower than expected school achievement in students with behavior disorders may result from an extrinsically motivated orientation to academic activities. Additionally, possessing an extrinsically motivated orientation may further intensify existing problems in achievement due to students' subaverage intelligence and emotional problems. An intrinsically motivated orientation to academic activities may compensate for students' subaverage intelligence and emotional problems and raise levels of school achievement scores. The expectation was that intrinsically motivated behavior disorder students would demonstrate higher levels of scholastic achievement in reading comprehension and mathematics achievement than extrinsically motivated behavior disorder students when IQ, age, and sex were statistically balanced.

A 2 (behavior disorder or group without behavior disorder) 2 (intrinsically or extrinsically motivated motivational orientation) multivariate analysis of covariance (MANCOVA) with IQ, Age, and Sex as covariates was used with reading comprehension and mathematics achievement as dependent measures. The results showed a main effect for group, indicating both higher mathematics and higher reading achievement for the students without behavior disorders compared to the students with behavior disorders. There also was a main effect for motivational orientation indicating that intrinsically motivated students had higher reading comprehension than did extrinsically motivated students. More important, there was an interaction between group and motivational orientation indicating that behavior disorder students exhibited significantly greater academic performance differences due to motivational orientation compared to their peers without behavior disorder. Intrinsically motivated behavior disorder students had both higher mathematics and higher reading achievement than did extrinsically motivated behavior disorder students, whereas there was no significant difference between the intrinsically and extrinsically motivated non-behavior-disorder students' mathematics and reading achievement. Individual differences in motivational orientation appear to affect the academic performance of behavior disorder students to a greater extent compared to their peers without behavior disorder. These achievement differences reveal that children in both groups who are more motivated by factors intrinsic to learning tend to achieve at a higher level than children who are motivated by extrinsic factors. While these academic performance differences due to motivation orientation appear to be significant in both groups of children, they are much more important in students formally identified as behavior disordered. Intrinsically motivated behavior disorder students had substantially higher math and reading achievement test scores than did extrinsically motivated behavior disorder students. The results of this study support previous research (Haywood 1968a, 1968b; Haywood & Switzky, 1986; Switzky & Heal, 1990) which suggests that the lower than expected school achievement observed in many exceptional students (mentally retarded or behavior disorder) is associated with having an extrinsically motivated orientation to academic activities which may further intensify existing problems in achievement due to the students' subaverage intelligence and emotional problems. Having more of an intrinsically motivated orientation to academic activities may compensate for many exceptional students' subaverage intelligence and emotional problems and raise levels of school achievement.

B. Interaction Between Motivational Orientation and Incentives

There is an interaction between motivational orientation and incentives such that one must match incentive systems to the unique motivational orientations of individuals, that is, the performance of intrinsically motivated individuals will be optimally reinforced by task-intrinsic incentives, whereas the performance of extrinsically motivated individuals will be optimally reinforced by task-extrinsic incentives. This original formulation of theory was first tested by Haywood and Weaver (1967), who showed that there was an interaction between the motivational orientation of institutionalized children and adults with mental retardation and the incentives that are effective in a simple task. Relatively intrinsically motivated and strongly extrinsically motivated retarded persons participated in a repetitive motor task under one of four incentive conditions: a 10-cent reward (strong extrinsically motivated incentive), a 1-cent reward (weak extrinsically motivated reward), the promise of an opportunity to do another task (strong intrinsically motivated reward), and no reward (control). Extrinsically motivated subjects performed most vigorously under the 10-cent condition and least well under the task-incentive condition, while intrinsically motivated subjects showed the opposite behavior, giving their best performance when offered only the opportunity to do another task and performing least well under the 10-cent incentive condition. In the control condition, intrinsically motivated subjects performed more vigorously than did extrinsically motivated subjects.

C. Internal Self-Monitored Reinforcement Systems

Intrinsically motivated persons are more sensitive to task-intrinsic incentives, have high performance standards of internal-self reward, and are more likely to self-reinforce their own behavior. Extrinsically motivated persons are characterized by dependence on external reinforcement systems that make them intensively outerdirected, have very low performance standards of internal self-reward, and are extremely sensitive to the external reinforcement environment.

This extension of the theoretical model of motivational orientation is my unique contribution, which was tested by a whole series of studies (Gambro & Switzky, 1988, 1991; Haywood & Switzky, 1975, 1985, 1986, 1992; Haywood, Tzuriel, & Vaught, 1992; Schultz & Switzky, 1990, 1993; Switzky, 1985; Switzky & Haywood, 1974, 1984, 1991, 1992; Switzky & Heal, 1990; Switzky & Schultz, 1988), and was interpreted in terms of Bandura's (1969, 1976, 1978, 1986a, 1993, 1997) social cognitive learning theories, especially his theory of self-reinforcement, and his formulation of the self-system which stressed the importance of internal self-system processes reciprocally interacting with the external demand characteristics of the environment and the individual's own behavior. In the social cognitive view people are neither driven by inner forces nor automatically shaped and controlled by external stimuli. Rather, human functioning is explained in terms of a model of transactional reciprocity in which behavior, cognitive, biological, and affective factors, and environmental events all operate as interacting determinants of each other (Bandura, 1986a, 1993, 1997).

Bandura's model of self-reinforcement (1969, 1993, 1997) is based on the notion that persons construct their own internal self-standards and self-incentives that are used to guide, motivate, and regulate their own behavior. Persons behave in such a manner to increase their self-satisfaction, self-reward, and self-worth and refrain from behaving in ways that violate their own internal standards to avoid self-censure.

In a study (Haywood & Switzky, 1975) that was performed during my postdoctoral fellowship at Peabody, evidence emerged which supported the idea that the behavior of intrinsically and extrinsically motivated school-age children may be interpreted in terms of Bandura's (1969, 1993, 1997) concept of self-reinforcement. We found that it was possible to condition the verbal expression of motivation in intrinsically and extrinsically motivated school-age children by contingent social reinforcement of statements that were counter to or supportive of the individual's own motivational orientation. Subjects in all contingent-reinforcement groups learned to discriminate intrinsically motivated from extrinsically motivated statements, with extrinsically motivated subjects demonstrating slightly more efficient learning, suggesting that the task-extrinsic verbal social reinforcement was more effective for them than for the intrinsically motivated children. In a noncontingent (control) condition, where responses were randomly reinforced, intrinsically motivated subjects increased their rate of intrinsically motivated verbalizations in spite of the lack of consistent external verbal social reinforcement, whereas extrinsically motivated subjects failed to show any significant change over trial blocks.

This led me to question the source of the reinforcement for the intrinsically motivated subjects in the noncontingent (control) condition that increased their performance. In an epiphany of insight worthy of Archimedes, I realized that it was self-reinforcement in the Bandurian sense. This was a turning point for me in my conception of the motivational system of low mental age groups both with and without mental retardation. If Bandura's (1969, 1993, 1997) concept of self-reinforcement was true, intrinsically motivated persons may be characterized by self-monitored reinforcement systems that make them less dependent on external reinforcement conditions, while extrinsically motivated persons may be characterized by dependence on external reinforcement systems. Within the boundaries of the study which was performed on school-age children, the extrinsically motivated children were differentially more responsive than were the intrinsically motivated children to social reinforcement and consequently showed more efficient learning under such task-extrinsic incentives. When task-extrinsic incentives were presented noncontingently, extrinsically motivated children should not show any change in performance, while intrinsically motivated children (who are more sensitive to task-intrinsic incentives and who are more likely to self-reinforce their own behavior) should show changes in performance in spite of the absence of contingent conditions. Thus, it is necessary to consider both the relative strengths of an individual's self-monitored and externally imposed reinforcement system as well as the nature of the reinforcers in order to understand and predict performance under different reinforcement operations in persons showing individual differences in motivational orientation. This analysis was dramatically confirmed in the next two studies in the series, one with grade school children (Switzky & Haywood, 1974) and the other with adults with mild mental retardation (Haywood & Switzky, 1985). A more recent study (Zewdie, 1995), with inner city African American adults with moderate mental retardation only partially replicated the results of the Haywood and Switzky (1985) study but showed the strong effects of having an intrinsically motivated orientation on work production and work supervisor's ratings.

Switzky & Haywood (1974) showed that in order to predict performance under different reinforcement operations in school children in Grades 2 through 5, it was necessary to consider: (a) the locus of control of the reinforcers, self-controlled or externally controlled, (b) individual differences in motivational orientation, and (c) the relative strengths of an individual's self-monitored and externally imposed reinforcement system. Bandura and Perloff (1967) had compared the motor performance of children under self-monitored and externally imposed reinforcement and found no significant differences between the two conditions. Both reinforcement conditions supported performance, but the control conditions did not. Adding the dimension of individual differences in motivational orientation, Switzky and Haywood (1974) divided their participants into intrinsically and extrinsically motivated groups and gave them the Bandura and Perloff task. Children were given a motor wheel-cranking task where it was possible to vary the number of cranks of the wheel required to turn on a light on a column of lights, as well as the number of lights that had to be turned on to get a token. Tokens could be exchanged for prizes. In the self-monitored reinforcement condition subjects determined their own schedules of reinforcement, that is, decided how many cranks were needed to turn on a light and how many lights had to be turned on to earn a token. For each of these subjects there was a yoked subject in the externally imposed reinforcement condition who had to follow the schedule of reinforcement selected by the self-monitored subject. We found a dramatic interaction between the reinforcement conditions and the motivational orientations of the participants: intrinsically motivated children worked harder, set leaner schedules of reinforcement, and maintained their performance longer than

did extrinsically motivated children under self-monitored reinforcement conditions; by contrast, extrinsically motivated children performed more vigorously and maintained their
performance longer under conditions of externally imposed reinforcement. Thus, Bandura and Perloff's (1967) failure to find differential effects of these reinforcement systems may have been
due to the cancelling effects of individual differences in motivational orientation, with very strong differential effects interacting
with such individual differences. These effects suggest that persons who are predominately intrinsically motivated are characterized by an internal self-regulatory system where they are able
to determine, choose, and pace their own behavior without direction or reliance from external environmental sources and if external environmental controlling conditions are imposed, they will
interfere with the operation of the intrinsically motivated individuals' self-regulatory system. This latter inference is supported by a
set of studies (Amabile, 1996; Deci, Koestner, & Ryan, 1999; Deci,
Nezlek & Sheinman, 1981; Deci & Ryan, 1985; Deci et al., 1991;
Flink, Boggiano, & Barrett, 1990; Grolnick & Ryan, 1987; Lepper,
1996; Lepper & Hodell, 1989; Morgan, 1984; Ryan & Grolnick,
1986; Utman, 1997) showing generally that, for individuals who
are already intrinsically motivated, task-extrinsic incentive
rewards interfere with task-intrinsic motivation. On the other
hand, individuals who are predominately extrinsically motivated
are primarily under the control of a strongly developed external
environmental reinforcement system and need external direction
from the environment in order to perform, which makes them
less inclined to engage in internally generated self-regulated
activities for their own sake. If forced to determine, choose, and
pace their own behavior without direction or reliance from external environmental sources, such individuals are unable to do so
and just shut down and perform very poorly under such internal-
demand conditions.

The Haywood and Switzky (1985) study with adults with mild
mental retardation was based on the ideas that self-regulation is
extremely important to the ability of persons with mental retardation to adjust to relatively independent living, and the response of
persons with mental retardation to expectations of self-regulation
or to expectations of externally imposed regulation depends upon
individual differences in task-intrinsic motivation. Since previous

studies had shown that persons with mental retardation are usually less intrinsically motivated than are persons without mental retardation, self-regulation might be difficult to produce in persons with mental retardation to the extent that motivational orientation and self-regulatory behavior are related. Additionally, we wanted to find out to what extent the incentive-system relationships previously established with normally developing schoolchildren were generalizable to lower levels of intrinsic motivation, specifically those lower levels typically found in persons with mental retardation.

The Haywood and Switzky (1985) experiment was designed as an analogue of the Bandura and Perloff motor task extending the Switzky and Haywood (1974) study to the work behavior of adults with mild mental retardation. The Haywood and Switzky (1985) study was designed to get evidence on the relative efficacy of self-monitored and externally imposed reinforcement to intrinsically and extrinsically motivated persons with mental retardation, specifically with response to their performance in work-related tasks. It was expected that because intrinsically motivated persons have a more highly developed self-reinforcement system compared to extrinsically motivated persons, that intrinsically motivated persons would maintain their performance under conditions of minimal external support. extrinsically motivated persons, on the other hand, were expected to be more responsive to and dependent upon the operation of externally imposed reinforcement. Specifically, it was expected that under conditions in which persons with mental retardation would set their own performance standards and reinforcement schedules, intrinsically motivated persons with mental retardation would set a higher standard for their performance, maintain their work longer, and set a leaner schedule of reinforcement than would extrinsically motivated persons with mental retardation. By contrast, a condition in which performance standards and reinforcement schedules were imposed externally should be more effective for extrinsically motivated persons with mental retardation than for intrinsically motivated persons with mental retardation in maintaining work. Finally, it was expected that under a no-reinforcement control condition, intrinsically motivated persons with mental retardation would show more sustained work than would extrinsically motivated persons with mental retardation.

The participants were 72 adults with mild mental retardation residing in a community-based intermediate care facility. They were divided into two groups constituting the top (intrinsically motivated) and the bottom (extrinsically motivated) quartiles of the distribution of intrinsic motivation scores. Their mean age was 40 years and their mean IQ was 69. Participants were assigned randomly to three conditions: self-regulated reinforcement, externally imposed reinforcement, and no-token control. Participants in the external-reinforcement group were matched individually to participants in the self-regulation group by sex, age, motivational orientation, and, in a yoked manner, schedule of reinforcement. Those in the control group were matched for sex, age, and motivational orientation with participants in the self-regulation group. All participants were given a work task consisting of placing a single flat or lock washer into each compartment of seven 18-compartment boxes placed side by side in a row. Work goals were set by placing a washer in the end-most compartment they intended to reach. Participants in the self-regulation condition set their own work goals and, after reaching the work goals, determined the number of tokens they should get for their work. They also determined how long they would work. Tokens were exchanged for prizes at the end of the experimental session. Selections made by the self-regulation participants were imposed on participants in the external-reinforcement condition. In the control condition, the experimenter set the work goals, participants worked as long as they wished with no indication of "pay" for their work and were given a prize at the end. The study consisted of a 2 (motivational orientation) × 3 (condition) factorial design. The principal dependent variable was the number of compartments filled (a measure of performance maintenance or task persistence). The analysis of variance revealed a main effect of motivational orientation. Intrinsically motivated participants with mental retardation worked harder (mean of 118 compartments filled) than did extrinsically motivated participants with mental retardation (mean of 80 compartments filled), confirming previous research with school-aged children without mental retardation (Switzky & Haywood, 1974). In addition, there was an interaction of condition and motivational orientation. In both the self-regulation and the control conditions, intrinsically motivated participants with mental retardation filled more compartments than did extrinsically motivated participants with mental retardation, while intrinsically and extrinsically motivated participants with mental retardation did not differ significantly under the external-reinforcement condition. Intrinsically motivated participants also filled more of the compartments under the self-regulation condition than they did under the external-reinforcement condition. A higher level of intrinsic motivation was associated with more self-regulatory behavior than was a lower level of intrinsic motivation, replicating the Switzky and Haywood (1974) findings with children without mental retardation and the Haywood and Weaver (1967) findings with adults with mental retardation. These differences in performance between intrinsically and extrinsically motivated persons are due to differences in their internal self-system characteristics. Intrinsically motivated persons appear to respond chiefly to internal, cognitive, self-regulatory processes, whereas extrinsically motivated persons appear to respond chiefly to external, environmental influences. Furthermore, intrinsically motivated persons appear to have a more strongly developed internal reinforcement system, whereas extrinsically motivated persons have a more strongly developed external reinforcement system.

The purpose of the Zewdie (1995) study was to replicate and extend the findings of the Haywood and Switzky (1985) study to get further evidence on the relative efficacy of self-monitored and externally imposed reinforcement for intrinsically and extrinsically motivated inner-city African American persons with moderate mental retardation regarding their performances on real-world subcontract work in a sheltered workshop. The Zewdie (1995) study was an attempt to extend the theory of motivational orientation to African American adults with mental retardation and to strengthen the ecological validity of the theory by observing the work performance of workers with mental retardation in the real-world setting of the sheltered workshop.

The participants were 72 primarily African American adults with moderate mental retardation. Their mean age was 34 years, their mean IQ was 55, and their mean length of employment and training in the workshop was 8 years. They were divided into two groups constituting the top (intrinsically motivated) and the bottom (extrinsically motivated) median split of the distribution of intrinsic motivation scores. Participants were assigned randomly to three conditions: self-regulated reinforcement, externally imposed reinforcement, and no token control. Participants in the external-reinforcement group were matched individually to participants in the self-regulation group by sex, age, motivational orientation, and, in a yoked manner, schedule of reinforcement. Those in the control group were matched for sex, age, and motivational orientation with participants in the self-regulation group. All participants were given a work task consisting of an 8-step relatively complex packing–assembly task involving packaging Chia Pets over four consecutive 30-minute sessions.

Subjects in the self-reinforcement condition were instructed that they were to perform and get tokens in addition to their regular pay. They were also informed that they would receive prizes in exchange for their acquired tokens and the more tokens they got, the better prize they would get. Subjects were told that they had to set their own goals by determining how many work units (Chia Pets) they would produce per trial. Whenever they reached their projected production goal, they could give themselves as many tokens from a nearby box as they thought their work was worth. Subjects worked as long as they wished and by themselves. Supervisors (who were blinded as to the motivational orientation) remained on the work floor with minimal contact with subjects at a distance of 2-m where they could unobtrusively keep track of the subjects' work goals and the number of tokens that subjects were awarding themselves. When subjects completed their work goal, they would inform the supervisor, at which time the subjects traded their acquired tokens for a prize commensurate in value to the number of tokens accumulated.

Subjects in the external reinforcement condition were yoked to subjects in the self-regulation condition in terms of the work goal and the number of tokens received. Subjects in this condition were given the same instructions as those in the self-regulation group. The only exception for the external group was that they were told that the supervisor would determine the work goal and the number of tokens that were dispensed. Subjects in this group were also allowed to work as long as they wished.

Subjects in the no-token condition were also yoked to subjects in the self-regulation condition in terms of the work goal. Supervisors set the work goal and subjects were allowed to work as long as they wished with no indication of "pay" for their work.

When subjects finished working, they were given an unexpected prize in appreciation of their work.

All subjects' work was also rated by supervisors blinded as to the motivational orientation of the subjects on the Workshop Supervisor Behavioral Rating Scale (WSBR), a 16–item scale that measured typical work skills and work behavior demands of sheltered workshop environments, which was specifically developed for this study. Cronbach's coefficient alpha was .87 and test-retest reliability was .72 on the WSBR. Principal component analysis with varimax rotation was performed on the WSBR. Four factors were extracted. Factor one was named independent work behavior and accounted for 46% of the variance. Items that loaded on factor one were ability to work independently, motivation to work, persistence and steadiness of work pace, speed, quality of work, initiating request for materials, working on monotonous work, and overall behavioral qualification. Factor two was named collaborative work behavior and accounted for 12% of the variance. Items that loaded on factor two were ability to follow directives, reaction to supervisor criticism, frustration tolerance, and odd or inappropriate behavior. Factor three was named work habits and accounted for 11% of the variance. Items that loaded on factor three were attendance, punctuality, and distractibility during work. Factor four was named appearance behavior at work and accounted for 7% of the variance. Only one item loaded on factor four, appearance and grooming.

The study consisted of a 2 (motivational orientation) × 3 (behavioral-regulation condition) × 4 (sessions) factorial mixed ANCOVA, with sessions as a repeated measures factor and age, IQ, and workshop experience as covariates. Two dependent variables, the mean number of production units completed and the mean total minutes of work performed, were used as a measure of performance maintenance and task persistence. Supervisor ratings on the WSRB were analyzed using the factor scores on the four factors extracted by factor analysis. Then, t tests were carried out in order to examine whether there where differences between intrinsically and extrinsically motivated groups.

The ANCOVA conducted on the mean number of production units revealed a main effect of motivational orientation. Intrinsically motivated African American workers with mental retardation produced more units ($M = 31.00$ units) than did extrinsically motivated African-American workers with mental retardation (M = 25.00 units), replicating the findings of the Haywood and Switzky(1985) study. However, there were no interaction effects of the motivational orientation and behavioral regulation condition. There was an interaction of session and behavioral regulation condition. The locus of the interaction showed that the self-regulation group dropped off in performance on the 4th session, whereas the control and external-reinforcement groups appeared to produce equivalently across all four sessions. The effect was small and was probably due to chance sampling error.

The ANCOVA conducted on the mean total minutes of work performed revealed a main effect of motivational orientation. Intrinsically motivated workers worked longer (M = 14.62 minutes) compared to extrinsically motivated workers (M = 13.20 minutes). There was also a main effect of behavioral regulation conditions. Workers in the self-reinforcement condition (M = 15.96 minutes) and in the external-reinforcement condition (M = 14.05 minutes) worked longer than workers in the no-token control condition (M = 11.85 minutes). There were no significant differences between workers in the two experimental conditions although there was an interaction between behavioral regulation conditions and sessions that mirrors the results for the dependent variable of the mean number of production units completed. Simply, the mean total minutes of work performed by the self-reinforcement group decreased from session three to session four, whereas the other two groups showed a stable pattern of endurance on the work task.

A series of t tests examining the difference in component factor scores derived from the Workshop Behavior Rating Scale (e.g., factor 1, independent work behavior; factor 2, collaborative work behavior; factor 3, work habits; and factor 4, appearance behavior at work) were carried out for the intrinsically and extrinsically motivated workers. There was a significant difference between intrinsically and extrinsically motivated workers on factor 1. Intrinsically motivated workers scored higher (M = .33 SD units) than did extrinsically motivated workers (M = -.32 SD units). No significant differences on other factor scores for the intrinsically motivated and extrinsically motivated workers were found. In general, the results replicate the Haywood and Switzky (1985) study and provide additional construct and ecological validity to the theory of motivational orientation in real-world workshop settings even though the expected interaction of motivational orientation and behavioral regulation condition was not obtained. Perhaps these African American adults with moderate mental retardation needed more training to understand the behavioral regulation conditions since the subjects in this experiment were considerably more mentally retarded than subjects in the previous studies.

However, the core idea that differences in performance between intrinsically and extrinsically motivated persons are due to differences in their internal self-system characteristics (e.g., intrinsically motivated persons appear to respond chiefly to internal, cognitive, self-regulatory processes and to have a more strongly developed internal reinforcement system, whereas extrinsically motivated persons appear to respond chiefly to external, environmental influences and extrinsically motivated to have a more strongly developed external reinforcement system) were strongly confirmed in the next set of studies which were designed to further test the validity of the motivational orientation construct by investigating the effects of internal self-system influences and the role of the external demand characteristics of the environment in the self-regulatory behavior of adults with mild retardation (Switzky & Haywood, 1991) and of young children without mental retardation (Gambro & Switzky, 1991; Switzky & Haywood, 1992).

In the Switzky and Haywood (1991) study, the effects of external (environmental) and internal (cognitive) self-influences of self-regulatory behavior were investigated in 60 adults with mild mental retardation (one half were relatively intrinsically motivated and one-half were relatively extrinsically motivated; mean age 37.3 years, mean IQ 66.4) residing in a community-based intermediate care facility. External environmental influences such as stringent, variable, and lenient demand conditions; instructional sets; performance standards; and schedules of self-reinforcement were varied. Intrinsically and extrinsically motivated participants were randomly assigned to three conditions of self-reinforcement task demands: stringent (instructed to set very high performance standards, instructed to work as hard and fast as they could on a work task, experimenter modeled a lean schedule of reinforcement), variable (not explicitly instructed as to how hard or fast to work, given choice of high or low performance standards, and experimenter modeled a schedule of reinforcement proportional in richness to the performance criterion chosen, i.e., more tokens for higher goals), or lenient (not explicitly instructed as to how hard or fast to work, but rather allowed to set lower performance standards and experimenter modeled a rich schedule of reinforcement). A motor–attention task was constructed varying in seven levels of difficulty, ranging from three to nine lines of geometric figures arranged randomly on a page. The seven sheets of geometric figures containing random combinations of squares, trapezoids, and heptagons were arranged in sequence from easy (three lines) to difficult (nine lines) in front of the participants. The performance task consisted of crossing out figures that matched a model (one initially crossed out) on each sheet. All participants were told to perform the task to get tokens that could be exchanged for prizes; the more tokens, the better the prize. After reaching their work goals (performance standards) they could pay themselves as many tokens from a nearby container as they thought their work had been worth. The dependent variables were: (1) total work (sum of standards chosen over trials); (2) average performance standard chosen; (3) percentage of modeled standard (goal chosen as a percentage of the goal modeled by the experimenter); (4) schedule of reinforcement (items of work accomplished divided by the number of tokens paid to self); and (5) percentage of modeled schedule of reinforcement (schedule of reinforcement as a percentage of the schedule of reinforcement modeled by the experimenter). The dependent variables were analyzed individually in terms of a 2 (motivational orientation) × 3 (instructional demands) factorial design.

It was expected that because internal self-influences interact with external environmental influences in determining behavior, intrinsically motivated persons with mild mental retardation residing in quasi-institutional settings would perform more vigorously than extrinsically motivated persons under all imposed conditions. This was because intrinsically motivated persons were believed to have a more highly developed self-reinforcement system and also an external reinforcement system as strongly developed as extrinsically motivated persons. These ideas were derived from theory and my own clinical experiences with persons with mental retardation since 1966, when I entered the field (see Switzky, 1995). Intrinsically motivated persons were expected to work harder, set higher performance standards, and set leaner schedules of self-reinforcement as compared to extrinsically motivated persons.

Results showed that the differential work performance of persons with mild mental retardation who differ in motivational orientation illustrated that both external-environmental conditions (task demand conditions) and internal-self characteristics (motivational orientation) had significant effects on the performance of the motor–attention task. Participants in the stringent-demand condition worked harder, set higher performance standards (higher goals), and arranged leaner schedules of self-reinforcement than did participants in the lenient demand condition. Intrinsically motivated participants worked harder, set higher performance standards (higher goals), and arranged leaner schedules of self-reinforcement than did extrinsically motivated participants over all demand conditions. Furthermore, intrinsically motivated subjects chose higher performance standards (higher goals) than had been demonstrated to them in the lenient-demand condition and also arranged leaner schedules of self-reinforcement over all demand conditions than had been demonstrated to them, while extrinsically motivated participants either copied the schedule set by the experimenter or set richer ones. Differences between intrinsically and extrinsically motivated participants were most pronounced in the lenient demand condition, suggesting that individual differences in motivational orientation will lead to the most divergent performances in situations where there is the least external support and guidance.

Internal self-system characteristics of persons with mental retardation appear to interact reciprocally with external demand characteristics of the environment to reveal substantial individual differences of self-reward behavior. These effects show that environmental (external) demand instructions do not operate in a vacuum. The recipients play an active role in selecting what information they extract from ongoing events and when and how they use that information and their own abilities. Persons do not simply react mechanically to situational influences; they actively process, interpret, and transfer the influences in support of Bandura's concept of the self-system in reciprocal determinism (Bandura, 1969, 1976, 1977, 1978, 1986a, 1993, 1997). The results of this study confirm modern conceptions of the self-system (Boekaerts, Pintrich, & Zeidner, 2000; Dweck, 1999; Harter, 1999) and affirm the role of self-evaluative reactions (Gollwitzer & Bargh, 1996; Skinner, 1995) in the self-regulation of behavior as applied to persons with mild mental retardation, as well as the previous theories and research of the Peabody-Vanderbilt group on the construct validity of motivational orientation (Haywood, 1992; Haywood & Switzky, 1986, 1992; Haywood et al., 1992; Schultz & Switzky, 1990; Switzky, 1997, 1999; Switzky & Heal, 1990; Switzky & Schultz, 1988). The results of the study which so strongly supported the theory of motivational orientation in persons with mental retardation were astounding.

Switzky and Haywood (1992) extended the Switzky and Haywood (1991) paradigm to 32 middle-class preschool children without mental retardation, one half of whom were relatively intrinsically motivated and the other half of whom were relatively extrinsically motivated (3.1 to 5.8 years, $M = 4.7$ years), in an attempt to investigate further the research validity of the motivational orientation construct by investigating the ontogenesis of intrinsic and extrinsic self-system characteristics and the interaction of ongoing behavior, with stringent and lenient environmental demand conditions in young children's self-reinforcing behavior. The interest was in determining at what age intrinsic and extrinsic motivational self-system characteristics are present and are functional in a population of young children. The effects of a stringent-demand condition, in the form of stringent instructional sets and criterion settings and lean schedules of self-reinforcement, and a lenient-demand condition in the form of very lenient instructional sets and criterion settings and a very rich schedule of reinforcement, were provided to maintain performance on a motor–attention task. A motor–attention task was constructed varying in four levels of difficulty, ranging from three to nine lines of geometric figures arranged randomly on a page (e.g., three, five, seven, or nine lines). The work task consisted of crossing out a geometric shape matching one initially crossed out on each sheet. The same dependent variables as in the Switzky and Haywood (1991) study were analyzed individually in terms of a 2 (motivational orientation) × 2 (instructional demands) factorial design. Again, both external and internal self-influences affected self-reinforcement performance on the motor–attention task. Children in the stringent-demand condition set a higher performance standard and arranged a leaner schedule of self-reinforcement than did children in the lenient-demand condition. Extrinsically motivated children outperformed intrinsically motivated children on measures reflecting the strength of performance (total work behavior and total time working), presumably because of the higher incentive value of the reinforcers for the extrinsically motivated children. In previous research (Haywood & Switzky, 1985; Switzky & Haywood, 1974, 1991), subjects were not shown the reinforcers that were to be exchanged for the tokens until the end of the experiment. In this experiment, reinforcers that were to be obtained by the exchange of the tokens were shown to the children at the very beginning of the experiment, thereby potentiating the incentive value of the reinforcers for the extrinsically motivated children. On measures reflecting internal standards of self-regulation, intrinsically motivated children set a higher performance standard in the lenient-demand condition than did extrinsically motivated children. Also intrinsically motivated children chose a higher performance standard than that modeled in the lenient-demand condition than did extrinsically motivated children. This experiment shows that in preschool-age children internal self-regulatory characteristics are present, well organized, and active, which interact with external demand characteristics of the environment to reveal substantial individual differences in the patterns of self-reward behavior.

The purpose of the Gambro & Switzky (1991) study was to further test the research validity of the motivational orientation construct and the ontogenesis of intrinsic and extrinsic motivational self-system characteristics and their interaction with external demand characteristics of the environment in 34 middle-class preschool children without mental retardation, one half of whom were relatively intrinsically motivated and the other half who were relatively extrinsically motivated (3.7 to 6.0 years, $M = 4.8$ years), by extending the Switzky & Haywood (1992) study in three ways: first, by including two tasks to test the durability of effects, second, by adding ecological validity through the use of more pragmatic tasks (letter recognition and object sorting) under lenient-demand conditions, and third, by not showing the children the reinforcers that were to be exchanged for the tokens until the end of the experiment, thereby not emphasizing the external reinforcers. It was expected since internal self-influences interact with external environmental influences in determining behavior, that intrinsically motivated young children would perform more vigorously under the lenient-demand condition for both tasks. This follows because intrinsically motivated children probably will have a more developed self-reinforcement system than would extrinsically motivated children.

A letter recognition task was constructed varying in three levels of difficulty, ranging from three to seven lines of upper case letters arranged randomly on a page (three, five, or seven lines). The pages were placed side by side in a line. The letter task consisted of crossing out the letters which matched the letter initially crossed out on the first line of each sheet. The sorting task, consisting of 900 blue, brown, and red craft sticks; 650 white and red cotton swabs; and 350 red and green bingo chips, was also constructed ranging in three levels of difficulty. Three piles of materials were placed side by side in a line. The first pile contained 250 blue craft sticks, 250 red craft sticks, and 250 brown craft sticks mixed randomly. The second pile contained 300 blue craft sticks, 300 red craft sticks, 300 brown craft sticks, 300 red cotton swabs, and 300 white cotton swabs mixed randomly. The third pile contained 350 blue craft sticks, 350 red craft sticks, 350 brown craft sticks, 350 red cotton swabs, 350 white cotton swabs, 350 red bingo chips, and 350 green bingo chips mixed randomly. The sorting task consisted of placing all the identical individual items of each category (e.g., blue craft sticks, green bingo chips, red cotton swabs, green craft sticks, etc.) into a corresponding container.

Only one task per day which was counterbalanced over the two days was attempted by each child. For all children, the experimenter explained and demonstrated each task and then allowed the children two demonstration practice trials. Children were told that they were performing a task for tokens, which could be exchanged for prizes. The more tokens they obtained, the more prizes they would receive. The reinforcement procedure was modeled by the experimenter. A low work goal was set by the experimenter by instructing the children to work on the easy pile in both tasks.

A 2 (motivational orientation) × 2 (task) factorial analysis of variance was performed with the dependent variable being the total time on the two tasks in minutes. The analysis revealed a main effect of motivational orientation. Intrinsically motivated children worked longer (M = 11.4 minutes) than extrinsically motivated children (M = 8.4 minutes), confirming expectations. The performance of young children with different motivational orientations showed significant individual differences in self-regulatory behavior when completing the two tasks under lenient demand conditions with little emphasis placed on external reinforcers. As expected, intrinsically motivated young children spent more time on the tasks when compared to extrinsically motivated young children. Intrinsically motivated young children did not rely on external cues, but rather worked until their internal self-standards were satisfied. Extrinsically motivated young children may have worked only until they felt they had earned enough tokens to obtain a prize. In the Switzky & Haywood (1992) study, external reinforcers were stressed, and the extrinsically motivated young children spent more time on tasks. In this study, external reinforcers were de-emphasized, more realistic tasks were utilized, and the lenient-demand condition encouraged young children to use their internal self-system with the result that the extrinsically motivated young children did not work as long because of their dependence on external environmental conditions for guiding their performance.

The Gambro and Switzky (1991) and Switzky and Haywood (1992) studies show that in children younger than 5 years of age, internal self-system characteristics of individuals are present and interact with external demand characteristics of the environment to reveal substantial individual differences in patterns of self-reward behavior, affirming the role of self-evaluative reactions in the self-regulation of behavior in very young children and extending and confirming the theoretical model of motivational orientation developed by the Peabody-Vanderbilt group regarding the construct validity of the motivational orientation concept to preschool children.

Taken together, these five studies (Gambro & Switzky, 1991; Haywood & Switzky, 1985; Switzky & Haywood, 1974, 1991, 1992) demonstrate that individual differences in motivational orientation are associated with important dimensions of self-regulation, incentive-selection, goal setting, work performance, and, perhaps most important, the satisfaction derived from the task itself, both in persons with and without mental retardation ranging from pre-school- and school-age children, to adults. Bandura's model of the self-system (1969, 1976, 1977, 1978, 1986a, 1993, 1997), especially his concept of reciprocal determinism, that is, the continuous reciprocal transactional interaction among the elements of behavior, internal cognitive processes, biological and affective factors that can affect perceptions and actions, and the external environment, deeply influenced the evolution of the motivational orientation construct of the Peabody-Vanderbilt group and their research agenda.

The research presented here supports Bandura's ideas and confirms related conceptions of the self-system, thus confirming the role of self-evaluative reactions in the self-regulation of behavior in persons with mild mental retardation and in normally developing preschool- and school-age children. Bandura (1986b, 1997) more recently wrote about personal agency, that is, the idea that individuals take responsibility for their actions and ascribe success and failure to the goals they choose, the resources they mobilize, and the effort they expend. Perceived self-efficacy, that is, beliefs concerning one's capabilities to organize and imple-ment actions necessary to attain designated levels of perform-ance, is one of the most important constructs in Bandura's (1986a, 1997) social-cognitive approach and a critical component of per-sonal agency because perceptions of one's ability to behave in a particular way establish one's expectations and motivation. A strong belief in one's ability to use specific actions effectively (high perceived self-efficacy) enhances successful performance, and enhances feelings of pride, satisfaction, self-respect, and sat-isfaction with one's efforts (Schunk, 1989a, 1989b, 1990, 1994; Schunk & Ertmer, 2000).

The theory of motivational orientation has also been strongly influenced by Feuerstein's theory of mediated learning experiences (Arbitman-Smith, Haywood, & Bransford, 1984; Feuerstein, Klein, & Tannenbaum, 1991; Feuerstein & Rand, 1974; Feuerstein, Rand, Hoffman, & Miller, 1980; Haywood, 1977; Hay-wood, Brooks, & Burns, 1986; Haywood & Tzuriel, 1992). Children acquire knowledge and understanding in two ways (Schultz & Switzky, 1990): (1) by teaching themselves by learning through natural exposure to environmental stimuli where, because of their inborn intrinsic motivation to learn, they independently acquire very complex skills and abilities, and (2) by learning from significant others in their lives, that is, acquiring from parents and teachers knowledge and understanding of complex skills that are not easily learned independently. Depending on how they communicate and interact with children when they are passing on knowledge and understanding of skills, teachers and parents play an important role in maintaining and further shaping the natural ability in children to learn intrinsically by creating mediational learning experiences which arouse in children vigilance, curiosity, and sensitivity to the mediated stimuli and create for and with the children temporal, spatial, and cause-effect relationships among stimuli (Schultz & Switzky, 1990; Tzuriel & Haywood, 1992). On the other hand, adult-child instructional interactions which lack this mediational quality tend to undermine the inborn intrinsic motivation that most children bring to the learning experiences they have with adults. Thus, problem-solving behavior reflects the interaction of affective-motivational processes such as motivational orientation (Haywood & Switzky, 1992) and cognitive processes including learned information processing components of intelligence, the internal or mental processes that underlie intelligent behavior: metacognitive and higher order control processes, performance components, and knowledge acquisition components (Borkowski & Kurtz, 1987; Borkowski et al., 1990, 1992; Carr, Borkowski, & Maxwell, 1991; Pressley, Borkowski, & Schneider, 1990; Sternberg, 1985), which allow individuals to use their fluid intelligence in an optimal fashion.

In order to qualify as mediated learning experiences interactions between children and the mediating adult must meet the following criteria (Feuerstein & Feuerstein, 1991; Haywood et al., 1986):

1. *Intentionality.* The mediating adult must intend to use the interactions to produce cognitive change in the child.
2. *Transcendence.* The intended change must be a generalizable one (i.e., a cognitive structural change that transcends the immediate situation and will permit children to apply new processes of thought in new situations).

3. *Communication of meaning and purpose.* The mediating adult communicates to children the long-range, structural, or developmental meaning and purpose of a shared activity or interaction (i.e., explains why one is doing a particular activity in cognitive terms).

4. *Mediation of a feeling of competence.* The mediating adult gives feedback on the children's performance by praising what is done correctly (i.e., by using correct or incorrect aspects of the children's performance and thus attributing the children's achievement to their own efforts and learning strategies).

5. *Promotion of the self-regulation of children's behavior.* Children's behavior is brought under control when they are able to focus attention on the problem or task at hand. Initially, operant controls may be needed to regulate the children's behavior; however, these controls need to be removed systematically (and gradually) so that behaviors are maintained with less direct extrinsic reinforcement.

6. *Sharing.* The children and the mediating adult share the quest for solutions to immediate problems and, more important, for the developmental change in the children's cognitive structures. The quest is shared because each has a defined role and function, and the interaction is characterized by mutual trust and confidence.

Of course, the more cognitive abilities, intrinsic motivation, and environmental opportunities children have, the more easily children learn, and the greater the proportion they learn naturally and independently, the lesser the need for repeated and intense mediated learning experiences. Therefore, the need to utilize instructional guidelines that create mediated learning experiences is exacerbated in children with problems that impede their cognitive or motivational development such as chaotic impoverished environments, mental retardation, learning disabilities, behavior disorders, and sensory and motoric disabilities. Basically (Haywood et al., 1992; Tzuriel, 1991), the affective-motivational factors are thought of as an essential substrate for the proposed relationships among the components of mediated learning experiences and cognitive modifiability which operate in a transactional fashion. That is, efficient mediation by parents can facilitate affective-motivational processes which in turn encourage the adult mediators to adjust both the quality and the quantity of their mediation to match their children's responses (e.g., reduce or increase efforts for children's engagement).

Moreover, mediational learning experiences need to be used with all children to facilitate their intrinsic motivation and their reliance on internal self-system processes. This will increase their knowledge acquisition and knowledge usage to expand their efficiency to solve problems. Mediated learning experiences will also decrease children's extrinsic motivation and their overreliance and overdependence on environmental feedback which will decrease their knowledge acquisition and knowledge use and make them less competent and less able to solve problems. Mediational learning experiences have been successfully used for normally developing, exceptional, and high-risk children and adult populations to facilitate learning and intrinsic motivation (Adams, Skuy, & Fridjhon, 1992; Burden, 1987; Egozi, 1991; Kahn, 1992; Kaniel & Tzuriel, 1992; Kaniel, Tzuriel, Feuerstein, Ben-Shachar, & Eitan, 1991; Keane, Tannenbaum, & Krapt, 1991; Klein, 1991, 1992; Kopp-Greenberg, 1991; Lidz, 1991a, 1991b; Marfo, 1992; Mintzker, 1991; Notari, Cole, & Mills, 1992; Savell, Twohig, & Rachford, 1986; Sewell & Price, 1991; Tannenbaum, 1991; Thoman, 1992; Tzuriel & Haywood, 1991).

The research of the Peabody-Vanderbilt group has been most productive in helping researchers understand the influence of effectance motivation and motivational orientation (intrinsic and extrinsic motivation) on the performance of persons with and without mental retardation ranging from preschool, school-age, and middle-school children without mental retardation to adults with mild mental retardation. There is much overlap between the ideas and constructs of the Yale group and the Peabody-Vanderbilt group regarding the operation of personality and motivational processes in persons with mental retardation. Together the ideas of these research groups form a complementary tapestry of overlapping ideas which will help researchers understand those historically overlooked motivational and environmental variables regarding individual differences in behavior in persons both with and without mental retardation.

3. PRACTICAL IMPLICATIONS OF THE THEORY OF MOTIVATIONAL ORIENTATION FOR PERSONS WITH MENTAL RETARDATION

Personality and motivational self-system processes are the energizing factors that underpin all other psychological, educational, and self-regulatory processes in all persons and are particularly important in facilitating and enhancing the performance of learning-inefficient persons such as persons with mental retardation to allow them to behave in a more adaptive and functional fashion in the real world. The theory of motivational orientation, though far from complete, may yield important suggestions to help improve the quality of life for persons with mental retardation.

This section reflects my professional and personal experiences with persons with mental retardation, which began more than 34 years ago when I entered the field as a teacher. Since then, I have been a service-provider, a teacher trainer, a clinical psychologist, a researcher, and an advocate (see Switzky, 1995, in press). One of the things that has amazed me throughout my career has been the breadth of individual differences that I have observed in persons with mental retardation, which probably led to my interests in personality and motivational self-system processes in an attempt to understand in some systematic way the underpinnings of these individual differences. Knowledge of an individual's psychometric intelligence is insufficient by itself to predict that individual's learning potential or problem-solving ability, hence the importance of those overlooked personality and motivational variables and the significance of viewing persons with mental retardation as whole people.

For over 30 years, the Peabody-Vanderbilt group has concentrated on trying to measure (however crudely) motivational orientation in a very difficult population, low mental-age individuals, and describing the consequences in performance of having an intrinsically or an extrinsically motivated motivational orientation. Exactly why individuals have an intrinsically or extrinsically motivated motivational orientation was never investigated, although we have speculated about those conditions which may facilitate one or the other of these orientations.

As anyone who has ever watched young children knows, they are constantly exploring, touching, looking, playing, and attempting to gain mastery and understanding over their worlds. If parents and other socializing agents (teachers) create an environmental context which is supportive of these independent attempts at mastery and understanding by the use of the principles of mediated learning where these teachers interact with children in order to explain, communicate, and point out to them in a dynamic social interaction detailed aspects of the environment so that the children can attribute their own achievements to their own attempts at mastery, this teaching strategy will be supportive to the emergence of an intrinsically motivated motivational orientation.

When my own children were young, we would often go to visit the elephants at the zoo. I would engage in a conversation with my five-year-old son Andrew and three-year-old daughter Rachel as follows:

Dad: Look, what do you see?
Andrew: It's big.
Rachel: It's very big and it has a long funny nose.
Dad: How smart you both are. Yes, that funny long nose is the elephant's trunk. What is the elephant doing with his trunk?
Andrew: The elephant is eating hay.
Rachel: The elephant is eating leaves.
Dad: What clever children I have. You are right, the elephant is using his trunk like a hand and is using his trunk to bring food into his mouth. What is the elephant doing now?
Andrew and Rachel: He is drinking water.
Dad: Yes, the elephant can use his trunk like a straw and can get water into his mouth.
Andrew: Can the elephant use his trunk like a hose and blow water out of it?
Dad: Let's stay awhile and see what happens. (Elephant does blow water out of his trunk).
Andrew: I was right, the elephant can use his trunk like a hose.
Dad: How proud I am of both of you for knowing so much.

Successful attempts at mastery will facilitate the emergence of an intrinsically motivated motivational orientation. For children with mental retardation, successful attempts at mastery may be less frequent and the teachers in their environment must create an environmental context which will encourage children with mental retardation to trust in themselves and not give up. Though it is true that many children with mental retardation have an extrinsically motivated motivational orientation, this is not an unalterable consequence of mental retardation as research has demonstrated. Moreover, it is important to know the teaching strategies that will prove useful in facilitating an intrinsically motivated orientation in children with mental retardation.

A student of mine came to me deeply troubled. His visiting aunt and uncle from Oregon were very upset because their school in rural Oregon was getting ready to move their 10-year-old son, Greg, into a very restrictive educational setting in a school not known for educational excellence. When I got out of my car to evaluate Greg, Greg came out to greet me. "Hello Greg," I said, "What a big boy you are. Do you want to help me carry my briefcase into the house?" Greg was smiling and happy to help carry my briefcase. I evaluated Greg's reading ability using the Woodcock-Johnson Psycho-Educational Battery (Woodcock & Johnson, 1989) in the kitchen. Sure enough, Greg had learned nothing regarding reading comprehension during his previous school years. I went over the test with Greg and when he made an error, I asked him why he picked the choice he did. I made him pay very close attention to what he was doing and I became very excited and complimented him when he made the right response and corrected him when he made the wrong response and asked him why the response was wrong. Greg was slowly learning the material. When our session ended, Greg carried my briefcase back to my car and I told Greg what a wonderful job he had done. I visited Greg weekly for about a month and, using the same teaching strategy, I noticed that Greg's learning rate started to accelerate. At the end of four weeks, Greg was testing at grade level. He was happy and more confident and his mother told me he had become more interested in reading and in books.

A few years ago my colleague Geofrey Schultz and I became interested in the Children's Analogical Thinking Modifiability (CATM) instrument (Tzuriel & Klein, 1985). The CATM is a set of analogical thinking problems in which flat blocks vary in terms of their color, shape, and size. The subject is presented with an analogical thinking problem, for example, small red square, small red circle, big red square, blank. The task is to pick the correct block which follows in the series from a matrix of 18 flat blocks varying in color (red, blue, yellow), shape (circle, square, triangle), and size (big, small). In the example, the subject would move the big red circle block onto the blank space. The test is constructed so that items become increasingly difficult. On level I, one dimension changes while the other two are held constant. On level II, two dimensions change and one dimension is held constant. On level III, all three dimensions change.

The subjects were 70 adult individuals with mild mental retardation residing at a community intermediate care facility (ICF). On the baseline phase we just asked the subjects to go through all the items on the CATM and provided no feedback, but just kept track of their correct and incorrect responses. Then we divided the group in half. One group went through all the items on the CATM again without any feedback (the control group), while for the second group, as they were going through all the items on the CATM, we asked them why they picked the item that they had picked but we provided no feedback regarding the correctness of the responses (the experimental group). All groups went through the CATM a third time with astounding differences. The control group showed no differences in the number of correct problems solved even though they had gone over the CATM items three times. The experimental group showed dramatic increases in the number of correct problems solved in the third block of CATM items. Subjects in the experimental group appeared to pay a lot of attention to what they were doing. You could almost see the smoke come out of their ears due to their intense concentration. The experiment was never completed totally, but we did determine that the increase in scores was uncorrelated with psychometric intelligence, gender, age, or years at the ICF. It is unfortunate that we did not determine the motivational orientation of the subjects, but since subjects were randomly assigned to conditions, we doubted that effects observed were simply due to differences in motivational orientation.

These three clinical anecdotal scenarios illustrate combinations of mediated learning teaching strategies and variants of interactive assessment strategies (Haywood & Tzuriel, 1992) which illustrate techniques that can facilitate an intrinsically motivated orientation in all learners. My own children, Andrew and Rachel, have grown up with what I believe is a strong intrinsically motivated orientation. Greg, though psychometrically mildly mentally retarded, could benefit from good teaching strategies based on the principles of mediated learning. It is unfortunate that Greg's teachers in rural Oregon were unfamiliar with mediated learning strategies, though many cognitive curriculums are currently available (Costa, 1991a, 1991b; Feuerstein, Klein, & Tannenbaum, 1991; Haywood, Brooks, & Burns, 1986). Our adventure with the CATM showed that encouraging and supporting adults with mild mental retardation just to pay attention to what they are doing in order to solve a problem has tremendous benefits in facilitating problem-solving performance and also in facilitating an intrinsically motivated orientation because these adults with mild mental retardation were so successful in solving relatively difficult analogical reasoning problems. These clinical anecdotes indicate the power of mediated learning strategies in facilitating performance and encouraging and supporting intrinsic motivation. Well-controlled longitudinal studies with young children with mental retardation using highly focused and explicit mediated learning strategies to determine what indeed are the variables that will lead to the emergence of an intrinsically motivated orientation are needed. At this time all that can be provided are best guesses, which may be very useful to parents, service providers, and teachers until the hard data are in (see Alderman, 1999; Brophy, 1998; Stipek, 1998, Wehmeyer, Agran, & Hughes, 1998).

I am often asked if it is possible to create more of an intrinsically motivated orientation in persons who clearly demonstrate an extrinsically motivated orientation. I do not know of any systematic set of studies that has demonstrated that this can be done in individuals with or without mental retardation. I did attempt to use social reinforcement (e.g., praise) to change the verbal statements of a group of institutionalized adults with mild mental retardation during sessions of social interaction during my postdoctoral fellowship at Peabody. There were two groups of five adults. One group (experimental) received extensive social praise whenever their verbal statements indicated themes indicative of intrinsic motivation (e.g., achievement, I like to learn more; challenge, I like to do hard things; creativity, I like to draw; and responsibility, I like to be in charge). Themes indicative of extrinsic motivation (e.g., ease, It would be easier; safety and health, It would be safer or healthier; and practicality aspects of the environment, I would like to have more money) were ignored. The other group (control) received extensive social praise regardless of whatever verbal statements they made connoting either intrinsic or extrinsic motivation. Additionally, all subjects prior to the intervention were exposed to a set of puzzles varying in complexity and difficulty and the amount of time subjects spent on each puzzle was noted. All sessions of group verbal interactions were tape-recorded, the protocols were typed, and verbal statements were classified as to the degree they connoted intrinsic or extrinsic motivational themes. After 4 weeks of meeting twice a week with the groups, all subjects were again exposed to the set of puzzles. The results were interesting. Indeed, the experimental group did show increases in verbal themes connoting intrinsic motivation, whereas the control group showed no increases in verbal themes. The verbal behaviors of the groups were unrelated to their performance on the puzzles. This little demonstration showed that it was indeed possible to condition the verbal expression of motivation in persons with mild mental retardation but these changes in verbal behavior were unrelated to changes in behavior. It was quite naive to do the study. Subjects were perceptive enough to see a link between the reinforcement operation and their own verbal performance but that would not be enough to change deep-seated personality and motivational self-system processes.

Some suggestions can be offered in order to create more of an intrinsically motivated orientation in persons who clearly demonstrate an extrinsically motivated orientation. Perhaps one has to return to the use of mediated learning principles, which can arouse in individuals vigilance, curiosity, feelings of competence, empowerment, and mastery. Of course, this is not easy. The earlier the process is started, the better. Over the years I have heard thousands of skilled and caring teachers who are aware of mediated learning principles complain of their own frustrations in being unable to change the extrinsic motivational orientation of their students and to improve their students' ability to succeed in learning new things. My only suggestion to these teachers is not to lose faith or give up too soon. In my 34 years as a teacher of exceptional children and adults, I have seen extrinsically motivated individuals become more intrinsically motivated by the use of the principles of mediated learning. Of course, what is needed is more systematic research.It can be argued that few realistic solutions have been forthcoming that offer relief to teachers faced with student academic dysfunction that is confounded by low motivation for self-directed mastery learning. Much of the applied research on the personality dimension of intrinsic motivation has focused on the learning and performance of populations without mental retardation. Important questions need to be answered regarding the development of personality dimensions that shape the approach persons with mental retardation take toward learning in the classroom, in the community, and on the job. There have been few attempts to discover how intrinsic motivation develops in persons with mental retardation (I am still amazed after 30 years of research that it develops at all in persons with mental retardation considering all the difficulties that exist in their world) or, perhaps more important, how it is possible to convert the typically extrinsically orientated person with mental retardation into an intrinsically motivated person. However, we are now in the 21st century and knowledge is accumulating rapidly. We are now much more aware of the importance of motivational and personality self-regulatory system processes. I believe that this volume will be the harbinger of new strategies of facilitating the intrinsic motivation of persons with mental retardation and will inspire new generations of researchers.

REFERENCES

Abhalter, D., & Switzky, H. N. (1992, February). *Measures of intrinsic and extrinsic motivation in elementary school students: A test of construct validity.* Paper read at the Third Conference of the International Association for Cognitive Education, University of California at Riverside, Riverside, CA.

Abramson, L. Y., Seligman, M. E. P., & Teasdale, J. D. (1978). Learned helplessness in humans: Critique and reformulation. *Journal of Abnormal Psychology, 87,* 49–74.

Adams, I., Skuy, M., & Fridjhon, P. (1992). Effectiveness of a home-based program of pre-school children in disadvantaged South African communities. *International Journal of Cognitive Education & Mediated Learning, 2*(1), 5–16.

Alderman, M. K. (1999). *Motivation for achievement: Possibilities for teaching and learning.* Mahwah, NJ: Lawrence Erlbaum Associates.

Amabile, T. M. (1996). *Creativity in context.* New York: Westview Press.

Ames, C., & Ames, R. (1985). *Research on motivation in education* (Vol. 2). Orlando, FL: Academic Press.

Ames, C., & Ames, R. (1989). *Research on motivation in education* (Vol 3). San Diego, CA: Academic Press.

Ames, R., & Ames, C. (1984). *Research on motivation in education* (Vol. 1). Orlando, FL: Academic Press.

Arbitman-Smith, R., Haywood, H. C., & Bransford, J. D. (1984). Assessing cognitive change. In P. Brooks, R. Sperber, & C. McCauley (Eds.), *Learning and cognition in the mentally retarded* (pp. 433–471). Hillsdale, NJ: Lawrence Erlbaum Associates.

Atkinson, J. (1964). *An introduction to motivation.* Princeton, NJ: Van Nostrand.

Balla, D., Butterfield, E., & Zigler, E. (1974). Effects of institutionalization on retarded children: A longitudinal, cross-institutional investigation. *American Journal of Mental Deficiency, 78,* 530–549.

Balla, D., & Zigler, E. (1979). Personality development in retarded persons. In N. R. Ellis (Eds.), *Handbook of mental deficiency* (2nd ed., pp. 143–168). Hillsdale, NJ: Lawrence Erlbaum Associates.

Bandura, A. (1969). *Principles of behavior modification.* New York: Holt.

Bandura, A. (1976). Self-reinforcement: Theoretical and methodological considerations. *Behaviorism, 4,* 135–155.

Bandura, A. (1977). *Social learning theory.* Englewood Cliffs, NJ: Prentice-Hall.

Bandura, A. (1978). The self-system in reciprocal determinism. *American Psychologist, 33,* 344–358.

Bandura, A. (1986a). *Social foundations of thought and action: A social cognitive theory.* Englewood Cliffs, NJ: Prentice-Hall.

Bandura, A. (1986b). From thought to action: Mechanisms of personal agency. *New Zealand Journal of Psychology, 15,* 1–17.

Bandura, A. (1993). Perceived self-efficacy in cognitive development and functioning. *Educational Psychologist, 28*(2), 117–148.

Bandura, A. (1997). *Self-efficacy: The exercise of control.* New York: W. H. Freeman and Company.

Bandura, A., & Perloff, B. (1967). Relative efficacy of self monitored and externally imposed reinforcement systems. *Journal of Personality and Social Psychology, 7,* 111–116.

Bialer, I., (1961). Conceptualization of success and failure in mentally retarded and normal children. *Journal of Personality, 29,* 303–320.

Blumenfeld, P., Pintrich, P., Meece, J., & Wessels, K. (1982). The formation and role of self-perceptions of ability in elementary classrooms. *Elementary School Journal, 82,* 401–420.

Boekaerts, M., Pintrich, P. R., & Zeidner, M. (Eds.). (2000). *Handbook of self-regulation.* San Diego, CA: Academic Press.

Boggiano, A. K., Main, D. S., & Katz, P. A. (1988). Children's preference for challenge: The role of perceived competence and control. *Journal of Personality and Social Psychology, 54,* 134–141.

Borkowski J. G., Carr, M., Rellinger, E., & Pressley, M. (1990). Self-regulated cognition: Interdependence of metacognition, attributions, and self-esteem. In B. F. Jones & L. Idol (Eds.), *Dimensions of thinking and cognitive instruction* (pp. 53–92). Hillsdale, NJ: Lawrence Erlbaum Associates.

Borkowski, J. G., Day, J. D., Saenz, D., Dietmeyer, D., Estrada, T. M., & Groteluschen, A. (1992). Expanding the boundaries of cognitive interventions. In B. Y. L. Wong (Ed.), *Contemporary intervention research in learning disabilities* (pp. 1–21). New York: Springer-Verlag.

Borkowski, J. G., & Kurtz, B. E. (1987). Metacognition and executive control. In J. G. Borkowski & J. D. Day (Eds.), *Cognition in special children* (pp. 123–152). Norwood, NJ: Ablex.

Brophy, J. (1998). *Motivating students to learn.* Boston: McGraw-Hill.

Bryan, J. H., & Bryan, T. H. (1983). The social life of the learning disabled youngster. In J. D. McKinney & L. Feagans (Eds.), *Current topics in learning disabilities* (Vol. 1, pp. 57–85). Norwood, NJ: Ablex.

Burack, J. A., Hodapp, R. M., & Zigler, E. (Eds.). (1998). *Handbook of mental retardation.* New York: Cambridge University Press.

Burden, R. (1987). Instrumental enrichment programme: Important issues in research and evaluation. *European Journal of Psychology of Education, 2*(1), 3–16.

Bybee, J., Ennis, P., & Zigler, E. (1990). Effects of institutionalization on the self-concept and outerdirectness of adolescents with mental retardation. *Exceptionality, 1,* 215–226.

Bybee, J., Glick, M., & Zigler, E. (1990). Differences across gender, grade level, and academic track in the content of the ideal self-image. *Sex Roles, 22,* 349–358.

Bybee, J., & Zigler, E. (1991). The self-image and guilt: a further test of the cognitive-developmental formulation. *Journal of Personality, 59,* 733–745.

Bybee, J., & Zigler, E. (1992). Is outerdirectedness employed in a harmful or beneficial manner by students with and without mental retardation? *American Journal of Mental Retardation, 96,* 512–521.

Call, R.J. (1968). *Motivation-hygiene orientation as a function of socioeconomic status, grade, race, and sex.* Unpublished master's thesis, Tennessee State University, Nashville.

Cantor, G. N. (1963). Hull-Spence behavior theory and mental deficiency. In N. R. Ellis (Ed.), *Handbook of mental deficiency* (pp. 90–133). New York: McGraw-Hill.

Carr, M., Borkowski, J. G., & Maxwell, S. E. (1991). Motivational components of underachievement. *Developmental Psychology, 27,* 108–118.

Castaneda, A., McCandless, B. R., & Palermo, D. S. (1956). The Children's Form of the Manifest Anxiety Scale. *Child Development, 27,* 317–326.

Cochran, I. L., & Cleland, C. C. (1963). Manifest anxiety of retardates and normals matched as to academic achievement. *American Journal of Mental Deficiency, 67,* 539–542.

Collins, H. A., & Burger, G. K. (1970). The self-concepts of adolescent retarded students. *Education and Training of the Mentally Retarded, 5,* 23–30.

Connell, J. P., & Ryan, R. M. (1985). *A theory of and assessment of children's self regulation within the academic domain.* Unpublished manuscript, University of Rochester., Rochester, NY.

Costa, A. L. (Ed.). (1991a). *Developing minds: A resource book for teaching thinking* (Rev. ed., Vol. 1). Alexandria, VA: Association for Supervision and Curriculum Development.

Costa, A. L. (Ed.). (1991b). *Developing minds: Programs for teaching thinking* (Rev. ed., Vol.2). Alexandria, VA: Association for Supervision and Curriculum Development.

Covington, M. V. (1987). Achievement motivation, self-attributions and exceptionality. In J. D. Day & J. G. Borkowski (Eds.), *Cognition in special children* (pp. 173–213). Norwood, NJ: Ablex.

Cromwell, R. L. (1963). A social learning approach to mental retardation. In N.R. Ellis (Ed.), *Handbook of mental deficiency* (pp. 41–91). New York: McGraw-Hill.

Cromwell, R. L. (1967). Success-failure reactions in mentally retarded children. In J. Zubin & G. A. Gervis (Eds.), *Psychopathology of mental development*. New York: Grune & Stratton.

DeCharms, R. (1968). *Personal causation: The interval affective determinants of behavior*. New York: Academic Press.

DeCharms, R. (1976). *Enhancing motivation: Change in the classroom*. New York: Irvington.

DeCharms, R. (1984). Motivating enhancement in educational settings. In R. Ames & C. Ames (Eds.), *Research on motivation in education: Vol 1. Student motivation* (pp. 275–310). Orlando, FL: Academic Press.

Deci, E. L., Eghrari, H., Patrick, B. C., & Leone, D. R. (1991). *Facilitating internalization: The self-determination theory perspective*. Unpublished manuscript, University of Rochester, Rochester, NY.

Deci, E. L., Hodges, R., Pierson, L. H., & Tomassone, J. (1992). Autonomy and competence and motivational factors in students with learning disabilities and emotional handicaps. *Journal of Learning Disabilities, 25*, 457–471.

Deci, E. L., Koestner, R., & Ryan, R. M. (1999). A meta-analytic review of experiments examining the effects of extrinsic rewards on intrinsic motivation. *Psychological Bulletin, 125*, 627–668.

Deci, E. L., Nezlek, J., & Sheinman, L. (1981). Characteristics of the rewarder and the intrinsic motivation of the rewardee. *Journal of Personality and Social Psychology, 40*, 1–10.

Deci, E. L., & Ryan, R. M. (1985). *Intrinsic motivation and self-determination in human behavior*. New York: Plenum.

Deci, E. L., & Ryan, R. M. (1991). A motivational approach to self: Integration in personality. In R. Dienstbier (Ed.), *Nebraska symposium on motivation: Vol. 38, Perspectives on motivation* (pp. 237–288). Lincoln: University of Nebraska Press.

Deci, E. L., & Ryan, R. M. (1995). Human autonomy: The basis for true self-esteem. In M. Kernis (Ed.), *Efficacy, agency, and self-esteem* (pp. 31–49). New York: Plenum.

126 SWITZKY

Deci, E. L., Schwartz, A. J., Scheinman. L., & Ryan, R. M. (1981). An instrument to assess adults' orientation toward control versus autonomy with children. *Journal of Educational Psychology, 73,* 642–650.

Dobbs, V. (1967). *Motivational orientation and programmed instruction achievement gains of educable mentally retarded adolescents.* Unpublished doctoral dissertation, George Peabody College, Nashville, TN.

Dweck, C. S. (1989). Motivation. In A. Lesgold & R. Glaser (Eds.), *Foundations for a psychology of education* (pp. 87–136). Hillsdale, NJ: Lawrence Erlbaum Associates.

Dweck, C. S. (1998). The development of early self-conceptions: Their relevance for motivational processes. In J. Heckhausen & C. S. Dweck (Eds.), *Motivation and self-regulation across the life span* (pp. 257–280). New York: Cambridge University Press.

Dweck, C. S. (1999). *Self-theories: Their role in motivation, personality, and development.* Philadelphia: Taylor & Francis.

Egozi, M. (1991). Instrumental enrichment and mediation. In R. Feuerstein., P. S. Klein, & A. J. Tannenbaum (Eds.), *Mediated learning experience (MLE): Theoretical, psychosocial and learning implications* (pp. 347–364). London: Freund.

Evans, D. W. (1998). Development of the self-concept in children with mental retardation: Organismic and contextual factors. In J. A. Burack, R. M. Hodapp, & E. Zigler (Eds.), *Handbook of mental retardation and development* (pp. 462–480). New York: Cambridge University Press.

Eysenck, S. B. G. (1965). Manual for the *Junior Eysenck Personality Inventory.* San Diego, CA: Educational and Industrial Testing Service.

Feuerstein, R., & Feuerstein, S. (1991). Mediated learning experience: A theoretical review. In R. Feuerstein., P. S. Klein, & A. J. Tannenbaum (Eds.), *Mediated learning experience (MLE): Theoretical, psychosocial and learning implications* (pp. 3–51). London: Freund.

Feuerstein, R., & Rand, Y. (1974). Mediated learning experiences: An outline of the proximal etiology for differential development of cognitive functions. *International Understanding, 9–10,* 7–37.

Feuerstein, R., Klein, P. S., & Tannenbaum, A. J. (Eds.). (1991). *Mediated learning experience (MLE): Theoretical, psychosocial and learning implications.* London: Freund.

Feuerstein, R., Rand, Y., Hoffman, M. B., & Miller, R. (1980). *Instrumental enrichment: intervention program for cognitive modifiability.* Baltimore: University Park Press.

Fitts, W. H. (1965). *Manual for the Tennessee Self-Concept Scale.* Nashville, TN: Counselor Recordings and Tests.

Flink, C., Boggiano, A. K., & Barrett, M. (1990). Controlling teaching strategies: Undermining children's self-determination and performance. *Journal of Personality and Social Psychology, 59,* 916–924.

Ford, M. E. (1992). *Motivating humans: Goals, emotions, and personal agency beliefs.* Newbury Park, CA: Sage Publications.

Ford, M. E. (1995). Motivation and competence development in special and remedial education. *Intervention in Schools and Clinics, 31,* 70–83.

Gambro, J. S., & Switzky, H. N. (1988). Motivational orientation and self-regulation in young children. *Reflections of Learning Research, 3,* 6–7.

Gambro, J. S., & Switzky, H. N. (1991). Motivational orientation and self-regulation in young children. *Early Child Development and Care, 70,* 45–51.

Glick, M. (1999). Developmental and experiential variables in the self-images of people with mild mental retardation. In E. Zigler & D. Bennett-Gates (Eds.), *Personality development in individuals with mental retardation* (pp. 47–69). New York: Cambridge University Press.

Glick, M., Bybee, J., & Zigler, E. (1997). [Self-images of adolescents with mild mental retardation]. Unpublished raw data.

Glick, M., & Zigler, E. (1985). Self-image: A cognitive-developmental approach. In R. Leahy (Ed.), *The development of the self* (pp. 1–53). New York: Academic Press.

Gollwitzer, P. M., & Bargh, J. A. (Eds.). (1996). *The psychology of action: Linking cognition and motivation to behavior.* New York: The Guilford Press.

Gorlow, L., Butler, A., & Guthrie, G. (1963). Correlates of self-attitudes of retardates. *American Journal of Mental Deficiency, 67,* 549–554.

Gottfried, A. E. (1985). Academic intrinsic motivation in elementary and junior high school students. *Journal of Educational Psychology, 20,* 205–215.

Gottfried, A. E. (1990). Academic intrinsic motivation in young elementary school children. *Journal of Educational Psychology, 82,* 525–538.

Grolnick, W., & Ryan, R. (1987). Autonomy in children's learning: An experimental and individual difference investigation. *Journal of Personality and Social Psychology, 52,* 890–898.

Gruen, G., & Zigler, E. (1968). Expectancy of success and the probability learning of middle-class, lower-class, and retarded children. *Journal of Abnormal Psychology, 73,* 343–352.

Harter, S. (1978). Effectance motivation reconsidered: Toward a developmental model. *Human Development, 6,* 34–64.

Harter, S. (1981a). A model of intrinsic motivation in children. In W. A. Collins (Ed.), *Minnesota Symposium on Child Psychology* (Vol. 14, pp. 215–255). Hillsdale, NJ: Lawrence Erlbaum Associates.

Harter, S. (1981b). A new self-report scale of intrinsic versus extrinsic orientation in the classroom: Motivational and informational components. *Developmental Psychology, 17,* 300–312.

Harter. S. (1982). The Perceived Competence Scale for Children. *Child Development, 53,* 87–97.

Harter, S. (1983). Developmental perspectives on the self-system. In E. M. Hetherington (Ed.), *Handbook of child psychology: Socialization, personality and social development* (Vol. 4, pp. 278–386). New York: Wiley.

Harter, S. (1985). Manual for the *Self-Perception Profile for Children.* Unpublished manuscript, University of Denver.

Harter, S. (1987). The determinants and mediational role of global self-worth in children. In N. Eisenberg (Ed.), *Contemporary topics in developmental psychology* (pp. 219–241). New York: Wiley.

Harter, S. (1990). Causes, correlates and the functional roles of global self-worth: A life span perspective. In R. Sternberg & J. Kolligian (Eds.), *Competence considered* (pp. 67–97). New Haven, CT: Yale University Press.

Harter, S. (1992). The relationship between perceived competence, affect, and motivational orientation within the classroom: Process and patterns of change. In A. Boggiano & T. Pittman (Eds.), *Achievement and motivation: A social-developmental perspective* (pp. 77–114). Cambridge, UK: Cambridge University Press.

Harter, S. (1993). Visions of self: Beyond the me in the mirror. *Nebraska Symposium on Motivation, 40,* 99–144.

Harter, S. (1999). *The construction of the self: A developmental perspective.* New York: Guilford

Harter, S., & Connell, J. (1984). A comparison of alternative models of the relationships between academic achievement and children's perceptions of competence, control, and motivational orientation. In J. Nicholls (Ed.), *The development of achievement-related conditions and behavior* (pp. 219–250). Greenwich, CT: JAI Press.

Harter, S., & Pike, R. (1984). The pictorial scale of perceived competence and social acceptance for young children. *Child Development, 55,* 1969–1982.

Harter, S., Whitesell, N., & Kowalski, P. (1992). Individual differences in the effects of educational transitions on young adolescent's perceptions of competence and motivational orientations. *American Educational Research Journal, 29,* 777–807.

Harter, S., & Zigler, E. (1968). Effectiveness of adult and peer reinforcement on the performance of institutionalized and noninstitutionalized retardates. *Journal of Abnormal Psychology, 73,* 144–149.

Harter, S., & Zigler, E. (1972). Effects of rate of stimulus presentation and penalty conditions on the discrimination learning of normal and retarded children. *Developmental Psychology, 6,* 85–91.

Harter, S., & Zigler, E. (1974). The assessment of effectance motivation in normal and retarded children. *Developmental Psychology, 10,* 169–180.

Haywood, H. C. (1968a). Motivational orientation of overachieving and underachieving elementary school children. *American Journal of Mental Deficiency, 72,* 662–667.

Haywood, H. C. (1968b). Psychometric motivation and the efficiency of learning and performance in the mentally retarded. In B. W. Richards (Ed.), *Proceedings of the First Congress of the International Association for the Scientific Study of Mental Deficiency* (pp. 276–283). Reigate, England: Michael Jackson.

Haywood, H. C. (1971). Individual differences in motivational orientation: A trait approach. In H. I. Day, D. E. Berlyne, & D. E. Hunt (Eds.), *Intrinsic motivation: A new direction in education.* Toronto: Holt, Rinehart & Winston.

Haywood, H. C. (1977). A cognitive approach to the education of retarded children. *Peabody Journal of Education, 54,* 110–116.

Haywood, H. C. (1992). The strange and wonderful symbiosis of motivation and cognition. *International Journal of Cognitive Education & Mediated Learning, 2,* 186–197.

Haywood, H. C., Brooks, P., & Burns, S. (1986). Stimulating cognitive development at developmental level: A tested, non-remedial preschool curriculum for preschool and older retarded children. In M. Schwebel & C. A. Maher (Eds.), *Facilitating cognitive development:*

Principles, practices, and programs (pp. 127–147). New York: Haworth Press.

Haywood, H. C., & Burke, W. P. (1977). Development of individual differences in intrinsic motivation. In I. C. Uzgiris & F. Weizman (Eds.), *The structuring of experience* (pp. 235–263). New York: Plenum.

Haywood, H. C., & Switzky, H. N. (1975). Use of contingent social reinforcement to change the verbal expression of motivation in children of differing motivational orientation. *Perceptual and Motor Skills, 86,* 356–365.

Haywood, H. C., & Switzky, H. N. (1985). Work response of mildly mentally retarded adults to self versus external regulation as a function of motivational orientation. *American Journal of Mental Deficiency, 90,* 151–159.

Haywood, H. C., & Switzky, H. N. (1986). Intrinsic motivation and behavioral effectiveness in retarded persons. In N. Ellis & N. Bray (Eds.), *International review of research in mental retardation* (Vol.14, pp. 1–46). New York: Academic Press.

Haywood, H. C., & Switzky, H. N. (1992). Ability and modifiability: What, how and how much? In J. S. Carlson (Ed.), *Advances in cognition and educational practice: Theoretical issues: Intelligence, cognition, and assessment* (Vol. 1, Part A, pp. 25–85). Greenwich, CT: JAI Press.

Haywood, H. C., Switzky, H. N., & Wright, W. (1974, June). *Symposium on the personality and motivational structure in the mentally retarded.* Annual meeting of the American Association on Mental Deficiency, Toronto, Ontario, Canada.

Haywood, H. C., & Tzuriel, D. (Eds.),(1992). *Interactive assessment.* New York: Springer-Verlag.

Haywood, H. C., Tzuriel, D., Vaught, S. (1992). Psychoeducational assessment from a transactional perspective. In H.C. Haywood, & D. Tzuriel (Eds.), *Interactive assessment* (pp. 38–63). New York: Springer-Verlag.

Haywood, H. C., & Wachs, T. D. (1966). Size discrimination learning as a function of motivation-hygiene orientation in adolescents. *Journal of Educational Psychology, 57,* 279–286.

Haywood, H. C., & Weaver, S. J. (1967). Differential effects of motivational orientation and incentive conditions on motor performance in institutionalized retardates. *American Journal of Mental Deficiency, 72,* 459–467.

Heckhausen, H. (1967). *The anatomy of achievement motivation.* New York: Academic Press.

Heckhausen, H. (1983). The development of achievement motivation. In W. W. Hartrup (Ed.), *Review of child development research* (pp. 600–668). Chicago: University of Chicago Press.

Heckhausen, H. (1991). *Motivation and action.* New York: Springer-Verlag.

Heckhausen, J., & Dweck, C. C. (Eds.). (1998). *Motivation and self-regulation across the lifespan.* New York: Cambridge University Press.

Herzberg, F. (1966). *Work and the nature of man.* Cleveland, OH: World.

Herzberg, F., & Hamlin, R. M. (1961). A motivation-hygiene concept of mental health. *Mental Hygiene, 47,* 394–401.

Herzberg, F., & Hamlin, R. M. (1963). The motivation-hygiene concept and psychotherapy. *Mental Hygiene, 47,* 384–397

Herzberg, F., Mausner, B., & Snyderman, B. B. (1959). *The motivation to work.* New York: Wiley.

Hill, K. (1984). Debilitating motivation and testing: A major educational problem, possible solutions, and policy applications. In R. Ames & C. Ames (Eds.), *Research on motivation in education, Vol 1: Student motivation* (pp. 245–272). Orlando, FL: Academic Press.

Hill, K., & Wigfield, A. (1984). Test anxiety: A major educational problem and what can be done about it. *The Elementary School Journal, 85,* 105–126.

Hobbs, N. (1963). Foreword. In N. R. Ellis (Ed.), *Handbook of mental deficiency* (pp. ix-x). New York: McGraw-Hill.

Hodapp, R. M., Burack, J. A., & Zigler, E. (Eds.). (1990). *Issues in the developmental approach to mental retardation.* New York: Cambridge University Press.

Hoffman, J., & Weiner, B. (1978). Effects of attributions for success and failure on the performance of retarded adults. *American Journal of Mental Deficiency, 82,* 449–452.

Horai, J., & Guarnaccia, V. J. (1975). Performance and attributions to ability, effort, task, and luck of retarded adults after success or failure feedback. *American Journal of Mental Deficiency, 79,* 690–694.

Hunt, J. McV. (1963). Motivation inherent in information processing and action. In O. J. Harvey (Ed.), *Motivation and social interaction: Cognitive determinants* (pp. 35–94). New York: Ronald.

Hunt, J. McV. (1965). Intrinsic motivation and its role in psychological development. In D. Levine (Ed.), *Nebraska symposium on motiva-*

tion (Vol. 13, pp. 189–282). Lincoln, NE: University of Nebraska Press.

Hunt, J. McV. (1966). The epigenesis of intrinsic motivation and early cognitive learning. In R. N. Haber (Ed.), *Current research in motivation* (pp. 355–370). New York: Holt.

Hunt, J. McV. (1971). Toward a history of intrinsic motivation. In H. I. Day, D. E. Berlyne, & D. E. Hunt (Eds.), *Intrinsic motivation: A new direction in education* (pp. 1–32). Toronto: Holt.

Kagan, J. (1964). Final progress report: Passivity and styles of thought in children. Unpublished manuscript, Fels Research Institute, Yellow Springs, OH.

Kahn, R. J. (1992). Mediated learning experiences during parent/infant play interactions. *International Journal of Cognitive Education & Mediated Learning, 2*(2), 131–146.

Kaniel, S., & Tzuriel, D. (1992). Mediated learning experience approach in the assessment and treatment of borderline psychotic adolescents. In H. C. Haywood & D. Tzuriel (Eds.), *Interactive assessment* (pp. 399–418). New York: Springer-Verlag.

Kaniel, S., Tzuriel, D., Feuerstein, R., Ben-Shachar, N., & Eitan, T. (1991). Dynamic assessment: Learning and transfer abilities of Ethiopian immigrants to Israel. In R. Feuerstein, P. S. Klein, & A. J. Tannenbaum (Eds.), *Mediated learning experience (MLE): Theoretical, psychosocial and learning implications* (pp. 179–209). London: Freund.

Katz, P., & Zigler, E. (1967). Self-image disparity: A developmental approach. *Journal of Personality and Social Psychology, 5,* 186–195.

Keane, K. J., Tannenbaum, A. J., & Krapf, G. F. (1992). Cognitive competence: Reality and potential in the deaf. In H. C. Haywood & D. Tzuriel (Eds.), *Interactive assessment* (pp. 300–316). New York: Springer-Verlag.

Klein, P. S. (1991). Motor assessment and parental intervention in infancy an early childhood: New evidence. In R. Feuerstein, P. S. Klein, & A. J. Tannenbaum (Eds.), *Mediated learning experience (MLE): Theoretical, psychosocial and learning implications* (pp. 213–239). London: Freund.

Klein, P. S. (1992). More intelligent and sensitive child (MISC): A new look at an old question. *International Journal of Cognitive Education & Mediated Learning, 2*(2), 105–116.

Kopp-Greenberg, K. H. (1991). A model for providing intensive mediated learning experience in preschool settings. In R. Feuerstein, P. S.

Klein, & A. J. Tannenbaum (Eds.), *Mediated learning experience (MLE): Theoretical, psychosocial and learning implications* (pp. 241–258). London: Freund.

Kounin, J. (1941a). Experimental studies of rigidity: I. The measurement of rigidity in normal and feebleminded persons. *Character and Personality, 9,* 251–272.

Kounin, J. (1941b). Experimental studies of rigidity: II. The explanatory power of the concept of rigidity as applied to feeblemindedness. *Character and Personality, 9,* 273–282.

Kovacs, M. (1983). *The Children's Depression Inventory: A self-rated depression scale for school-aged youngsters.* Unpublished Manuscript, University of Pittsburgh School of Medicine.

Kuhl, J. (1987). Action control: The maintenance of motivational states. In F. Halisch & J. Kuhl (Eds.), *Motivation, intention and volition* (pp. 279–291). Berlin: Springer-Verlag.

Kuhl, J. (2000). A functional-design approach to motivation and self-regulation: The dynamics of personality systems and interactions. In M. Boekaerts, P. R. Pintrich, & M. Zeidner (Eds.), *Handbook of self-regulation* (pp.111–169). San Diego, CA: Academic Press.

Kunca, D. F., & Haywood, N. P. (1969). The measurement of motivational orientation in low mental age subjects. *Peabody Papers in Human Development, 7*(2).

Lambert, N. M. & McCombs, B. L. (Eds.). (1998). *How students study: Reforming schools through learner-centered education.* Washington, DC: APA Books.

Leahy, R., Balla, D., & Zigler, E. (1982). Role taking, self-image and imitativeness in mentally retarded and nonretarded individuals. *American Journal of Mental Deficiency, 86,* 372–379.

Leahy, R. L. (Ed.). (1985). *The development of the self.* Orlando, FL: Academic Press.

Lepper, M. (1996). Intrinsic motivation and extrinsic rewards: A commentary on Cameron and Pierce's meta-analysis. *Review of Educational Research, 66,* 5–32.

Lepper, M. R., & Hodell, M. (1989). Intrinsic motivation in the classroom. In C. Ames & R. Ames (Eds.), *Research on motivation in education* (Vol. 3, pp. 73–105). San Diego, CA: Academic Press.

Lewin, K. (1936). *A dynamic theory of personality.* New York: McGraw-Hill.

Licht, B. G., & Kistner, J. A. (1986). Motivational problems of learning-disabled children: Individual differences and their implications for treatment. In J. K. Torgesen & B. W. L. Wong (Eds.), *Psychological and educational perspectives on learning disabilities* (pp. 225–255). Orlando, FL: Academic Press.

Lidz, C. S. (1991a). MLE components and their roots in theory and research. In R. Feuerstein, P. S. Klein, & A. J. Tannenbaum (Eds.), *Mediated learning experience (MLE): Theoretical, psychosocial and learning implications* (pp. 271–291). London: Freund.

Lidz, C. S. (1991b). *Practitioner's guide to dynamic assessment.* New York: Guilford Press.

Lipman, R. S. (1960). Children's manifest anxiety scale in retardates and approximately equal M.A. normals. *American Journal of Mental Deficiency, 64,* 1027–1028.

Lipman, R. S. (1963). Learning: Verbal, perceptual-motor, and classical conditioning. In N.R. Ellis (Ed.), *Handbook of mental deficiency* (pp. 391–423). New York: McGraw-Hill.

Lipman, R. S., & Griffith, B. C. (1960). Effects of anxiety level on concept formation: a test of drive theory. *American Journal of Mental Deficiency, 65,* 342–348.

Lustman, N., & Zigler, E. (1982). Imitation by institutionalized and non-institutionalized mentally retarded and nonretarded children. *American Journal of Mental Deficiency, 87,* 252–258.

Luthar, S., & Zigler, E. (1988). Motivational factors, school atmosphere, and SES: Determinants of children's probability task performance. *Journal of Applied Developmental Psychology, 9,* 477–494.

MacMillan, D. L. (1975). Effect of experimental success and failure on the situational expectancy of EMR and nonretarded children. *American Journal of Mental Deficiency, 80,* 90–95.

MacMillan, D. L., & Keogh, B. K. (1971). Normal and retarded children's expectancy for failure. *Developmental Psychology, 4,* 343–348.

Maehr, M., & Pintrich, P. R. (1991). *Advances in motivation and achievement: Goals and self-regulatory processes* (Vol. 7). Greenwich, CT: JAI.

Marfo, K.(1992). Interaction-focused early intervention: Current approaches and contributions from the mediated learning experience paradigm. *International Journal of Cognitive Education & Mediated Learning, 2*(2), 85–104.

Markus, H., & Nurius, P. (1986). Possible selves. *American Psychologist, 41,* 954–969.

Markus, H., & Wurf, E. (1987). The dynamic self-concept: A social psychological perspective. *Annual Review of Psychology, 38,* 299–337.

Marsh, H., Barnes, J., Cairns, L., & Tidman, M. (1984). Self-description questionnaire: Age and sex effects in the structure and level of self-concept for preadolescent children. *Journal of Educational Psychology, 76*, 940–956.

Marsh, H. W., & Hattie, J. (1996). Theoretical Perspectives on the structure of self-concept. In B. A. Bracken (Ed.), *Handbook of self-concept* (pp. 38–90). New York: Wiley.

Marsh, H. W., & Holms, I. W. M. (1990). Multidimensional self-concepts: Construct validation of responses by children. *American Educational Research Journal, 27*, 89–118.

Marsh, H. W., & Shavelson, R. (1985). Self-concept: Its multifaceted, hierarchical structure. *Educational Psychologist, 20*, 107–123.

McCombs, B. L. (1988). Motivational skill training: combining metacognitive, cognitive, and affective learning strategies. In C. E. Weinstein, E. T. Goetz, & P. A. Alexander (Eds.), *Learning and study strategies: Issues in assessment, instruction, and evaluation* (pp. 141–169). New York: Academic Press.

McCombs, B. L. (1989). Self-regulated learning and academic achievement: A phenomenological view. In B. J. Zimmerman & D. H. Schunk (Eds.), *Self-regulated learning and academic achievement* (pp. 51–82). New York: Springer-Verlag.

McCombs, B. L., & Marzano, R. J. (1990). Putting the self in self-regulated learning: The self in regulating will and skill. *Educational Psychologist, 25*, 51–69.

McCombs, B. L., & Whisler, J. S. (1989). The role of affective variables in autonomous learning. *Educational Psychologist, 24*, 277–306.

McCombs, B. L., & Whisler, J. S. (1997). *The learner-centered classroom and school: Strategies for increasing student motivation and achievement.* San Francisco: Jossey-Bass.

McManis, D. L., & Bell, D. R. (1968). Risk-taking by reward-seeking, punishment-avoiding, or mixed-orientation retardates. *American Journal of Mental Retardation, 73*, 267–272.

McManis, D. L., Bell, D. R., & Pike, E. O. (1969). Performance of reward-seeking and punishment-avoiding retardates under reward and punishment. *American Journal of Mental Deficiency, 73*, 906–911.

Merighi, J., Edison, M., & Zigler, E. (1990). The role of motivational factors in the functioning of mentally retarded individuals. In R. M. Hodapp, J. A. Burack, & E. Zigler (Eds.), *Issues in the developmental approach to mental retardation* (pp. 114–134). New York: Cambridge University Press.

Miller, J. O. (1965). The Children's Locus of Evaluation and Control Scales. *Abstracts of Peabody Studies on Mental Retardation, 3, No. 23.*

Miller, M. B. (1961). *Locus of control, learning climate, and climate shift in serial learning with mental retardates.* Ann Arbor, MI: University Microfilms.

Miller, M. B., Haywood, H. C., & Gimon, A. T. (1975). Motivational orientation of Puerto Rican children in Puerto Rico and the U.S. mainland. In G. Marin (Ed.), *Proceedings of the 15th Interamerican Congress of Psychology.* Bogota: Sociedad Interamericana de Psicologia.

Mintzker. Y. (1991). When the baby does not smile back: Obstacles to successful mediated learning experience. In R. Feuerstein, P. S. Klein, & A. J. Tannenbaum (Eds.), *Mediated learning experience (MLE): Theoretical, psychosocial and learning implications* (pp. 259–269). London: Freund.

Morgan, M. (1984). Reward-induced decrements and increments in intrinsic motivation. *Review of Educational Research, 54,* 5–30.

Moss, J.W. (1958). *Failure-avoiding and success-striving behavior in mentally retarded and normal children.* Ann Arbor, MI: University Microfilms.

Nicholls, J. G. (1984). Achievement motivation: Conceptions of ability, subjective experience, task choice, and performance. *Psychological Review, 91,* 328–346.

Nicholls, J. G. (1989). *The competitive ethos and democratic education.* Cambridge, MA: Harvard University Press.

Nicholls, J. G. (1990). What is ability and why are we mindful of it? A developmental perspective. In R. Sternberg & J. Kolligen, Jr. (Eds.), *Competence considered* (pp. 11–40). New Haven, CT: Yale University Press.

Nicholls, J. G., & Miller, A. (1984a). Reasoning about the ability of self and others: A developmental study. *Child Development, 55,* 1990–1999.

Nicholls, J. G., & Miller, A. (1984b). Development and its discontents: The differentiation of the concept of ability. In J. Nicholls (Ed.), *Advances in motivation and achievement: Vol. 3, The development of achievement motivation* (pp. 185–218). Greenwich, CT: JAI Press.

Notari, A., Cole, K., & Mills, P. (1992). Facilitating cognitive and language skills of young children with disabilities: The mediated learning program. *International Journal of Cognitive Education & Mediated Learning, 2*(2), 169–179.

Piers, E. V., & Harris, D. B. (1964). Age and other correlates of self-concept in children. *Journal of Educational Psychology, 55,* 91–95.

Piers, E. V., & Harris, D. B. (1969). Manual for the *Piers-Harris Children's Self-Concept Scales.* Nashville, TN: Counselor Recordings and Tests.

Pintrich, P. R. (2000). The role of goal-orientation in self-regulated learning. In M. Boekaerts, P. R. Pintrich, & M. Zeidner (Eds.), *Handbook of self-regulation* (pp. 452–502). San Diego, CA: Academic Press.

Pintrich, P. R., Anderman, E. M., & Klobucar, C. (1994). Intraindividual differences in motivation and cognition in students with and without learning disabilities. *Journal of Learning Disabilities, 27,* 360–370.

Pintrich, P. R., & Schrauben, B. (1992). Students' motivational beliefs and their cognitive engagement in classroom academic tasks. In D. Schunk & J. Meece (Eds.), *Student perceptions in the classroom: Cause and consequences* (pp. 149–183). Hillsdale, NJ: Lawrence Erlbaum Associates.

Porter, R. B., Cattell, R. B., & Ford, J. J. (1968). Manual for the *Children's Personality Questionnaire.* Champaign, IL: Institute for Personality and Ability Training.

Pressley, M., Borkowski, J. G., & Schneider, W. (1990). Good information processing: What it is and how education can promote it. *International Journal of Educational Research, 2,* 857–867.

Raven, J. C. (1956). *Guide to using the Colored Progressive Matrices (1967) Sets A, Ab, B, Revised.* London: Lewis.

Raven, J. C. (1960). *Guide to using the Standard Progressive Matrices (1956) Sets A, B, C, D, E, Revised.* London: Lewis.

Renick, J., & Harter, S. (1989). Impact of social comparisons on the developing self-perceptions of learning disabled students. *Journal of Educational Psychology, 81,* 631–638.

Ringness, T. A. (1961). Self-concept of children of low, average, and high intelligence. *American Journal of Mental Deficiency, 65,* 453–462.

Rogers, C. (1947). Some observations on the organization of personality. *American Psychologist, 2,* 358–368.

Rotter, J. (1954). *Social learning and clinical psychology.* New York: Prentice-Hall.

Ryan, R. M. (1995). Psychological needs and the facilitation of integrative processes. *Journal of Personality, 63,* 397–427.

Ryan, R. M. (1998). Commentary: Human psychological needs and the issues of volition, control, and outcome focus. In J. Heckhausen & C. S. Dweck (Eds.), *Motivation and self-regulation across the life span* (pp. 114–133). New York: Cambridge University Press.

Ryan, R. M., Connell, J. P., & Deci, E. L., (1985). A motivational analysis of self-determination and self-regulation. In C. Ames & R. Ames (Eds.), *Research on motivation in the classroom: Vol. 2. The classroom milieu* (pp. 13–51). Orlando, FL: Academic Press.

Ryan, R. M., & Deci, E. L. (2000). Self-determination theory and the facilitation of intrinsic motivation, social development, and well-being. *American Psychologist, 55,* 68–78.

Ryan, R. M., Deci, E. L., & Grolnick, W. S. (1995). Autonomy, relatedness, and the self: Their relationship to development and psychopathology. In D. Cicchetti & D.J. Cohen (Eds.), *Developmental Psychopathology: Vol. 1, Theory and methods* (pp. 618–655). New York: Wiley.

Ryan, R., & Grolnick, W. (1986). Origins and pawns in the classroom: Self-report and projective assessments of individual differences in children's perceptions. *Journal of Personality and Social Psychology, 50,* 350–358.

Sarason, S., Davidson, K., Lighthall, F., Waite, R., & Ruebusch, B. (1960). *Anxiety in elementary school children.* New York: Wiley.

Savell, J. M., Twohig, P. T., & Rachford, D. L. (1986). Empirical status of Feuerstein's "Instrumental Enrichment" (FIE) technique as a method of teaching thinking skills. *Review of Educational Research, 56*(4), 381–409.

Schultz, G. F., & Switzky, H. N. (1990). The development of intrinsic motivation in students with learning problems. *Preventing School Failure, 34,* 14–20.

Schultz, G. F., & Switzky, H. N. (1993). The academic achievement of elementary and junior high school students with behavior disorders and their nonhandicapped peers as a function of motivational orientation. *Learning & Individual Differences, 5,* 31–42.

Schunk, D. H. (1989a). Self-efficacy and cognitive skill learning. In C. Ames & R. Ames (Eds.), *Research on motivation in education: Vol. 3. Goals and cognitions* (pp. 13–44). San Diego: Academic Press.

Schunk, D. H. (1989b). Social cognitive theory and self-regulated learning. In B. J. Zimmerman & D. H. Schunk (Eds.), *Self-regulated learning and academic achievement* (pp. 83–119). New York: Springer-Verlag.

Schunk, D. H. (1990). Goal setting and self-efficacy during self-regulated learning. *Educational Psychologist, 25*(1), 71–86.

Schunk, D. H. (1991). Self-efficacy and academic achievement. *Educational Psychologist, 16*(3 & 4), 207–231.

Schunk, D. H. (1994). Self-regulation of self-efficacy and attributions in academic settings. In D. H. Schunk & B. J. Zimmermann (Eds.), *Self-regulation of learning and performance: Issues and educational applications* (pp. 75–99). Hillsdale, NJ: Lawrence Erlbaum Associates.

Schunk, D. H., & Ertmer, P. A. (2000). Self-regulation and academic learning: Self-efficacy enhancing interventions. In M. Boekaerts, P. R. Pintrich, & M. Zeidner (Eds.), *Handbook of self-regulation* (pp. 631–649). San Diego, CA: Academic Press.

Schwarz, R. H., & Jens, K. G. (1969). The expectation of success as it modifies the achievement of mentally retarded adolescents. *American Journal of Mental Deficiency, 73,* 946–949.

Sewell, T. W., & Price, V. D. (1991). Mediated learning experience: Implications for achievement motivation and cognitive performance in low socio-economic and minority children. In R. Feuerstein, P. S. Klein, & A. J. Tannenbaum (Eds.), *Mediated learning experience (MLE): Theoretical, psychosocial and learning implications* (pp. 295–314). London: Freund.

Silon, E. L., & Harter, S. (1985). Assessment of perceived competence, motivational orientation, and anxiety in segregated and main-streamed educable mentally retarded children. *Journal of Educational Psychology, 77,* 217–230.

Skinner, E. A. (1995). *Perceived control, motivation, & coping.* Thousand Oaks, CA: Sage Publications.

Snygg, D., & Combs, A. V. (1949). *Individual behavior: A new frame of reference for psychology.* New York: Harper.

Sonnenschein, J. L. (1983). *Basic Achievement Skills Individual Screener.* Cleveland: The Psychological Corporation.

Spielberger, C. (1972). Anxiety as an emotional state. In C. Spielberger (Ed.), *Anxiety: Current trends in theory and research* (Vol. 1, pp. 23–49). New York: Academic Press.

Sternberg, R. J. (1985). *Beyond IQ: A triarchic theory of human intelligence.* Cambridge: Cambridge University Press.

Sternberg, R. J., & Berg, C. A. (Eds.), (1992). *Intellectual development.* New York: Cambridge University Press.

Stevenson, H. W., & Zigler, E. (1958). Probability learning in children. *Journal of Experimental Psychology, 56,* 185–192.

Stipek, D. J. (1984). The development of achievement motivation. In R. Ames & C. Ames (Eds.), *Research on motivation in education: Vol. 1, Student motivation* (pp. 145–174). Orlando, FL: Academic Press.

Stipek, D. J. (1998). *Motivation to learn* (3rd ed.), Boston: Allyn and Bacon.

Switzky, H. N. (1985). Self-reinforcement schedules in young children: A preliminary investigation of the effects of motivational orientation and instructional demands. *Reflections of Learning Research, 1,* 3–18.

Switzky, H. N. (1995). The changing role of psychologists: The influence of paradigm shifts and their implications for clinical practice, service, and research in the area of mental retardation and developmental disabilities. In O. Karen & S. Greenspan (Eds.), *Community rehabilitation services for people with disabilities* (pp. 399–419). Newton, MA: Butterworth and Heinemann.

Switzky, H. N. (1996). Issues in the developmental approach to mental retardation [Review of the book *Issues in the developmental approach to mental retardation*]. *American Journal on Mental Retardation, 100,* 428–430.

Switzky, H. N. (1997). Individual differences in personality and motivational systems in persons with mental retardation. In W. E. MacLean, Jr. (Ed.), *Ellis' handbook of mental deficiency, psychological theory and research* (3rd ed., pp. 343–377). Hillsdale, NJ: Lawrence Erlbaum Associates.

Switzky, H. N. (1999). Intrinsic motivation and motivational self-system processes in persons with mental retardation. In E. Zigler & D. Bennett-Gates (Eds.), *Personality development in individuals with mental retardation* (pp. 70–106). New York: Cambridge University Press.

Switzky, H. N. (in press). The cognitive-motivational perspective on mental retardation. In H. N. Switzky & S. Greenspan (Eds.), *What is mental retardation: Ideas for an evolving disability.* Washington, DC: AAMR Press.

Switzky, H. N., & Hanks, R. S. (1973, May). *Some possible predictors of vocational success among mentally retarded and physically handicapped sheltered workshop trainees.* Paper read at the annual meeting of the American Association on Mental Deficiency, Washington, D.C.

Switzky, H. N., & Haywood, H. C. (1974). Motivational orientation and the relative efficacy of self-monitored and externally imposed reinforcement schedules. *Journal of Personality and Social Psychology, 30,* 360–366.

Switzky, H. N., & Haywood, H. C. (1984). Bio-social ecological perspectives on mental retardation. In N. S. Endler & J. McV. Hunt (Eds.),

Personality and the behavior disorders (2nd ed., Vol. 2, pp. 851–896). New York: Wiley.

Switzky, H. N., & Haywood, H. C. (1991). Self-reinforcement schedules in persons with mild mental retardation: Effects of motivational orientation and instructional demands. *Journal of Mental Deficiency Research, 35,* 221–230.

Switzky, H. N., & Haywood, H. C. (1992). Self-reinforcement schedules in young children: Effects of motivational orientation and instructional demands. *Learning & Individual Differences, 4,* 59–71.

Switzky, H. N., Haywood, H. C., & Isett, R. (1974). Exploration, curiosity, and play in young children: Effects of stimulus complexity. *Developmental Psychology, 10,* 321–329.

Switzky, H. N., & Heal, L. (1990). Research methods in special education. In R. Gaylord-Ross (Ed.), *Issues and research in special education* (Vol. 1., pp. 1–81). New York: Teachers College Press.

Switzky, H. N., Ludwig, L., & Haywood, H. C. (1979). Exploration, curiosity, and play in young children: Effects of object complexity and age. *American Journal of Mental Deficiency, 86,* 637–646.

Switzky, H. N., & Schultz, G. F. (1988). Intrinsic motivation and learning performance implications for individual educational programming for the mildly handicapped. *Remedial & Special Education, 9,* 7–14.

Tannenbaum, A. J. (1991). Unmasking and unmaking achievement among the gifted. In R. Feuerstein, P. S. Klein, & A. J. Tannenbaum (Eds.), *Mediated learning experience (MLE): Theoretical, psychosocial and learning implications* (pp. 315–346). London: Freund.

Thoman, E. B. (1992). A mediated learning experience for very youngest: Premature infants. *International Journal of Cognitive Education & Mediated Learning, 2*(2), 117–129.

Tzuriel, D. (1991). Cognitive modifiability, mediated learning experience and affective motivational processes: A transactional approach. In R. Feuerstein, P. S. Klein, & A. J. Tannenbaum (Eds.), *Mediated learning experience (MLE): Theoretical, psychosocial and learning implications* (pp. 95–120). London: Freund.

Tzuriel, D., & Haywood, H. C. (1992). The development of interactive-dynamic approaches to assessment of learning potential. In H. C. Haywood & D. Tzuriel (Eds.), *Interactive assessment* (pp. 3–37). New York: Springer-Verlag.

Tzuriel, D., & Klein, P. S. (1985). Analogical thinking modifiability is disadvantaged, regular, special education, and mentally retarded children. *Journal of Abnormal Child Psychology, 13,* 539–552.

Utman, C. H. (1997). Performance effects of motivational states: A meta-analysis. *Personality and Social Psychological Review, 1,* 170–182.

Wehmeyer, M. L., Agran, M., & Hughes, C. (1998). *Teaching self-determination to students with disabilities.* Baltimore: Brookes.

Weiner, B. (1986). *An attributional theory of motivation and emotion.* New York: Springer-Verlag.

Weiner, B. (1990). History of motivational research in education. *Journal of Educational Psychology, 82,* 616–622.

Weiner, B. (1994). Integrating social and personal theories of achievement strivings. *Review of Educational Research, 64,* 557–573.

Weisz, J. R. (1999). Cognitive performance and learned helplessness in mentally retarded persons. In E. Zigler & D. Bennett-Gates (Eds.), *Personality development in individuals with mental retardation* (pp. 17–46). New York: Cambridge University Press.

White, R. H. (1959). Motivation reconsidered: The concept of competence. *Psychological Review, 66,* 297–333.

Woodcock, R. W., & Johnson, M. B. (1989). *Woodcock-Johnson psycho-educational battery: Revised.* Allen, TX: DLM Teaching Resources.

Wooldridge, R. (1966). *Motivation-hygiene orientation and school achievement in mentally subnormal children.* Unpublished EdS Study, George Peabody College, Nashville, TN.

Yerkes, R. M., & Dodson, J. O. (1908). The relation of strength of stimulus to rapidity of habit formation. *Journal of Comparative Neurology and Psychology, 18,* 459–482.

Yussen, S., & Kane, P. (1985). Children's conception of intelligence. In S. R. Yussen (Ed.), *The growth of reflection in children* (pp. 207–241). Orlando, FL: Academic Press.

Zeidner, M. (1995). Personality correlates of intelligence. In D. H. Saklofske & M. Zeidner (Eds.), *International handbook of personality and intelligence* (pp. 299–319). New York: Plenum.

Zewdie, A. (1995). *Work performances of afro-american adults with mild and moderate mental retardation to self versus external regulation as a function of intrinsic versus extrinsic motivation.* Unpublished doctoral dissertation, Northern Illinois University, Dekalb.

Zigler, E. (1961). Social deprivation and rigidity in the performance of feebleminded children. *Journal of Abnormal and Social Psychology, 62,* 413–421.

Zigler, E. (1966a). Mental retardation: Current issues and approaches. In L. W. Hoffman & M. L. Hoffman (Eds.), *Review of child development research* (Vol. 2, pp. 107–168). New York: Russell Sage.

Zigler, E. (1966b). Research on personality structure in the retardate. In N. R. Ellis (Ed.), *International review of research in mental retardation* (Vol. 1, pp. 77–108). New York: Academic Press.

Zigler, E., & Balla, D. (1981). Issues in personality and motivation in mentally retarded persons. In M. J. Begab, H. C. Haywood, & H. L. Garber (Eds.), *Psychosocial influences in retarded performance* (Vol. 1, pp. 197–218). Baltimore, MD: University Park Press.

Zigler, E., & Balla, D. (Eds.). (1982). *Mental retardation: The developmental-difference controversy.* Hillsdale, NJ: Lawrence Erlbaum Associates.

Zigler, E., Balla, D., & Watson, N. (1972). Developmental and experiential determinants of self-image disparity in institutionalized and non-institutionalized retarded and normal children. *Journal of Personality and Social Psychology, 23,* 81–87.

Zigler, E., & Bennett-Gates, D. (1999). (Eds.), *Personality development in individuals with mental retardation.* New York: Cambridge University Press.

Zigler, E., Butterfield, E. C., & Goff, G. A. (1966). A measure of preinstitutional social deprivation for institutionalized retardates. *American Journal of Mental Deficiency, 70,* 873–885.

Zigler, E., & Glick, M. (1986). *A developmental approach to adult psychopathology.* New York: Wiley.

Zigler, E., & Hodapp, R. M. (1991). Behavioral functioning in individuals with mental retardation. *Annual Review of Psychology, 42,* 29–50.

Zimmerman, B. J. (2000). Attaining self-regulation: A social cognitive perspective. In M. Boekaerts, P. R. Pintrich, & M. Zeidner (Eds.), *Handbook of self-regulation* (pp. 13–39). San Diego, CA: Academic Press.

Zimmerman, B. J., & Schunk, D. H. (Eds.). (1989). *Self-regulated learning and academic achievement.* New York: Springer-Verlag.

Zoeller, C., Mahoney, G., & Weiner, B. (1983). Effects of attribution training on the assembly task performance of mentally retarded adults. *American Journal of Mental Deficiency, 88,* 109–112.

Part II

New Directions

3

Self-Determination and Mental Retardation: Assembling the Puzzle Pieces

Michael L. Wehmeyer

The University of Kansas

INTRODUCTION

Since 1990, my colleagues and I have conducted research and model demonstration projects to define, examine, and promote self-determination for people with mental retardation. Our research began at the end of an eventful era in the emergence of theories of personality as they relate to people with mental retardation. Switzky (1997) observed the following:

> Over the past 30 years there has been a veritable explosion of research on persons with mental retardation that has described the complex interplay of personality and motivational processes within a developmental perspective. This new conceptualization of mental retardation is consistent with mainstream psychological thought concerning the development of human beings as active problem solvers and reflects the accelerating integration of a psychology of mental retardation and a developmental psychology of human growth for all human beings. (p. 343)

Switzky also noted that conceptions of personality and motivational processes in persons with mental retardation prior to the 1960s:

> were only loosely related to theoretical models derived from mainstream psychological thought, and virtually none of the available knowledge was based on any sustained systematic study of mentally retarded persons. Researchers were concerned primarily with identifying the cognitive deficits that characterized persons with mental retardation. (p. 343)

Merighi, Edison, and Zigler (1990) noted this focus placed inordinate emphasis on the construct of intelligence and its role in the lives of people with mental retardation. Despite evidence that personality and motivational aspects were equally important to positive outcomes for people with mental retardation, "there remained a tendency to overemphasize the importance of intellect in the adjustment of retarded persons" (Merighi et al., 1990, p. 124). These authors concluded "more work is needed on the relationship between IQ, personality-motivation, and life success (Merighi et al., 1990, p. 128).

Progress in the fields of education, psychology, and rehabilitation have provided anecdotal evidence that IQ and life success are not as strongly correlated as previously presumed and have spurred a de-emphasis on the primacy of intelligence as a determinant of positive outcomes for people with mental retardation. For example, the supported employment movement of the 1980s (Wehman & Moon, 1988) provided supports and accommodations that enabled people with severe and profound mental retardation to work in competitive employment settings. In addition, advances in assistive technology have enabled more people with significant disabilities to participate in their community, while the passage of legislative and civil protections affording equal opportunity and protection have ensured access to these communities. These changes have emphasized the fact that people with mental retardation, like other human beings, live and must function in a world that demands active problem-solving and goal driven, task-attainment oriented behavior and have the right to express preferences, make choices, and participate in decisions that impact their lives. This, in turn, has brought to the forefront the importance of self-determination in the lives of people with mental retardation, indeed people with disabilities in general, and emphasized the need to understand better how to achieve the outcome that people with mental retardation become self-determined individuals.

Assembling the Puzzle Pieces

In their widely used introductory text on theories of personality, Hall and Lindzey (1957) made the following observations about personality theories and theorists:

1. Personality theories are functional in their orientation. They are concerned with questions that make a difference in the adjustment of the organism (p. 4).
2. Personality theorists have customarily assigned a crucial role to the motivational process (p. 5).
3. Related to this interest in the functional and motivational is the personality theorist's conviction that an adequate understanding of human behavior will evolve only from the study of the whole person (see Zigler, chap. 1). Most personality psychologists insisted that the subject should be viewed from the vantage of the entire functioning person in his or her natural habitat. They pleaded strongly for the study of behavior in context, with each behavioral event examined and interpreted in relation to the rest of the individual's behavior (p. 6).

Hall and Lindzey concluded that as a consequence of these factors:

One of the most distinctive features of personality theory is its function as an *integrative theory*. While psychologists in general have shown increased specialization, leading to the complaint that they were learning more and more about less and less, the *personality theorist accepted at least partial responsibility for bringing together and organizing the diverse findings of specialists* [italics added]. The personality psychologist was, in this sense, more concerned with reconstruction or integration than he was with analysis or the segmental study of behavior. From these considerations comes the somewhat romantic conception of the personality theorist as the individual who will put together the jigsaw puzzle provided by the discrete findings of the separate studies within the various specialties that make up psychology. (pp. 6–7)

While one can certainly argue that in the more than 40 years since the publication of this text the field of personality psychology has matured and expanded to such a degree that theories in this area are not accurately characterized by the assemblage of parts identified by other theorists and that theorists working in this area have, like much of the rest of psychology, moved toward increased specialization. However, despite the fact that their description of personality theories and theorists is dated, there remains an important role for the type of theoretical activities described by Hall and Lindzey. That is, there is heuristic and practical value to theoretical activities that assemble the jigsaw puzzle pieces of more specialized research and theory development in order to explain human behavior and, primarily, provide impetus for practice. This chapter describes just such an effort.

THEORETICAL CONCEPTUALIZATIONS
OF SELF-DETERMINATION

At the end of the 1980s, when the call for self-determination for individuals with disabilities was first sounded, the term had two primary conceptualizations, both having some shared meaning, but addressing very different issues and purposes.

The first of these conceptualizations, and the earliest use of the term self-determination, referred to the right of nations and peoples to self-governance. In his examination of national self-determination, Heater (1994) attributed much of the notoriety for self-determination, and its relative importance in 20th century politics, to Woodrow Wilson's famous "Fourteen Points" speech to a joint session of Congress on January 8, 1918. In this speech, Wilson outlined 14 points for a postwar settlement that would lead to world peace. Six of the 14 points referred specifically to ensuring that nations who were defeated in the war would be ensured the opportunity for national self-determination. Heater noted that the 20th century preference for national self-determination emerged from twin 18th century notions that the people, not monarchs, are sovereign and that the people are to be thought of as "the nation." Throughout the 19th century, the belief that a people should have the right and opportunity to determine their own government spread and gained wide acceptance, and by the 20th century it had become a principal of international justice.

Self-Determination as a Personal Construct

The second use of the term self-determination was as a personal construct, referring not to the right of a nation or peoples to self-governance, but to the right and capacity of people to self-govern their lives. For much of the past half century, a guiding principle of social work has been the client's right to self-determination (Biestek & Gehrig, 1978; McDermott, 1975). Owing much to the sense of the term as a national or political right, the emphasis in social work on client self-determination became a principle that guided the way in which services should be provided by social workers. More than just a right of people in general, however, the use of the construct in social work embodies a respect and value for the rights of individuals to make choices and decisions and to, in essence, live autonomous lives.

The construct as a personal trait, disposition or characteristic has been most extensively explored, however, in the field of psychology, and specifically within theories of personality and, later, motivation. The earliest conceptualizations of self-determination within the personality literature used the term as it related to the determination of one's own fate or course of action without compulsion. For example, in his early text titled *Foundations for a science of personality*, Angyal (1941) proposed that an essential feature of a living organism is its autonomy, where autonomous means self-governing or governed from inside. According to Angyal (1941), an organism "lives in a world in which things happen according to laws which are heteronomous (e.g., governed from outside) from the point of view of the organism" (p. 33). Angyal stated that "organisms are subjected to the laws of the physical world, as is any other object of nature, with the exception that it can oppose self-determination to external determination" (p. 33). Angyal exhibited the trademark characteristic of a personality theorist, stating that "one has to study life as a dynamic whole" (p. 21). He suggested that the important task for developing a science of personality was the identification of principle(s) of the *biological total process*—the movement of organisms from undifferentiated parts to an organized whole. Angyal typified an organismic-developmental orientation in which the assumption, later termed the orthogenetic principle (Werner and Kaplan, 1965), was that "organisms are naturally directed towards a series of transformations reflecting a tendency to move from a state of relative globality and undifferentiatedness towards states of increasing differentiation and hierarchic organization" (p. 7).

Ultimately, Angyal (1941) defined the biological total process as a trend toward autonomy and argued that the science of personality is, in essence, the study of two essential components or determinants to behavior, autonomous determination (or self-determination) and heteronomous determination (other-determined). He noted that "in the realm of 'organismic happenings' we find neither entirely autonomous nor entirely heteronomous determinants" (p. 21) and suggested a psychology of individual differences by noting that, within nature, there are marked variations in the importance and balance of autonomous and heteronomous determinants to behavior. Nonetheless, Angyal (1941) placed primary importance for laying the foundation for a science of personality in the fact that a central process of an organism is the movement toward autonomous determination. He showed this by stating:

> It would probably be generally agreed that without autonomy, without self-government, the life process could not be understood. Selection, choice, self-regulation, adaptation, regeneration are phenomena which logically imply the autonomy of the organism. Selection, that is the search for certain environmental conditions, is only possible in a being capable of self-directed activity. (p. 34)

It is worthy to note one other corollary of Angyal's (1941) thesis of the centrality of self-determination to personality study; that is, behavior is neither exclusively internally nor externally determined. He noted:

> the autonomy of the organism is not an absolute one. Self-determination is restricted by outside influences which, with respect to the organism, are heteronomous. The organism

lives in a world in which processes go on independent of it. The organism asserts itself against the heteronomous surroundings. (p. 38) Among the first uses of the term in the mental retardation literature was in a chapter by Nirje (1972), in Wolfensberger's (1972) classic text on the principle of normalization. Nirje (1972) titled his chapter "The Right to Self-Determination" and in the opening paragraph stated the following:

One major facet of the normalization principle is to create conditions through which a handicapped person experiences the normal respect to which any human being is entitled. Thus the choices, wishes, desires, and aspirations of a handicapped person have to be taken into consideration as much as possible in actions affecting him. To assert oneself with one's family, friends, neighbors, co-workers, other people, or vis-à-vis an agency is difficult for many persons. It is especially difficult for someone who has a disability or is otherwise perceived as devalued. But in the end, even the impaired person has to manage as a distinct individual, and thus has his identity defined to himself and to others through the circumstances and conditions of his existence. Thus, the road to self-determination is both difficult and all important for a person who is impaired. (p. 177)

Nirje's use of the term suggests, at the least, familiarity with self-determination as a personality construct and resembles the use of the construct within the field of social work. His use of the term, while still pertaining to the rights of a particular group of people (e.g., people with mental retardation), is nonetheless a call for individual or personal self-determination or self-governance. Nirje (1972) identified making choices, asserting oneself, self-management, self-knowledge, decision making, self-advocacy, self-efficacy, self-regulation, autonomy, and independence (although often not using those terms) as the salient features of this individual or personal self-determination. His is a call for a wide range of actions that enable people to control their lives and their destinies.

Historically, then, self-determination refers fundamentally to self-governance. Theories of personal self-determination are, in essence, theories of how or why people become self-governing and exert control over their lives. With a few exceptions, the bulk of the theoretical work in this area has not used the term self-determination, per se, but instead focused on components that contribute to self-determination, including human control and causality, self-efficacy and outcome expectations, self-regulation, achievement, effectance and mastery motivation, interpersonal cognitive problem solving, goal setting and attainment, and so forth. The theories that explain and predict human behavior in these diverse areas include personality and motivation theories and theories of learning and cognition, and emerged from numerous disciplines, including (in addition to personality psychology), cognitive, developmental, social, experimental, and community psychology. These varied theoretical perspectives provide the pieces to the jigsaw puzzle of promoting self-determination for individuals with disabilities.

Deci's Self-Determination Theory

One theoretical perspective that addressed self-determination specifically is the work of Edward Deci and his colleagues (Deci & Ryan, 1985). Deci and his colleagues built on earlier conceptualizations of self-determination forwarded by Angyal (1941) and others, to propose a theory of intrinsic motivation that incorporates a central role for self-determination. Based largely on White's (1959) classic proposal of an innate, intrinsic energy source, referred to by White as effectance motivation and which was theorized to motivate a wide variety of human behavior, and also building on work by cognitive theorists on personal causation and perceived locus of causality (deCharms, 1968; Heider, 1958), Deci (Deci, 1975; Deci & Ryan, 1985), proposed that intrinsic motivation and self-determination were "necessary concepts for an organismic theory" [of motivation] (Deci & Ryan, p. 7). In 1975, Deci forwarded a theory to explain empirical findings concerning the effects of external events on intrinsic motivation. This theory, called cognitive evaluation theory (Deci, 1975), contained three primary propositions: (1) people have an intrinsic need to be self-determining; (2) people have an intrinsic need to be competent and to master optimal challenges; and (3) events relevant to the initiation and regulation of behavior have three aspects (informational, controlling, and amotivating) that are differentially salient to different people (Deci & Ryan, 1985, p. 62). Deci and his colleagues (Deci & Ryan, 1985) later expanded their original conceptualization and this expanded theory is called self-determination theory. Briefly, Deci (1992) summarized self-determination theory as:

> distinguish[ing] between the motivational dynamics underlying activities that people do freely and those that they feel coerced or pressured to do. To be self-determining means to engage in an activity with a full sense of wanting, choosing, and personal endorsement. When self-determined, people are acting in accord with, or expressing, themselves. (p. 44)

Within self-determination theory, Deci and Ryan define self-determination as:

> the capacity to choose and to have those choices, rather than reinforcement contingencies, drives, or any other forces or pressures, to be the determinants of one's actions. But self-determination is *more than a capacity, it is also a need* [italics added]. We have posited a basic, innate propensity to be self-determining that leads organisms to engage in interesting behaviors. (p. 38)

Self-Determination as Empowerment

Prior to detailing our theoretical perspective of self-determination, it is important to consider one more meaning or intent to the term as used in the disability field. Inherent in the initial attention to the topic of self-determination as it pertained to people with disabilities was its association, primarily by disability advocates and policymakers, with empowerment. In a speech at the National Conference on Self-Determination, an event organized in 1989 by the U.S. Department of Education's Office of Special Education Programs (Ward, 1996), Robert Williams (1989) effectively captured this link between self-determination and empowerment, stating:

> But, without being afforded the right and opportunity to make choices in our lives, we will never obtain full, first class

American citizenship. So we do not have to be told what self-determination means. We already know that it is just another word for freedom. We already know that self-determination is just another word for describing a life filled with rising expectations, dignity, responsibility, and opportunity. That it is just another word for having the chance to live the American Dream. (p. 16)

It is evident from Williams' remarks, and from the comments of other people with disabilities, that for many people in the disability community the use of the term is as a call for the right to personal self-governance, more related, perhaps, to the meaning of the term as the right of a nation to self-governance than as a motivational or personality construct. Like Nirje's call from 20 years earlier, however, the use of the term as a right mixes the meaning of the term as both a national right and a personal entity.

A FUNCTIONAL MODEL OF SELF-DETERMINATION

It is within this smorgasbord of meaning and intent that we began our work in the area of self-determination. From the onset, we viewed this effort much as that described by Hall and Lindzey (1957); our intent was to draw on the theoretical foundations laid by researchers from a wide range of psychological disciplines that had explored the topic of personal control and causation, though mainly from the realm of personality, social, and developmental psychology, in order to construct a theory of self-determination that would explain and help promote self-determination for individuals with mental retardation. This is not a theory of self-determination specific only to mental retardation, a developmental psychopathology of self-determination as it were, but a theory of self-determination that views people with mental retardation as actors in their own lives, just as people without disabilities are actors in their own lives. Although largely untested with individuals without disabilities, we approached the definitional and theoretical development activities from the perspective of explaining human behavior, not just the behavior of people with mental retardation.

Deci's self-determination theory (Deci & Ryan, 1985) is a theory of motivation in that it posits that people engage in behaviors that are interesting, make choices, and express preferences because of an innate need of the human organism for competence and self-determination. Our work was not explicitly conducted to address the "why" of behavior, and thus is not a motivation theory, as is Deci's, but is instead a personality theory, both in its focus (e.g., concerned with function of the individual in the natural context; see Hall and Lindzey (1957) and in the nature of its construction. There is, however, some implicit proposal of motivational aspects based upon the various theoretical perspectives from which we have selected the puzzle pieces. The following section describes self-determination as a dispositional characteristic of individuals, the empirical examination of that theoretical framework with people with mental retardation, and examines a model of the development of self-determination based on this theoretical framework.

Defining Self-Determination

Self-determination has been defined in a number of ways in the disability literature, particularly: (a) as a basic human right, (b) as a specific response class, and (c) as based on functional properties of the response class. Self-determination as a basic human right was discussed previously, and while it has utility for advocacy and policy efforts, such a conceptualization has limited utility, if any, for explaining and predicting human behavior. Attempts to describe self-determination strictly as a specific response class, (e.g., as a set of behaviors), although potentially more useful for explaining behavior, have not been successful in actually defining the construct. It is quite easy to describe what self-determined people do. For example, Martin and Marshall (1995) summarized the evolving definition of self-determination in the special education literature as describing individuals who:

> know how to choose—they know what they want and how to get it. From an awareness of personal needs, self-determined individuals choose goals, then doggedly pursue them. This involves asserting an individual's presence, making his or her needs known, evaluating progress toward meeting goals,

adjusting performance and creating unique approaches to solve problems. (p. 147)

However, although infinitely simpler, defining self-determination by a response class (e.g., by a set of behaviors or actions) is problematic because virtually any behavior can be construed as exerting control over one's life and both the occurrence and the nonoccurrence of a behavior can be self-determined behavior (Wehmeyer, 1996b). The first point has a parallel in defining, for example, stereotyped or self-stimulatory behaviors exhibited by some people with mental retardation. Virtually any motor behavior can be exhibited in a stereotyped manner, and thus stereotyped behavior cannot be defined by a specific response class (rocking behavior, hand flapping, etc.). This is equally true for self-determination and self-determined behavior. Almost any human action or behavior can be exhibited as a means to exert control over one's life.

This leads to the second point, that defining self-determination by a set of behaviors is impossible because that list will eventually have to include behaviors that, definitionally, are mutually exclusive. For example, there are many times when assertively speaking up for oneself and for one's rights is a necessary act and can be identified as a self-determined behavior. On the other hand, there are times when not speaking up for one's own rights might, in fact, also be an expression of self-determined behavior if the person decides that the most effective course of action might be to remain quiet. A third problem with defining self-determination by a response class is that this leads to a tautology (e.g., we know that self-determination is such and such behaviors because self-determined people exhibit those behaviors).

It becomes necessary, therefore, to define self-determination according to the function of a response class, or, more simply, by the function of the person's actions or behaviors. Wehmeyer (1996a) defined self-determination as "acting as the primary causal agent in one's life and making choices and decisions regarding one's quality of life free from undue external influence or interference" (p. 24). Self-determined behavior refers to actions that are identified by four essential characteristics: (a) The person acted autonomously; (b) the behavior(s) are self-regulated; (c) the person initiated and responded to the event(s) in a psychologically empowered manner; and (d) the person acted in a self-realizing manner. People who consistently engage in self-determined behaviors can be described as self-determined, where self-determined refers to a dispositional characteristic. *Dispositional characteristics* involve the organization of cognitive, psychological, and physiological elements in such a manner that an individual's behavior in different situations will be similar (though not identical). Eder (1990) described dispositional states as frequent, enduring tendencies that are used to characterize people and are used to describe important differences between people. As such, people are self-determined based on the functional characteristics of their actions or behaviors.

The concept of causal agency is central to this definition and our theoretical perspective. Broadly defined, *causal agency* implies that it is the individual who makes or causes things to happen in his or her life. However, since one's physical presence or the exhibition of behaviors which are exclusively autonomic can likewise result in changes in the person's immediate environment, it is necessary to go beyond simply the effect of the individual on the environment to examine issues of intent to imply agency. An agent is a person or thing through which power is exerted or an end is achieved. Causal agency, as opposed to implying strictly that the individual caused something to happen, implies that the action was purposeful or performed to achieve an end.

Bandura (1997) addresses these issues when describing the nature of human agency. He stated:

> people can exercise influence over what they do. Most human behavior, of course, is determined by many interacting factors, and so people are contributors to, rather than the sole determiners of, what happens to them. In evaluating the role of intentionality in human agency, one must distinguish between the personal production of action for an intended outcome, and the effects that carrying out that course of action actually produce. Agency refers to acts done intentionally. (p. 3)

A *causal agent* is, then, someone who makes or causes things to happen in his or her life. Self-determined people act as the causal agent in their lives. They act with intent to shape their futures and their destiny.

We have opted to frame causal agency within the concept of quality of life. Quality of life is a complex construct which has gained increasing importance as a principle in human services. Schalock (1996) suggested that quality of life is best viewed as an organizing concept to guide policy and practice to improve the life conditions of all people. He proposed eight core dimensions of quality of life: emotional well-being, interpersonal relations, material well-being, personal development, physical well-being, self-determination, social inclusion, and rights. Schalock emphasized that quality of life is composed of the same factors for and is important to all people (independent of disability status), is experienced when a person's basic needs are met, and is enhanced by integration and by enabling individuals to participate in decisions that impact their lives.

Third, we have suggested that self-determination means acting as a causal agent without undue interference and influence. As Angyal (1941) noted, human beings are not completely autonomous or independent but are *interdependent*; our lives intermingle with the lives of many others, seen and unseen. For all people, choices are frequently constrained and rarely represent optimal options. We are dependent upon numerous others in our decisions, from close relatives and spouses to medical professionals or financial advisors. Our plans are interfered with by the plans or actions of others, sometimes to our benefit! In short, self-determination does not reflect an absence of influence or even interference. Instead, it reflects choices and decisions made without undue interference or influence. The term *undue* remains intentionally subjective and contextual as what may be perceived by one individual to be an acceptable level of influence may appear to another as an unacceptable level of interference. This varies both between individuals and between cultures.

From this framework, my colleagues and I described the development of component elements of self-determined behavior in order to design instructional activities for students across their school career (Wehmeyer, 1997; Wehmeyer, Sands, Doll, & Palmer, 1997). We also suggested a model (depicted in Fig. 3.1) in which three primary factors impact the emergence of self-determination: (a) individual capacity, as influenced by learning and

FIG. 3.1.   *Functional model of self-determination.*

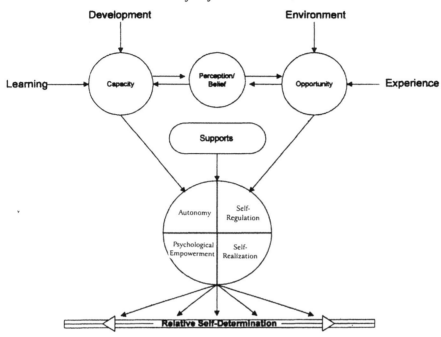

development; (b) opportunity, as influenced by environments and experiences; and (c) supports and accommodations.

Napoleon Bonaparte is reported to have said that ability is of little account without opportunity, and while much of our work focused on enhancing the capacity of individuals with disabilities, we recognize the important role of opportunity in this process. The environments in which people live and work influence the way supports are provided and have an impact on the opportunities many people with mental retardation have to experience and enhance their self-determination and improve their quality of life, as well as prescribe, to a certain extent, the degree to which personalized, independent supports can be provided.

Recently, for example, Wehmeyer and Bolding (1999) conducted a study in which research participants matched by age, level of intelligence, and gender but who worked or lived in one of three environments (community-based independent, community-based congregate, non-community-based congregate). Individuals who lived or worked in congregate settings, either community based (group homes, sheltered workshops) or non-community-based (institutions, day activity programs, nursing homes) were significantly less self-determined than peers (again, matched by IQ, age, and gender) who were supported in their community (worked competitively or in a supported employment, lived on one's own or with spouse or peer). In this case, the working or living environments did not provide adequate opportunities for individuals to make choices, experience options, and so forth.

Essential Characteristics of Self-Determined Behavior

People who are self-determined act autonomously, self-regulate their behavior, and are psychologically empowered and self-realizing. The term essential characteristic implies that an individual's actions must reflect, to some degree, each of these four characteristics. Age, opportunity, capacity and circumstances may impact the degree to which any of the essential characteristics are present and, as such, the relative self-determination expressed by an individual will likely vary, sometimes over time and other times across environments. Nonetheless, these essential elements need to be present—each characteristic is a necessary but not sufficient characteristic of self-determined behavior.

Behavioral Autonomy. Our use of the term autonomy and its subsequent use within the theoretical framework draws from two primary sources: (a) autonomy as synonymous with individuation from the developmental psychology literature, and (b) functional or behavioral autonomy as roughly synonymous with independence, drawn primarily from the disability-intervention literature. Developmental psychologists view the process of individuation, the formation of the person's individual identity (Damon, 1983), as a critical component of social and personality development. Sigafoos, Feinstein, Damond, and Reiss (1988) defined individuation as "a progression from dependence on others for care and guidance to self-care and self-direction" (p. 432), the outcome of which is autonomous functioning or, when describing the actions of individuals achieving this outcome, behavioral autonomy. Behavioral autonomy, therefore, is the outcome of the process of individuation, and encompasses, fundamentally, actions in which people act (a) according to their own preferences, interests and/or abilities; and (b) independently, free from undue external influence or interference. Sigafoos et al. (1988) identified four behavioral categories contributing to autonomous functioning: (a) self- or family-care activities; (b) management activities; (c) recreational or leisure activities; and (d) social or vocational activities. Self- or family-care activities include routine personal care and family-oriented functions such as meal preparation, care of possessions, performing household chores, shopping, home repairs, and other activities of daily living. Management activities refer to the degree to which a person independently handles interactions with the environment. These activities involve the use of community resources and the fulfillment of personal obligations and responsibilities. Recreational activities reflecting behavioral autonomy are not specific actions, but the degree to which an individual uses personal preferences and interests to choose to engage in such activities. Likewise, social and vocational activities include social involvement, vocational activities, and the degree to which personal preference and interests are applied in these areas.

Self-Regulated Behavior. Self-regulation is critical to self-governance, and people who are self-determined self-regulate their behaviors. Whitman (1990) defined self-regulation as:

> a complex response system that enables individuals to examine their environments and their repertoires of responses for coping with those environments to make decisions about how to act, to act, to evaluate the desirability of the outcomes of the action, and to revise their plans as necessary. (p. 373)

Self-regulated behaviors include the use of self-management strategies (including self-monitoring, self-instruction, self-evaluation, and self-reinforcement), goal setting and attainment behaviors, problem-solving and decision-making behaviors, and observational learning strategies (Agran, 1997).

Psychological Empowerment. While self-determination is presented in this theoretical framework as a dispositional characteristic where functional characteristics of a person's actions define his or her relative self-determination, this does not minimize the contribution of individual cognitions and perceptions to the performance of such behaviors. Just as there are people who do not act in a self-determined manner because they lack certain skills, so too are there people who possess such skills and the opportunity to use them who still do not act in a self-determined manner, usually because they have come to believe they cannot adequately perform the behavior or because they believe that doing so would be fruitless.

The inclusion of psychological empowerment and self-realization as essential elements for self-determined behavior illustrates the importance of both cognitive and behavioral contributions to this theoretical framework. As Bandura (1977) noted, a "theory of human behavior cannot afford to neglect symbolic activities" (p. 13). Similarly, Agran (1997) noted the importance of cognitive behaviors in achieving self-regulation, including the use of metacognitive, self-instruction, self-reinforcement, and observational learning strategies. Psychological empowerment is a term emanating from the community psychology literature and referring to the multiple dimensions of perceived control, including its cognitive (personal efficacy), personality (locus of control), and motivational domains (Zimmerman, 1990). Community psychology involves theory, research, and practice relevant to the reciprocal relationships between individuals and the social system which constitute the community context. Zimmerman (1990) proposed a model in which positive perceptions of control (psychological empowerment) are an outcome of *learned hopefulness.* He defined learned hopefulness as the "process of learning and utilizing problem-solving skills and the achievement of perceived or actual control" (p. 72). Zimmerman's model of learned hopefulness "suggests that experiences that provide opportunities to enhance perceived control will help individuals cope with stress and solve problems in their lives" (pp. 7273). In a factor-analytic study of perceptions of control and community involvement, Zimmerman (1990) found that measures of three elements of perceived control (e.g., cognitive [self-efficacy], personality [locus of control] and motivation [motivation to control]) formed a single discriminant function which distinguished between individuals who scored low and individuals who scored high on a measure of hopelessness or alienation, including indicators of powerlessness and social isola-tion. The construct of psychological empowerment was for-warded to describe this factor. Thus, according to Zimmerman, through the process of learning and using problem-solving skills and achieving perceived or actual control in one's life (e.g., learned hopefulness), individuals develop a perception of *psychological empowerment* which, in turn, enables them to achieve desired outcomes such as social inclusion and involvement in the community.

Self-Realization. The term self-realization was originally used by Gestalt psychologists to refer to the intrinsic purpose in the life of the person, but also has a more global meaning related to the "tendency to shape one's life course into a meaningful whole" (Angyal, 1941, p. 355). Though not frequently used any longer in the psychology literature, the term captures some nuances or an essence of self-determination missed by other con-ceptualizations. Basically, this essence is that self-determined people know what they do well and act accordingly.

The two most frequently mentioned alternatives to the term self-realization are *self-actualization* and *self*-awareness, but both have limited utility. Self-actualization, as conceptualized by Maslow (1943), adequately captures the essence of a self-deter-mined person's actions as capitalizing on his or her best assets and becoming all that one is capable of becoming. However, in addition to problems with Maslow's definition and the theoretical underpinnings of self-actualization (see, for example, Heylighen, 1992), Maslow conceptualized self-actualization as being attained only by a small proportion of the population. Conceptualizing self-determination within the construct of self-actualization implies that only a select number of individuals become self-determined, and people with mental retardation are, almost cer-tainly, not among that select group.

Alternatively, the construct of self-awareness fails to capture the sense that self-determined people act on their knowledge about themselves to capitalize on their strengths. As such, people who are self-determined are self-realizing in that they use a com-prehensive, and reasonably accurate, knowledge of themselves and their strengths and limitations to act in such a manner as to capitalize on this knowledge. This self-knowledge and self-understanding forms through experience with and interpretation of one's environment and is influenced by evaluations of significant others, reinforcement, and attributions of one's own behavior.

Empirical Examination of the Theoretical Framework

The theoretical framework we have described and have used to examine self-determination was initially formulated based on a comprehensive review of the pertinent literature (Wehmeyer, 1992a) and the outcomes of focus group discussions with people with mental retardation (Wehmeyer, 1992b). The essential characteristics and component elements of this framework appear in similar efforts by other researchers (Abery, 1993; Field & Hoffman, 1994; Martin & Marshall, 1995), providing limited construct validity for the theory. However, to empirically validate the theory we conducted a national research project with individuals with mental retardation that examined the contribution of the proposed essential characteristics of self-determined behavior to the achievement of behavioral outcomes closely associated with self-determination (Wehmeyer, Kelchner, & Richards, 1996).

The sample for this study included 407 individuals (mean age was 36 years) with mental retardation from self-advocacy groups (consumer organized and run advocacy organizations for people with mental retardation) across the nation. We collected data from self-report measures of each of the essential characteristics, usually in the context of a self-advocacy group meeting. Autonomy was measured using a self-report form of the Autonomous Functioning Checklist (AFC; Sigafoos et al., 1988; Wehmeyer & Kelchner, 1995a). A second measure of autonomy was the Life Choices Survey (LCS; Kishi, Teelucksingh, Zollers, Park-Lee, & Meyer, 1988). The LCS has 10 items measuring major life decisions and daily choices, is completed in an interview format, and yields a score reflecting total amount of choice.

Self-regulation was measured using the means-ends problem solving (MEPS) technique (Platt & Spivack, 1989), which examines interpersonal cognitive problem solving. The MEPS procedure uses a series of story items portraying situations where a need is introduced at the beginning of a story and satisfied at the end. Respondents complete the story by filling in events that might have occurred to fulfill the need (Platt & Spivack, 1989). Stories are scored according to the number of means, no means, irrelevant means, or no responses provided by the respondent. A mean was defined as "any relevant unit of information designed to reach the goal or to overcome an obstacle, a purposeful action taken by someone with the intent to reach a goal" (Platt & Spivack, 1989). The number of relevant means were tallied for each story and added to compute the total relevant means score for each participant. A second measure of self-regulation was the Assertiveness Inventory (Ollendick, 1984) a 14-item, yes–no measure assessing the degree to which someone initiates interactions, gives and receives compliments, stands up for his or her own rights, and refuses unreasonable requests. Psychological empowerment was measured using a locus of control scale and two related measures of social self-efficacy and outcome expectancy. The Adult version of the Nowicki-Strickland Internal-External Scale (ANS-IE; Nowicki & Duke, 1974) is a widely used measure of locus of control. People who see themselves as in control of outcomes in their lives have an internal locus of control, while people who perceive outcomes as controlled by others, fate, or chance hold an external locus of control. The ANS-IE consists of 40 items answered with a "yes" or "no" and higher scores reflect more external orientations. Although normed with adults without disabilities, the instrument has been used to determine locus of control orientation for individuals with cognitive limitations (Wehmeyer, 1994a). Moreover, it was determined (Wehmeyer, 1993, 1994b) that the factor structure of the ANS-IE when used with individuals with mental retardation was comparable to that for youth and adults without disabilities and that the scale was reliable for use with individuals with mental retardation.

Self-efficacy and outcome expectancy were measured by two related scales. The Self-Efficacy for Social Interactions Scale (Ollendick, Oswald, & Crowe, 1986) measures how sure a respondent is that he or she could perform a set of socially related behaviors, and the Outcome Expectancy Measure (Ollendick et al., 1986) replicates questions on the self-efficacy measure, focusing instead on the expected outcome if the student performed the described behavior.

The final essential characterization, self-realization, was measured using the short version of the Personal Orientation

Inventory (Jones & Crandall, 1986), a 15-item measure of an individual's understanding of his or her emotions, abilities, and limitations and the degree to which he or she is influenced by others or by their own motivations and principles.

The relative self-determination of participants was measured using the National Consumer Survey (NCS; Jaskulski, Metzler, & Zierman, 1990), used previously to examine the self-determination of people with mental retardation (Wehmeyer & Metzler, 1995). Participants responded to a series of questions concerning the degree to which they had control over their lives in several domains, including: (a) home and family living; (b) employment; (c) recreation and leisure; (d) transportation; and (e) money management. They were also asked to respond to a set of questions pertaining to their personal advocacy and leadership experiences. Wehmeyer, Kelchner, and Richards (1995) determined that this survey had adequate structural and concurrent validity and internal stability. Total scores for the survey correlated strongly with self-reported estimates of the level of caregiving a person needed and his or her level of independence, with respondents who scored more positively on the survey requiring less support in caregiving and indicating greater independence.

To identify essential characteristics that distinguished between people with mental retardation or developmental disabilities who were self-determined and those who were not, we conducted a multiple discriminant function analysis, forming two dichotomous groups based on NCS total scores. Scores below the midpoint (e.g., more self-determined) were assigned to a high self-determination group and scores above the midpoint were assigned to a low self-determination group.

Univariate statistics generated by the discriminant function analysis procedure indicated differences between predictor variables based on group membership. Nine of the 11 predictor variables reached significance ($p < .05$) when examining differences between groups and in each of those cases the direction of the difference was more favorable for individuals in the high self-determination group. Figure 3.2 shows scores from each measure converted to a z-score for each group.

Measures of autonomy, particularly the management, social and vocational activities, and self- and family-care subscales, were the primary variables distinguishing between groups. Mea-

FIG. 3.2. *Z-scores (converted from raw test scores) of measures of essential characteristics of self-determined behavior.*

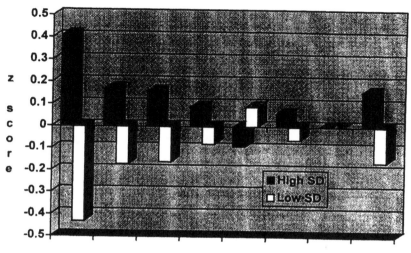

Measure of Essential Characteristic

sures of self-awareness (Personal Orientation Inventory), self-regulation (assertiveness and problem solving), and psychological empowerment (locus of control) followed in importance. The correlation between total self-determination and level of disability scores for the high and low self-determination groups were both statistically significant, but low ($r = .19$, $p = .006$ for the high group; $r = .22$, $p = .002$ for the low group), representing less than 5% of common variation in both groups, suggesting that results were not just a function of level of ability.

These findings supported our hypothesis that people who were more autonomous, self-regulating, psychologically empowered, and self-realizing are, in fact, more self-determined than people who are not. This research has subsequently been supported by research examining the importance of self-determination in the lives of adults and students with cognitive disabilities, as measured using these four essential characteristics. Based on findings from this broad examination of self-determination, we developed a self-report measure of self-determination that provides an indication of total self-determination and subscale scores for each of the essential characteristics (Wehmeyer &

Kelchner, 1995b). This scale, titled The Arc's Self-Determination Scale, was normed with 500 students with and without cognitive disabilities enrolled in secondary education programs. A factor-analytic study provided evidence of construct validity for the measure. Using this scale, we measured the self-determination of 80 students with cognitive disabilities who were in their final year of school. One year out of school we contacted students and determined where they were living, if and where they were working, whether they were involved in a postsecondary education program, and other indicators of adult outcomes. Controlling for level of intelligence, we divided the sample into two groups, high and low self-determination, and used chi-square analyses to determine relative differences on adult outcomes based on self-determination status. Students who were in the high self-determination group were more likely to be employed and when employed earned more money; more likely to have taken responsibility and control over their finances, arrangements for transportation, and daily living activities; and more likely to have a plan to move from their parents' home. The study both supported the importance of self-determination for success as an adult and provided construct validity for our theoretical framework.

Component Elements of Self-Determined Behavior

The essential characteristics that define self-determined behavior emerge through the development and acquisition of multiple, interrelated component elements. Table 3.1 lists these elements. Although not intended as an exhaustive list, these component elements are particularly important to the emergence of self-determined behavior.

Each of these component elements has a unique developmental course or is acquired through specific learning experiences (Doll, Sands, Wehmeyer, & Palmer, 1996; Wehmeyer et al., 1997). The development and acquisition of these component elements is lifelong and begins when children are very young. It is at this level, as mentioned previously, that intervention occurs. This section briefly discusses each component element.

Choice Making. Perhaps more emphasis has been placed on this component element as critical to self-determination and a

TABLE 3.1
Component Analysis of Self-Determined Behavior

Choice-making skills
Decision-making skills
Problem-solving skills
Goal-setting and attainment skills
Self-observation, self-evaluation and self-reinforcement skills
Self-instruction skills
Self-advocacy and leadership skills
Internal locus of control
Perceptions of self-efficacy and outcome expectancy
Self-awareness
Self-knowledge

positive quality of life for people with disabilities than most of the other elements combined, particularly for individuals with significant disabilities. There have been training programs developed to teach choice making and increase choice-making behaviors (Gothelf, Crimmins, Mercer, & Finocchiaro, 1994; Parsons, McCarn, & Reid, 1993; Reid, Parsons, & Green, 1991; Warren, 1993), efforts to increase the diversity of choices for people with disabilities (Brown, Belz, Corsi, & Wenig, 1993), discussions about the importance to people with disabilities of making choices (Ficker-Terrill & Rowitz, 1991; Guess, Benson, & Siegel-Causey, 1985; Shevin & Klein, 1984; West & Parent, 1992), procedures developed to assess individual preferences and choices (Mithaug & Hanawalt, 1978; Stancliffe, 1995), and research efforts to determine the degree to which people with disabilities express choices and preferences (Houghton, Bronicki, & Guess, 1987; Kishi et al., 1988; Stancliffe & Wehmeyer, 1995; Wehmeyer et al., 1995; Wehmeyer & Metzler, 1995).

Guess et al. (1985) proposed three levels of choice making: (a) choice as indicating preferences, (b) choice as a part of the decision-making process, and (c) choice as an expression of autonomy and dignity. Reid et al. (1991) identified the instruction of choice making as consisting of two basic components: the act of choosing and the identification of a preference. The first component involves "emitting specific behaviors necessary to select one item or event from two or more alternatives" (Reid et al., 1991, p. 3), while the second directs that action toward the selection of preferred outcomes.

The limited body of research on choice making suggests that too frequently the preferences of individuals with disabilities are ignored or not acknowledged (Houghton et al., 1987; Kishi et al., 1988; Stancliffe & Wehmeyer, 1995; Wehmeyer et al., 1995; Wehmeyer & Metzler, 1995). This finding is ironic because increased opportunities and capacities to express preferences and make choices have been linked to reductions in problem behaviors exhibited by individuals with severe disabilities (Gardner, Cole, Berry, & Nowinski, 1983; Grace, Cowart, & Matson, 1988; Munk & Repp, 1994), increased participation in appropriate or adaptive tasks (Koestner, Ryan, Bernieri, & Holt, 1984; Swann & Pittman, 1977; Realon, Favell, & Lowerre, 1990), and more positive educational or achievement outcomes (Koenigs, Fielder, & deCharms, 1977).

Decision Making.   There is, in theory and in practice, considerable overlap between choice making and decision making. There is further overlap with the third essential element, problem solving. All three are critical to becoming autonomous and self-regulating. Choice making refers to a process of selecting between alternatives based on individual preferences. Decision-making skills refer to a broader set of skills that incorporate choice making as but one component. Beyth-Marom, Fischhoff, Jacobs Quadrel, and Furby (1991) suggested that most models of decision making incorporate the following steps: (a) listing relevant action alternatives, (b) identifying possible consequences of those actions, (c) assessing the probability of each consequence occurring (if the action were undertaken), (d) establishing the relative importance (value or utility) of each consequence, and (e) integrating these values and probabilities to identify the most attractive course of action (p. 21).

Baron and Brown (1991) proposed that "deficient decision-making is a serious problem throughout society at large and [this] problem needs addressing in childhood or adolescence" (p. 8). Self-determined individuals need to know how to define the issue or problem about which a specific decision is to be made, collect information about their specific situation, and become able to use this information to identify options for consideration. Once these options are clarified, individuals need to be able to identify and evaluate the consequences and outcomes of actions based on the various options. When those consequences have been detailed, choice-making skills can be applied to select a specific alternative. Finally, individuals must implement this plan of action.

Problem Solving. The third component element is problem-solving skills. Decision making is a process of weighing the adequacy of various solutions. A problem, on the other hand, is "a task whose solution is not immediately perceived" (Beyth-Marom et al., 1991, p. 20). More specifically, a problem "is a specific situation or set of situations to which a person must respond in order to function effectively in his environment" (D'Zurilla & Goldfried, 1971, p. 108).

Until recent years, problem-solving skills were studied almost entirely from an impersonal context (Platt & Hermalin, 1989). Most researchers focused on an individual's ability to complete puzzles and anagrams or solve mathematical problems. Such problems typically have only one correct solution with answers remaining the same over time (Wheeler, 1991). In contrast, problems involving interactions between people are complex with multiple processing demands and decision points and have numerous possible solutions that may vary according to time or setting. For example, the way an individual would greet a coworker if that person was recently demoted would differ greatly from a greeting if one knows that the person was promoted. Likewise, how one greets a coworker in front of a supervisor might be very different from how one might routinely greet that person. Researchers in the area of problem solving became increasingly concerned that "conceptualizing problem-solving as removed from real-world interactions and applications failed to capture the complexity of social and personal problem-solving and was not applicable to practitioners in counseling and education" (Spivack & Shure, 1974).

Consequently, research investigating problem-solving skills within a social context emerged and theorists working in this area began to describe and define social problem solving as a metacognitive process (Elliot, Godshall, Shrout & Witty, 1990). For the first time, questions began to be asked about how a person approached problems. As a result, research in problem solving began to more closely reflect the complexity of social interactions. For example, Heppner and Peterson (1982) suggested that successful social problem solving had three dimensions beyond just a repertoire of behavioral strategies: (a) confidence in one's ability to solve problems, (b) one's approach-avoidance style, and (c) perceptions of personal control.

Platt and Hermalin (1989) were among the earliest researchers to link effective social problem solving with more positive emotional and social outcomes. They proposed that in order to deal with real-life problems and stay well-adjusted a person must utilize a set of adaptive social problem-solving skills which include: (a) recognition of the problem, (b) optional thinking or the generation of alternatives, (c) causal thinking, (d) means-end thinking or step-by-step planning, (e) consequential thinking, and (f) role-taking or metarepresentation.

Like research efforts with individuals without disabilities, investigations of problem solving for individuals with disabilities, particularly mental retardation, have moved from impersonal to personal contexts. Much of this research has examined the capacity of individuals with mental retardation to solve problems. This research has suggested that people with mental retardation exhibit a largely inflexible pattern of problem-solving skills (Ellis, Woodley-Zanthos, Dulaney, & Palmer, 1989; Ferretti & Butterfield, 1989; Ferretti & Cavalier, 1991; Short & Evans, 1990). This pattern, labeled cognitive rigidity by Gestalt psychologists, "is characterized by repetition of past strategies to solve current problems without adapting to new stimuli or new task demands" (Short & Evans, 1990, p. 95). Wehmeyer and Kelchner (1994) examined the social problem-solving skills of adults with mental retardation and found that this group generated fewer potential solutions to social problems and that a greater proportion of solutions generated were irrelevant. Healey and Masterpasqua (1992) examined the social problem solving of elementary school students with mental retardation as a function of their adjustment to regular education classrooms. These researchers hypothesized that strong social problem-solving skills would be related to more positive peer relations and behavioral adjustment in the classroom. They found that this was indeed the case and that classroom adjustment could be predicted by interpersonal cognitive problem-solving skills.

There have been several studies showing that individuals with mental retardation can acquire effective problem-solving strategies. Castles and Glass (1986) found that training improved social problem-solving skills of youth with mild and moderate mental retardation. Browning and Nave (1993) used an interactive, video-based curriculum to teach social problem-solving skills to youth with mild mental retardation and learning disabilities.

Park and Gaylord-Ross (1989) found that there is a need to pair social skills training with social problem-solving training if individuals with mental retardation are to succeed. These researchers compared social skills training without problem-solving training to a general social program that incorporated problem-solving training for youth with developmental disabilities. They found that the social problem-solving training procedure increased generalization and maintenance of the targeted social behaviors.

As in the choice-making process, problem-solving skills are embedded into virtually all decision-making procedures. The first step in decision-making models is to identify the issue at hand or the problem. As it is conceptualized by most researchers, however, the decision-making process begins with the listing of already identified options. Practically, one must first engage in problem solving before decision making can occur. Problem-solving models typically include three focal points: (a) problem identification, (b) problem explication and analysis, and (c) problem resolution.

Goal Setting and Attainment.   To become the causal agent in his or her life, a person needs to learn the skills necessary to plan, set, and achieve goals. Goal setting theory is built on the underlying assumption that goals are regulators of human action. The effects of goal setting on behavior are a function of goal difficulty and specificity as well as previous experiences with the activity or action. Goal attainment is typically a function of two related aspects of goals: content and intensity. Goal content refers to the topic of the goal while goal intensity reflects that goal's priority in the person's hierarchy of goals. There are considerable between-individual differences in these aspects, and goal attainment or achievement will be affected by the salience and importance of the topic and the intensity of the individual's desire to achieve the goal.

Although self-determined behaviors are goal-directed, it is incorrect to assume that self-determined and goal-directed behaviors are always successful or attain the intended goal. Self-determined behavior cannot be judged by the relative success of the action, just as goal-directed action cannot be determined by the achievement of the specific target or objective.

Self-Observation, Self-Evaluation, Self-Instruction, and Self-Reinforcement Skills. Self-regulated behavior includes, at the very least, employing the skills of self-observation or self-monitoring, self-evaluation, self-instruction, and self-reinforcement. Self-monitoring strategies involve assessing, observing, and recording one's own behavior and the utilization of these strategies have been shown to improve work-related activities of people with mental retardation, such as attention to task, task completion, and task accuracy (Hughes, Korinek, & Gorman, 1991).

Self-evaluation involves the use of systematic strategies that enable an individual to track and evaluate his or her own progress on activities, including self-selected goals and objectives. Self-recording procedures are a type of self-evaluation activity in which the individual graphs, charts, or otherwise documents progress on a goal or objective. Individuals with mental retardation can be taught to score worksheets, identify the occurrence of a target behavior, track time intervals for the occurrence or nonoccurrence of a target behavior, and record this information in a graphic or chart format or using some other means of tracking, including the use of tokens.

A third aspect of self-regulation is the use of self-reinforcement strategies. Agran (1997) defined self-reinforcement as the self-administration of consequences, either positive or negative, contingent on the occurrence of a target behavior, and suggested that self-reinforcement should have two functions: self-identification of reinforcers and delivery of this reinforcer. Self-reinforcement can be more effective than having another person deliver the reinforcer, not the least because self-reinforcement can almost always be immediate (Agran, 1997).

Self-instructional strategies involve individuals "providing their own verbal prompts for solving a problem" (Hughes et al., 1991, p. 292). These skills have been shown to enable people with mental retardation to successfully solve work-related problems (Agran, Fodor-Davis, & Moore, 1986; Hughes & Rusch, 1989) and have been used to teach social skills critical to independence (Agran, Salzberg, & Stowitschek, 1987; Hughes & Agran, 1993).

Self-Advocacy and Leadership Skills. Self-advocacy skills are those skills individuals need to, quite literally, advocate on their own behalf. To advocate means to speak up or defend a cause or person. By definition, then, efforts to promote self-advocacy will focus on two common threads: how to advocate and what to advocate. Areas of emphasis related to how to advocate include (a) becoming assertive but not aggressive; (b) how to communicate effectively in one-on-one, small group, and large group situations; (c) how to negotiate, compromise, and use persuasion; (d) how to be an effective listener; and (d) how to navigate through systems and bureaucracies. It is evident that each of these is closely tied to the acquisition and emergence of other self-determination skills. For example, a reliable understanding of one's strengths and weaknesses is an important component if one is to actually use strategies such as negotiation and compromise to achieve an outcome.

Internal Locus of Control. The final component elements of self-determined behavior focus not on skill areas, but on the beliefs and perceptions that enable individuals to use acquired skills. Since psychological empowerment refers to the multiple aspects of perceived control, component elements contributing to acting in a psychologically empowered manner involve, logically, the acquisition of adaptive perceptions of control. The first of these is the construct of locus of control. Rotter (1966) introduced the construct and defined locus of control as the degree to which a person perceives contingency relationships between his or her actions and outcomes. Mercer and Snell (1977) described the construct as such when describing its efficacy for students with mental retardation:

> When a person is characterized as having an internal locus of control, he views reinforcement as primarily the consequences of one's own actions; whereas, if a person is characterized as having an external locus of control, reinforcement is viewed as the result of outside forces, e.g., luck, fate, chance and/or powerful others (p. 183).

The locus of control construct has proven to be a powerful heuristic for explaining, at least partially, individual and group differences in motivation, personality, and learning. Internal locus of control has been linked to adaptive outcomes, including positive educational and achievement outcomes and increased time and attention to school-related tasks (Lefcourt, 1976). External orientations have, conversely, been linked to increased impulsivity in decision making, distractibility, and sociometric ratings of rejection from peers (Ollendick, Greene, Francis, & Baum, 1991; Ollendick & Schmidt, 1987). In other words, individuals who feel in control of their lives and their destiny behave in ways that are more functional and adaptive than do individuals who feel that other people or circumstances dictate their lives.

Research that my colleagues and I have conducted examining the locus of control of individuals with mental retardation suggests that they tend to hold more external locus of control orientations than same age peers without disabilities or, indeed, than peers with other cognitive disabilities, such as learning disabilities. This research has examined locus of control orientations for more than 2,000 adolescents and adults with mental retardation, and individuals consistently score in a more external direction (Wehmeyer, 1993, 1994a; Wehmeyer & Palmer, 1997), even when inflated scores due to acquiescence are taken into account (Wehmeyer, 1994b). Additionally, while there is a general trend in typical child development with locus of control orientations becoming increasingly internal as children enter adolescence and young adulthood (Hertz-Lazarowitz, & Sharan, 1979; Knoop, 1981; Sherman, 1984), this trend does not appear to occur for children and youth with mental retardation (Wehmeyer, 1994a). Instead, the perceptions of adolescents and young adults with mental retardation remain largely external, changing little across time.

We have suggested (Wehmeyer, 1994a; Wehmeyer & Palmer, 1997) that individuals with mental retardation are *causal unrealists*, holding unrealistic understandings of causality and excessively external global perceptions of control. These perceptions of control probably "reflect both an overreliance on luck and chance inherent in less mature beliefs and understanding about ability, effort and circumstances and an inability to effectively judge competence and ability in themselves and others" (Wehmeyer, 1994a, p. 19) and result theoretically from the limited opportunities these individuals have had to experience control and choice in their lives.

Perceptions of Self-Efficacy and Positive Outcome Expectancies. Self-efficacy and efficacy expectations are two related constructs introduced by Bandura (1977). In a recent summary of self-efficacy research, Bandura (1997) defined perceived self-efficacy as referring to "beliefs in one's capabilities to organize and execute the courses of action required to produce given attainments" (p. 3). As a theory of human control and as an agent through which people can take greater control over their destiny, Bandura places central prominence on beliefs of personal efficacy, stating that "among the mechanisms of agency, none is more central or pervasive than beliefs of personal efficacy. Unless people believe they can produce desired effects by their actions, they have little incentive to act" (Bandura, 1997, p. 3). More specifically, he states, "Beliefs of personal efficacy constitute the key factor of human agency. If people believe they have no power to produce results, they will not attempt to make things happen (Bandura, 1997, p. 3).

Perceived self-efficacy and locus of control differ, according to Bandura, in that locus of control is primarily concerned with causal beliefs about the relationship between actions and outcomes and not with personal efficacy per se (Bandura, 1997). Bandura proposed an additional component to beliefs of personal efficacy, outcome expectancies. Perceived self-efficacy is the "judgement of one's ability to organize and execute given types of performances" (Bandura, 1997, p. 21), where outcome expectation "is a judgement of the likely consequence such performances will produce" (Bandura, 1997, p. 21).

It should be evident that the two are individually necessary but not sufficient for behavior such as goal-directed and self-determined actions. Simply put, a person has to believe that he or she can perform a specific behavior needed to achieve a desired outcome and that if that behavior is performed it will result in the desired outcome. If a person does not believe that he or she can perform a given behavior (independent of the validity of that belief), then consequently he or she will not perform that action. However, a person may believe that he or she is capable of performing a given behavior, but due to past experience may not believe that a desired outcome will occur even if that behavior is exhibited and, subsequently, will not perform the action.

Very little research has examined the self-efficacy and efficacy expectations of individuals with disabilities. Most of the extant literature in the area of learning disabilities focuses on changing self-efficacy and efficacy expectations through environmental or instructional modifications (Schunk, 1989). In 1994, I (Wehmeyer, 1994a) found that individuals with mental retardation held less adaptive attributions of efficacy and expectancy than did their nondisabled peers and that such attributions became less adaptive as the student got older, a trend not consistent with typical developmental functions for these attributes, but consistent with similar findings for this population on locus of control orientations.

Self-Awareness and Self-Knowledge. In order for a person to act in a self-realizing manner, he or she must possess a basic understanding of his or her strengths, weaknesses, abilities, and limitations as well as knowledge about how to utilize these unique attributions to beneficially influence his or her quality of life. This process is not one of pure introspection, however, and does not focus exclusively or even primarily on an understanding of limitations. There is very little research related to the self-awareness and self-knowledge held by people with mental retardation.

The Developmental of Self-Determination

This theory provides the basis for a model of the development of self-determination, based largely upon findings in developmental psychology related to the development of component elements of self-determined behavior. This section will describe this model of development.

Self-determination is usually associated with adolescence or adulthood. There are valid societal and developmental reasons young children are not seen as self-determined. As mentioned previously, the emergence of self-determination is part of the process of individuation, e.g., the formation of an individual's personal identity and the development of "one's sense of self and the forging of a special place for oneself within the social order" (Damon, 1983; p. 2). Just as there are identifiable developmental progressions in the emergence of cognitive processes or moral reasoning, so too are there developmental progressions to the emergence of self-determination. And, just as children who have not attained critical milestones in some cognitive abilities cannot be expected to use fully mature cognitive schemas, so too children who have not achieved critical milestones in the development of self-determination cannot be expected to be self-determined (Wehmeyer, 1996b). Because young children are not yet allowed or developmentally capable of being autonomous and self-regulating does not, however, abrogate the need to enable all children, including children with disabilities, to learn and develop the attitudes and abilities they will need to achieve this outcome. Self-determination may be primarily an adult outcome, but it is only achieved if there is a lifelong focus on its development and acquisition (Sands & Wehmeyer, 1996).

Doll and colleagues (1996) collapsed the component elements listed previously into five developmental domains important to self-determination: self-awareness and self-knowledge, self-evaluation and attributions of efficacy, choice making and decision making, metarepresentation, and goal setting and task performance. This section discusses development within each of these domains as a means of describing the development of self-determination.

Self-Awareness and Self-Knowledge

The first developmental milestone in this domain is the acquisition of a categorical sense of self, usually mature by 18 months of age (DeCasper & Spence, 1986; Lewis & Brooks-Gunn, 1979). Subsequently, infants display an interest in and act intentionally toward caregivers and other social objects. This intentional behavior is the catalyst for infants' recognition that they are a person, distinct from caregivers and others (8–10 months) and that they can control or cause specific outcomes through their own action.

The emergence of self-awareness and self-knowledge also requires an understanding of emotions, feelings, and other within-person states common to all individuals. Children have a rudimentary understanding of their own internal states by 3 years of age and begin to understand that others experience these as well at roughly the same age (Bretherton & Beeghy, 1982; Eder, 1989). By age 7, children can label multiple emotional states and, with age and experience, become more accurate in predicting the affect of other persons (Selman, 1980).

The next developmental step is to understand and use dispositional states to predict future behavior. Dispositional states, as noted previously, are frequent, enduring tendencies used to characterize people and to describe important differences between people. Understanding dispositional states emerges in its most simple form around 3 years of age (Eder, 1990) when children understand that people familiar to them have characteristic ways of acting that are stable over time. By age 8, children have developed a more complex understanding of these characteristics and by age 9 or 10 use them to predict behavior.

Another milestone in the development of this domain is the acquisition of metacognitive self-knowledge. This refers to the ability of children to reflect upon their own mental processes and take control over the cognitive processes they use. The accuracy of children's metacognitive self-knowledge increases with age. Preschoolers and kindergartners do not attend to their own thinking and do not always notice when they are being either ineffective or effective, and so tend not to revise or fine-tune their cognitive approaches to tasks, even when they are unsuccessful (Forrest & Walker, 1980; Ghatala, 1986; Paris & Lindauer, 1982). It is not until the early elementary years that children can actually match their skills and understanding to a task, judge their task success, and plan for task completion (Forrest & Walker, 1980). By 6th grade, students actively seek information so they can judge their task success and adjust their task approach as necessary (Ruble & Flett, 1988).

Self-Evaluation and Attributions of Efficacy

Acting in a psychologically empowered manner requires that self-determined people recognize their own actions and their outcomes clearly and without bias (self-evaluation). Such self-evaluations begin very early, although young children's self-descriptions and self-evaluations are inaccurate and often inconsistent from one task to another (Frey & Ruble, 1987). In the early elementary grades, children's estimates of their own ability become stable and global across tasks (Dweck & Elliot, 1983; Rholes & Ruble, 1984). By age 6 or 7, children begin to understand that these task abilities might be the basis for comparisons among children or skill domains (e.g., normative standards; Renick & Harter, 1989), even though they are unlikely to use normative comparisons spontaneously until the age of 10 (Nicholls, 1978; Ruble, Boggiano, Feldman, & Loebl, 1980). By the middle elementary years, students' spontaneous self-evaluations are stable across time and settings and are relatively accurate, and students are capable of judging their performance against a mastery standard (e.g., comparing work against a teacher's example).

Over time children's self-evaluations become less optimistic (e.g., unrealistic) and more congruent with their actual task performance. Concurrent with their increasingly accurate self-evaluations, children's development of perceptions of control and efficacy contribute to their acquired understanding of causality, including an understanding of contingency relationships and the different roles that effort, ability, and luck play in determining outcomes (Skinner, 1990). Young children (5–6) attribute excessive importance to effort for producing success and preventing failure. By age 8 or 9, children begin to distinguish between effort and luck, and by age 12 children can determine the relative contribution of each to a given outcome.

Choice and Decision Making

Developmental aspects of choice making focus on children's capacities to identify and communicate preferences. Once a child develops these capacities, the maturation of choice-making ability relies on children's opportunities to make selections and experience the outcomes of these choices. Children then apply these choice-making skills to acquire the capacity for systematic decision making and effective problem solving. The capacity to indicate preference is present at birth (Fantz, 1961; Haith, 1980; Stern, 1985). Indicating a preference requires that the child designate a specific option from between two or more choices, which in turn requires the emergence of intentional communication. Infants as young as 4 to 5 months indicate preferences through cries, smiles, or eye gaze, while the advent of motor skills at 10 months of age and on provide children with more ways of communicating (crawling to desired object, pointing, etc.). As children develop more advanced verbal skills at age 3, they typically use language to indicate preferences.

The organization of preferences and choice making into decision-making and problem-solving skills takes more time. Although information about the development of these skills is limited, as early as third grade, students can decide what support they need after assessing their own performance. Students at the elementary and secondary level can often make autonomous decisions regarding scholastic interventions (Deci, Schwartz, Sheinman, & Ryan, 1981), and the decisions of adolescents have been shown to be very similar to those of adults (Kaser-Boyd, Adelman, & Taylor, 1985). Older adolescents are typically superior to younger adolescents in their strategies to generate options to solve problems and make decisions and their anticipation of the consequences of their decisions (Ormond, Luszcz, Mann, & Beswick, 1991).

Metarepresentation

Metarepresentation skills refer to understanding or thinking about others' representation of the external world and their actions, intentions, and perspectives (Flavell, 1985). Metarepresentation skills enable a person to acquire and employ the social skills he or she needs to interact with other people (Kendall, 1984; Moore, 1979). Children younger than 5 or 6 years tend to use the "same situation = same viewpoint" rule, expecting others to respond just as they would (Selman, 1980). Only after ages 5–9 do children actually realize that other people might have a different perspective and begin to take that into account in social situations. Moore (1979) found that by age 7, children realize that other people see, hear, and think differently from themselves. Shantz (1975) reported that although 4-year-olds could not, 5-year olds were able to consider the intentions of the other person in assessing blame. However, other researchers have found that there is some evidence of the understanding of intentions, memories, feelings, and images in the plans of children as early as 3 or 4 years (Perner, Frith, Leslie, & Leekham, 1989; Perner & Wimmer, 1985).

Metarepresentation skills are linked to children's and adolescents' capacity for interpersonal social problem solving and self-regulation (Wehmeyer & Kelchner, 1994). Early elementary years are particularly important for these skills. Scarr, Weinberg, and Levine (1986) found that 7-year-olds were able to describe twice as many solutions as 5-year-olds.

Goal Setting and Task Performance

Children younger than age 4 do not associate specific actions with a goal or objective. At age 4, some children can recognize a goal plan as illustrated in a series of pictured events (Trabasso, Stein, Rodkin, Park, & Baughn, 1992). By 5 years of age, most children can link goals and specific actions that could be taken to reach that goal; however, until age 11 or older, children continue to need a great deal of ongoing support to set goals and identify how to achieve them.

CONCLUSIONS

Our efforts to define and explain self-determination were driven by a very practical agenda: the necessity of teaching students and adults with mental retardation to become self-determined. Pearl Buck, Pulitzer Prize winning author and herself the parent of a daughter with severe mental retardation, once stated that "none who have always been free can understand the terrible fascinating power of the hope of freedom to those who are not free" (Buck, 1943). She was basing her observation on her experiences in China in the first half of the 1900s, but her quote captures the intensity of emotion and feeling with which people with disabilities have demanded their right to self-determination. People with disabilities, and particularly people with mental retardation, have been among the most disenfranchised and discriminated against persons in our society and, in fact, are among those who have had the least amount of control in their lives. The overwhelming presumption for the majority of the past century, vestiges of which remain intact today, was that people with mental retardation were not capable of self-governance and should be, indeed had to be, watched over and cared for. As Buck's quote illustrates, the desire for self-governance for people who have had virtually no control over their lives is, most likely, beyond the conception of those of us who have had the chance to become self-determined.

The response to such an intense demand consists of parallel activities, including legislative and civil protections enabling people with disabilities to be protected from discrimination, systemic changes in the ways people with disabilities are supported and served by human services agencies, and chances to acquire the skills and beliefs that enable one to take advantage of opportunities to exert control and be self-governing.

Our theoretical construction has enabled us to develop assessment instruments (Wehmeyer, 1996c; Wehmeyer & Kelchner, 1995b) that enable us to examine the relationship between self-determination and successful adult functioning (Wehmeyer & Schwartz, 1997) and quality of life (Wehmeyer & Schwartz, 1998), to examine the relationship between environments and individual characteristics (Wehmeyer, Kelchner, & Richards, 1995) in order to promote greater control and choice, and to design models of instruction (Wehmeyer, Palmer, Agran, Mituaug, & Martin, 2000) and identify extant educational practices (Wehmeyer, Agran, & Hughes, 1998) that enable teachers to promote self-determination. By using the theoretical framework to construct a model of the development of self-determination (Doll et al., 1996; Wehmeyer et al., 1997), we are able to identify practices and environments that promote the acquisition and development of this outcome.

These activities can contribute both to the understanding of the behavior of people with mental retardation and to the changing perspective of people with mental retardation as actively involved in their lives. Even at this early stage, it is evident that people with mental retardation can become self-determined and can assume greater control over their lives.

REFERENCES

Abery, B. (1993). A conceptual framework for enhancing self-determination. In M. Hayden and B. Abery (Eds.), *Challenges for a service system in transtion: Ensuring quality community experiences for persons with developmental disabilities* (pp. 345–380). Baltimore: Paul H. Brookes.

Agran, M. (1997). *Student-directed learning: Teaching self-determination skills.* Pacific Grove, CA: Brooks/Cole.

Agran, M., Fodor-Davis, J., & Moore, S. (1986). The effects of self-instructional training on job-task sequencing: Suggesting a problem-solving strategy. *Education and Training in Mental Retardation, 21,* 273–281.

Agran, M., Salzberg, C.L., & Stowitschek, J.J. (1987). An analysis of the effects of a social skills training program using self-instructions on the acquisition and generalization of two social behaviors in a work setting. *Journal of the Association for Persons with Severe Disabilities, 12,* 131–139.

Angyal, A. (1941). *Foundations for a science of personality.* Cambridge, MA: Harvard University Press.

Bandura, A. B. (1977). Self-efficacy: Toward a unifying theory of behavioral change. *Psychological Review, 84,* 191–215.

Bandura, A. B. (1997). *Self-efficacy: The exercise of control.* New York: W.H. Freeman.

Baron, J., & Brown, R.V. (1991). Introduction. In J. Baron & R.V. Brown (Eds.), *Teaching Decision Making to Adolescents.* Hillsdale, NJ: Lawrence Erlbaum Associates.

Beyth-Marom, R., Fischhoff, B., Jacobs Quadrel, M., & Furby, L. (1991). Teaching decision-making to adolescents: A critical review. In J. Baron & R.V. Brown (Eds.), *Teaching Decision Making to Adolescents.* Hillsdale, NJ: Lawrence ErlbaumAssociates.

Biestek, F. P., & Gehrig, C.C. (1978). *Client self-determination in social work: A fifty-year history.* Chicago: Loyola University Press.

Bretherton, I., & Beeghly, M. (1982). Talking about internal states: The acquisition of an explicit theory of mind. *Developmental Psychology, 18,* 906–921.

Brown, F. Belz, P., Corsi, L., &Wenig, B. (1993). Choice diversity for people with severe disabilities. *Education and Training in Mental Retardation, 28,* 318–326.

Browning, P., & Nave, G. (1993). Teaching social problem solving to learners with mild disabilities. *Education and Training in Mental Retardation, 28*, 309–317.

Buck, P. (1943). *What America means to me.* New York: Columbia University Press.

Castles, E. E., & Glass, C. R. (1986). Training in social and interpersonal problem-solving skills for mildly and moderately mentally retarded adults. *American Journal of Mental Deficiency, 91*, 35–42.

Damon, W. (1983). *Social and personality development.* New York: W.W. Norton.

DeCasper, A. J., & Spence, M. J. (1986). Prenatal maternal speech influences newborns' perception of speech sounds. *Infant Behavior and Development, 9*, 133–150.

deCharms, R. (1968). *Personal causation: The internal affective determinants of behavior.* New York: Academic Press.

Deci, E. L. (1975). *Intrinsic motivation.* New York: Plenum Press.

Deci, E. L. (1992). The relation of interest to the motivation of behavior: A self-determination theory perspective. In K. A. Renninger, S. Hidi, & A. Krapp (Eds.), *The role of interest in learning and development* (pp. 43–70). Hillsdale, NJ: Lawrence Erlbaum Associates.

Deci, E. L., & Ryan, R. (1985). *Intrinsic motivation and self-determination in human behavior.* New York: Plenum Press.

Deci, E. L., Schwartz, A. J., Sheinman, L., & Ryan, R. M. (1981). An instrument to assess adults' orientations toward control versus autonomy with children: Reflections on intrinsic motivation and perceived competence. *Journal of Educational Psychology, 73*, 642–650.

Doll, B., Sands, D. J., Wehmeyer, M. L., & Palmer, S. (1996). Promoting the development and acquisition of self-determined behavior. In D. J. Sands & M. L. Wehmeyer (Eds.), *Self-determination across the life span: Independence and choice for people with disabilities* (pp. 63–88). Baltimore: Paul H. Brookes.

Dweck, C. S., & Elliott, E. S. (1983). Achievement motivation. In E. M. Hetherington (Ed.) & P. H. Mussen (Series Ed.), *Handbook of child psychology: Vol. 3, Socialization, personality and social developments* (4th ed., pp. 643–691). New York: John Wiley.

D'Zurilla, T. J., & Goldfried, M. R. (1971). Problem-solving and behavior modification. *Journal of Abnormal Psychology, 78*, 107–126.

Eder, R. (1989). The emergent personologist: The structure and content of 3–, 5–, and 7–year-olds' concepts of themselves and other persons. *Child Development, 60,* 1218–1228.

Eder, R. (1990). Uncovering young children's psychological selves: Individual and developmental differences. *Child Development, 61,* 849–863.

Elliot, T. R., Godshall, F., Shrout, J. R., & Witty, T. E. (1990). Problem-solving appraisal, self-reported study habits, and performance of academically at risk college students. *The Journal of Counseling Psychology, 37,* 203–207.

Ellis, N. R., Woodley-Zanthos, P., Dulaney, C. L., & Palmer, R. L. (1989). Automatic effortful processing and cognitive inertia in persons with mental retardation. *American Journal on Mental Retardation, 93,* 412–423.

Fantz, R. (1961). The origin of form perception. *Scientific American, 204,* 66–72.

Ferretti, R. P., & Butterfield, E. C. (1989). Intelligence as a correlate of children's problem-solving. *American Journal on Mental Retardation, 93,* 424–433.

Ferretti, R. P., & Cavalier, A. R. (1991). Constraints on the problem solving of persons with mental retardation. In N. W. Bray (Ed.), *International Review of Research in Mental Retardation* (Vol. 17, pp. 153–192). San Diego, CA: Academic Press.

Ficker-Terrill, C., & Rowitz, L. (1991). Choices. *Mental Retardation, 29,* 63–64.

Field, S., & Hoffman, A. (1994). Development of a model for self-determination. *Career Development for Exceptional Individuals, 17,* 159–169.

Flavell, J. H. (1985). *Cognitive development* (2nd ed.). Englewood Cliffs, NJ: Prentice Hall.

Forrest, D. L., & Walker, T. G. (1980, April). *What do children know about their reading and study skills?* Paper presented at the annual meeting of the American Educational Research Association, Boston.

Frey, K. S., & Ruble, D. N. (1987). What children say about classroom performance: Sex and grade differences in perceived competence. *Child Development, 58,* 1066–1078.

Gardner, W. I., Cole, C. L., Berry, D. L., & Nowinski, J. M. (1983). Reduction of disruptive behaviors in mentally retarded adults: A self-management approach. *Behavior Modification, 7,* 76–96.

Ghatala, E. S. (1986). Strategy-monitoring training enables young learners to select effective strategies. *Educational Psychologist, 21,* 43–54.

Gothelf, C. R., Crimmins, D. B., Mercer, C. A., & Finocchiaro, P. A. (1994). Teaching choice-making skills to students who are deaf-blind. *Teaching Exceptional Children, 26,* 13–15.

Grace, N., Cowart, C., & Matson, J. L. (1988). Reinforcement and self-control for treating a chronic case of self-injury in Lesch-Nyhan syndrome. *The Journal of the Multihandicapped Person, 1,* 53–59.

Guess, D., Benson, H. A., & Siegel-Causey, E. (1985). Concepts and issues related to choice making and autonomy among persons with severe disabilities. *Journal of the Association for Persons with Severe Handicaps, 10,* 79–86.

Haith, M. (1980). *Rules that babies look by: The organization of newborn visual activity.* Hillsdale, NJ: Lawrence Erlbaum Associates.

Hall, C. S., & Lindzey, G. (1957). *Theories of personality.* New York: John Wiley.

Healey, K., & Masterpasqua, F. (1992). Interpersonal cognitive problem-solving among children with mild mental retardation. *American Journal on Mental Retardation, 96,* 367–372.

Heater, D. (1994). *National self-determination: Woodrow Wilson and his legacy.* New York: St. Martin's Press.

Heider, F. (1958). *The psychology of interpersonal relations.* New York: John Wiley.

Heppner, P. P., & Petersen, C. H. (1982). The development and implications of a personal problem-solving inventory. *The Journal of Counseling Psychology, 29,* 66–75.

Hertz-Lazarowitz, R., & Sharan, S. (1979) Self-esteem, locus of control and children's perception of social climate: A developmental perspective. *Contemporary Educational Psychology, 4,* 154–161.

Heylighen, F. (1992). A cognitive-systemic reconstruction of Maslow's theory of self-actualization. *Behavioral Science, 37,* 39–58.

Houghton, J., Bronicki, G. J. B., & Guess, D. (1987). Opportunities to express preferences and make choices among students with severe disabilities in classroom settings. *Journal of the Association for Persons with Severe Handicaps, 10,* 79–86.

Hughes, C., & Agran, M. (1993). Teaching persons with severe disabilities to use self-instruction in community settings: An analysis of applications. *Journal of the Association for Persons with Severe Handicaps, 18,* 261–274.

Hughes, C., & Rusch, F. R. (1989). Teaching supported employees with severe mental retardation to solve problems. *Journal of Applied Behavior Analysis, 22,* 365–372.

Hughes, C. A., Korinek, L., & Gorman, J. (1991). Self-management for students with mental retardation in public school settings: A research review. *Education and Training in Mental Retardation, 26,* 271–291.

Jaskulski, T., Metzler, C., & Zierman, S. A. (1990). *Forging a new era: The 1990 reports on people with developmental disabilities.* Washington, D.C.: National Association of Developmental Disabilities Councils.

Jones, A., & Crandall, R. (1986). Validation of a short index of self-actualization. *Personality and Social Psychology Bulletin, 12,* 63–73.

Kaser-Boyd, N., Adelman, H. S., & Taylor, L. (1985). Minor's ability to identify risks and benefits of therapy. *Professional Psychology: Research and Practice, 16,* 411–417.

Kendall, P. C. (1984). Social cognition and problem-solving: A developmental and child-clinical interface. In B. Gholson & T. L. Rosenthal (Eds.), *Applications of cognitive developmental theory* (pp. 115–147). New York: Academic Press.

Kishi, G., Teelucksingh, B., Zollers, N., Park-Lee, S., & Meyer, L. (1988). Daily decision-making in community residences: A social comparison of adults with and without mental retardation. *American Journal on Mental Retardation, 92,* 430–435.

Koenigs, S., Fielder, M., & deCharms, R. (1977). Teacher beliefs, classroom interaction and personal control. *The Journal of Applied Social Psychology, 7,* 95–114.

Koestner, R., Ryan, R. M., Bernieri, F., & Holt, K. (1984). The effects of controlling versus informational limit-setting styles on children's intrinsic motivation and creativity. *Journal of Personality, 52,* 233–248.

Knoop, R. (1981). Age and correlates of locus of control. *The Journal of Psychology, 108,* 103–106.

Lefcourt, H. M., (1976). *Locus of control.* Hillsdale, NJ: Lawrence Erlbaum Associates.

Lewis, M., & Brooks-Gunn, J. (1979). *Social cognition and the acquisition of the self.* New York: Plenum.

Martin, J. E., & Marshall, L. H. (1995). Choice Maker: A comprehensive self-determination transition program. *Intervention in School and Clinic, 30,* 147–156.

Maslow, A. H. (1943). A theory of human motivation. *Psychological Review, 50,* 370–396.

McDermott, F. E. (1975). *Self-determination in social work.* London, UK: Routledge and Kegan Paul.

Mercer C. D., & Snell, M. E. (1977). *Learning theory research in mental retardation: Implications for teaching.* Columbus, OH: Charles E. Merrill.

Merighi, J., Edison, M., & Zigler, E. (1990). The role of motivational factors in the functioning of mentally retarded individuals. In R. M. Hodapp, J. A. Burack, & E. Zigler (Eds.), *Issues in the developmental approach to mental retardation* (pp. 114–134). New York: Cambridge University Press.

Mithaug, D. E., & Hanawalt, D. A. (1978). The validation of procedures to assess prevocational task preferences in retarded adults. *Journal of Applied Behavior Analysis, 11,* 153–162.

Moore, S. G. (1979). Social cognition: Knowing about others. *Young Children, 34,* 54–61.

Munk, D. D., & Repp, A. C. (1994). The relationship between instructional variables and problem behavior: A review. *Exceptional Children, 60,* 390–401.

Nicholls, J. G. (1978). The development of the concepts of effort and ability, perceptions of academic attainment, and the understanding that difficult tasks require more ability. *Child Development, 49,* 800–814.

Nirje, B. (1972). The right to self-determination. In W. Wolfensberger (Ed.), *Normalization: The principle of normalization* (pp. 176–200). Toronto: National Institute on Mental Retardation.

Nowicki, S., & Duke, M. P. (1974). A locus of control scale for non-college as well as college adults. *Journal of Personality Assessment, 38,* 136–137.

Ollendick, T. H. (1984). Development and validation of the Children's Assertiveness Inventory. *Child and Family Behavior Therapy, 5,* 1–15.

Ollendick, T. H., Greene, R. W., Francis, G., & Baum, C. G. (1991). Sociometric status: Its stability and validity among neglected, rejected and popular children. *Journal of Child Psychology and Psychiatry, 32,* 525–534.

Ollendick, T. H., Oswald, D., & Crowe, H. P. (1986). *The development and validation of the self-efficacy scale for social skills in children.* Unpublished manuscript.

Ollendick, T. H., & Schmidt, C. R. (1987). Social learning constructs in the prediction of peer interaction. *Journal of Clinical Child Psychology, 16,* 80–87.

Ormond, C., Luszcz, M. A., Mann, L., & Beswick, G. (1991). A metacognitive analysis of decision making in adolescence. *Journal of Adolescence, 14,* 275–291.

Paris, S. G., & Lindauer, B. K. (1982). The development of cognitive skills during childhood. In B. Wolman (Ed.), *Handbook of developmental psychology* (pp. 333–349). Englewood Cliffs, NJ: Prentice Hall.

Park, H. S., & Gaylord-Ross, R. (1989). A problem-solving approach to social skills training in employment settings with mentally retarded youth. *Journal of Applied Behavior Analysis, 22,* 373–380.

Parsons, M. B., McCarn, J. E., & Reid, D. H. (1993). Evaluating and increasing meal-related choices throughout a service setting for people with severe disabilities. *Journal of the Association for Persons with Severe Handicaps, 18,* 253–260.

Perner, J., Frith, U., Leslie, A. M., & Leekham, S. (1989). Exploration of the autistic child's theory of mind: Knowledge, belief and communication. *Child Development, 60,* 689–700.

Perner, J., & Wimmer, H. (1985). John thinks that Mary thinks that: Attribution of second-order beliefs by 5– to 10–year old children. *Journal of Experimental Child Psychology, 39,* 437–471.

Platt, J. P., & Hermalin, J. (1989). Social skill deficit interventions for substance abusers. *Psychology of Addictive Behaviors, 3,* 114–133.

Platt, J., & Spivack, G. (1989). *The MEPS procedure manual.* Philadelphia: Department of Mental Health Sciences, Hahnemann University.

Realon, R. E., Favell, J. E., & Lowerre, A. (1990). The effects of making choices on engagement levels with persons who are profoundly mentally handicapped. *Education and Training in Mental Retardation, 25,* 248–254.

Reid, D. H., Parsons, M. B., & Green, C. W. (1991). *Providing choices and preferences for persons who have severe handicaps.* Morganton, NC: Habilitative Management Consultants.

Renick, M. J., & Harter, S. (1989). Impact of social comparisons on the developing self- perceptions of learning disabled students. *Journal of Educational Psychology, 81,* 631–638.

Rholes, W. S., & Ruble, D. N. (1984). Children's understanding of dispositional characteristics of others. *Child Development, 55,* 550–560.

Rotter, J. B. (1966). Generalized expectancies for internal versus external control of reinforcement. *Psychological Monographs, 80*(1, Whole No. 609).

Ruble, D. N., Boggiano, A. K., Feldman, N. S., & Loebl, J. M. (1980). A developmental analysis of the role of social comparison in self-evaluation. *Developmental Psychology, 16,* 105–115.

Ruble, D. N., & Flett, G. L. (1988). Conflicting goals in self-evaluative information seeking: Developmental and ability level analyses. *Child Development, 59,* 97–106.

Sands, D. J., & Wehmeyer, M. L. (1996). Future directions in self-determination: Articulating values and policies, organizing organizational structures, and implementing professional practices. In D.J. Sands & M.L. Wehmeyer (Eds.), *Self-determination across the life span: Independence and choice for people with disabilities* (pp. 331–344). Baltimore: Paul H. Brookes.

Scarr, S., Weinberg, R. A., & Levine, A. (1986). *Understanding development.* San Diego: Harcourt Brace Jovanovich.

Schalock, R. L. (1996). Reconsidering the conceptualization and measurement of quality of life. In R. Schalock (Ed.), *Quality of life: Conceptualization and measurement* (Vol. I, pp. 123–139). Washington, DC: American Association on Mental Retardation.

Schunk, D. H. (1989). Self-efficacy and cognitive achievement: Implications for students with learning problems. *Journal of Learning Disabilities, 22,* 14–22.

Selman, R. L. (1980). *The growth of interpersonal understanding.* New York: Academic Press.

Shantz, C. U. (1975). The development of social cognition. In E.M. Heterington (Ed.), *Review of child development research* (Vol. 5, pp. 257–323). Chicago: University of Chicago Press.

Sherman, I. W. (1984). Development of children's perceptions of internal locus of control: A cross-sectional and longitudinal analysis. *Journal of Personality, 52,* 338–354.

Shevin, M., & Klein, N. K. (1984). The importance of choice-making skills for students with severe disabilities. *Journal of the Association for Persons with Severe Handicaps, 9,* 159–166.

Short, F. J., & Evans, S. W. (1990). Individual differences in cognitive and social problem-solving skills as a function of intelligence. In N. W. Bray (Ed.), *International review of research in mental retardation* (Vol. 16, pp. 89–123). San Diego, CA: Academic Press.

Sigafoos, A. D., Feinstein, C. B., Damond, M., & Reiss, D. (1988). The measurement of behavioral autonomy in adolescence: The Autonomous Functioning Checklist. In C. B. Feinstein, A. Esman, J. Looney, G. Orvin, J. Schimel, A. Schwartzberg, A. Sorsky & M. Sugar (Eds.), *Adolescent psychiatry* (Vol. 15, pp. 432–462). Chicago: University of Chicago Press.

Skinner, E. A. (1990). Age differences in the dimensions of perceived control during middle childhood: Implications for developmental conceptualizations and research. *Child Development, 61,* 1882–1890.

Spivack, G., & Shure, M. (1974). *Social adjustment of young children.* San Francisco: Jossey-Bass.

Stancliffe, R. (1995). Assessing opportunities for choice making: A comparison of self-report and staff reports. *American Journal on Mental Retardation, 99,* 418–429.

Stancliffe, R., & Wehmeyer, M. L. (1995). Variability in the availability of choice to adults with mental retardation. *Journal of Vocational Rehabilitation, 5,* 319–328.

Stern, D. (1985). *The interpersonal world of the infant.* New York: Basic Books.

Swann, W. B., & Pittman, T. S. (1977). Initiating play activity of children: The moderating influence of verbal cues on intrinsic motivation. *Child Development, 48,* 1128–1132.

Switzky, H. N. (1997). Individual differences in personality and motivational systems in persons with mental retardation. In W.E. MacLean (Ed.), *Ellis' handbook of mental deficiency, psychological theory and research* (3rd ed., pp. 343–377). Hillsdale, NJ: Lawrence Erlbaum Associates.

Trabasso, T., Stein, N., Rodkin, P., Park, M., & Baughn, C. (1992). Knowledge of goals and plans in the on-line narration of events. *Cognitive Development, 7,* 133–170.

Ward, M. J. (1996). Coming of age in the age of self-determination: A historical and personal perspective. In D. J. Sands & M. L. Wehmeyer (Eds.), *Self-determination across the life span: Independence and choice for people with disabilities* (pp. 1–16). Baltimore: Paul H. Brookes.

Warren, B. (1993). *The right to choose: A training curriculum.* New York: New York State Office of Mental Retardation and Developmental Disabilities.

Wehman, P. & Moon, C. (1988). *Vocational rehabilitation and supported employment.* Baltimore: Paul H. Brookes.

Wehmeyer, M. L. (1992a). Self-determination and the education of students with mental retardation. *Education and Training in Mental Retardation, 27,* 302–314.

Wehmeyer, M. L. (1992b). Self-determination: Critical skills for outcome-oriented transition services. *The Journal for Vocational Special Needs Education, 39,* 153–163.

196   WEHMEYER

Wehmeyer, M. L., (1993). Perceptual and psychological factors in career decision-making of adolescents with and without cognitive disabilities. *Career Development for Exceptional Individuals, 16,* 135–146.

Wehmeyer, M. L. (1994a). Perceptions of self-determination and psychological empowerment of adolescents with mental retardation. *Education and Training in Mental Retardation and Developmental Disability, 29,* 9–21.

Wehmeyer, M. L., (1994b). Reliability and acquiescence in the measurement of locus of control with adolescents and adults with mental retardation. *Psychological Reports, 75,* 527–537.

Wehmeyer, M. L. (1996a). Self-determination as an educational outcome: Why is it important to children, youth and adults with disabilities? In D. J. Sands & M. L. Wehmeyer (Eds.), *Self-determination across the life span: Independence and choice for people with disabilities* (pp. 15–34). Baltimore: Paul H. Brookes.

Wehmeyer, M. L., (1996b). Self-determination for youth with significant cognitive disabilities: From theory to practice. In L. Powers, G. H. S. Singer, & J. Sowers (Eds.), *On the road to autonomy: Promoting self-competence in children and youth with disabilities* (pp. 115–133). Baltimore: Paul H. Brookes.

Wehmeyer, M. L. (1996c). A self-report measure of self-determination for adolescents with cognitive disabilities. *Education and Training in Mental Retardation and Developmental Disabilities, 31,* 282–293.

Wehmeyer, M. L. (1997). Self-determination as an educational outcome: A definitional framework and implications for intervention. *Journal of Developmental and Physical Disabilities, 9,* 175–209.

Wehmeyer, M. L., Agran, M., & Hughes, C. (1998). *Teaching self-determination to youth with disabilities Basic skills for successful transition.* Baltimore: Paul H. Brookes.

Wehmeyer, M. L., & Bolding, N. (1999). Self-determination across living and working environments: A matched-samples study of adults with mental retardation. *Mental Retardation, 37,* 353–363.

Wehmeyer, M. L., & Kelchner, K. (1994). Interpersonal cognitive problem-solving skills of individuals with mental retardation. *Education and Training in Mental Retardation, 29,* 265–278.

Wehmeyer, M. L., & Kelchner, K. (1995a). Measuring the autonomy of adolescents and adults with mental retardation: A self-report form of the Autonomous Functioning Checklist. *Career Development for Exceptional Individuals, 18,* 3–20.

Wehmeyer, M. L., & Kelchner, K. (1995b). *The Arc's self-determination scale.* Arlington, TX: The Arc National Headquarters.

Wehmeyer, M. L., Kelchner, K., & Richards, S. (1995). Individual and environmental factors related to the self-determination of adults with mental retardation. *Journal of Vocational Rehabilitation, 5,* 291–305.

Wehmeyer, M. L., Kelchner, K., & Richards. S. (1996). Essential characteristics of self-determined behaviors of adults with mental retardation and developmental disabilities. *American Journal on Mental Retardation, 100,* 632–642.

Wehmeyer, M. L., & Metzler, C. A. (1995). How self-determined are people with mental retardation? The National Consumer Survey. *Mental Retardation, 33,* 111–119.

Wehmeyer, M. L., & Palmer, S. B. (1997). Perceptions of control of students with and without cognitive disabilities. *Psychological Reports, 81,* 195–206.

Wehmeyer, M. L., Palmer, S., Agran, M. Mithaug, D., & Martin, J. (2000). Promoting casual agency: The Self-Determined Learning Model of Instruction. *Exceptional Children, 66,* 439–453.

Wehmeyer, M. L., Sands, D. J., Doll, B., & Palmer, S.B. (1997). The development of self-determination and implications for educational interventions with students with disabilities. *International Journal of Disability, Development, and Education, 44,* 212–225.

Wehmeyer, M. L., & Schwartz, M. (1997). Self-determination and positive adult outcomes: A follow-up study of youth with mental retardation or learning disabilities. *Exceptional Children, 63,* 245–255.

Wehmeyer, M. L., & Schwartz, M. (1998). The relationship between self-determination and quality of life for adults with mental retardation. *Education and Training in Mental Retardation and Developmental Disabilities, 33,* 3–12.

Werner, H., & Kaplan, B. (1965). *Symbol formation.* Hillsdale, NJ: Lawrence Erlbaum Associates.

West, M. D., & Parent, W. S. (1992). Consumer choice and empowerment in supported employment services: Issues and strategies. *Journal of the Association for Persons with Severe Handicaps, 17,* 47–52.

Wheeler, D. (1991). Metaphors for effective thinking. In J. Baron & R. Brown (Eds), *Teaching decision making to adolescents* (pp. 309–327). Hillsdale, NJ: Lawrence Erlbaum Associates.

White, R. W. (1959). Motivation reconsidered: The concept of competence. *Psychological Review, 66,* 297–333.

Whitman, T. L. (1990). Self-regulation and mental retardation. *American Journal on Mental Retardation, 94,* 347–362.

Williams, R. R. (1989). Creating a new world of opportunity: Expanding choice and self-determination in lives of Americans with severe disability by 1992 and beyond. In R. Perske (Ed.), *Proceedings from the National Conference on Self-Determination* (pp. 16–17). Minneapolis, MN: Institute on Community Integration.

Wolfensberger, W. (1972). *Normalization: The principle of normalization.* Toronto: National Institute on Mental Retardation.

Zimmerman, M. A. (1990). Toward a theory of learned hopefulness: A structural model analysis of participation and empowerment. *Journal of Research in Personality, 24,* 71–86.

4

The Role of Motivation in the Decision Making of People With Mental Retardation

Linda Hickson and Ishita Khemka

Teachers College, Columbia University, New York

INTRODUCTION

On March 1, 1989, a 17–year-old girl with mental retardation was shooting baskets by herself at a playground near her home in Glen Ridge, New Jersey. Initially, she refused when asked by a group of popular, high-school athletes, some of whom had made fun of her in the past, to come with them to one of their homes. Insistent, one of them put his arm around her and promised her a date with his older brother if she would come. He led her to his friends' basement, where she was sexually assaulted repeatedly with a variety of objects—including a bat and a broomstick—in the presence of 13 laughing, cheering male onlookers. Although six of the onlookers left the scene early because they felt "uncomfortable," none made any effort to help the young woman to escape from the situation (Lefkowitz, 1997).

In a recent study (Hickson, Golden, Khemka, Urv, & Yamusah, 1998), adults with and without mental retardation were asked to respond to a brief vignette based on the above situation. In the vignette, Jeff approached Emily who was shooting baskets in the park and asked her to come with him to his friends' house. When she initially refused, "Jeff, who had often made fun of Emily in the past, put his arm around Emily and promised her a date with his handsome older brother" if she would come with him. When asked what Emily should do, all but one of the respondents without mental retardation said that Emily should not go with Jeff. However, only one third of the respondents with mental retardation said that Emily should not go with Jeff.

Along with opportunities for community inclusion, people with mental retardation often encounter situations involving exploitation and abuse. The particular vulnerability of these individuals to victimization is exemplified in the widely publicized Glen Ridge, New Jersey case described above and in numerous other well-known incidents in which people with intellectual disabilities fail to make self-protective decisions. In one such case, described by Greenspan (1996), Richard LaPointe, a man with Dandy-Walker syndrome, was sentenced to life in prison after being tricked, during a grueling and deceptive police interrogation, into confessing to a murder that many believe he did not commit. According to Greenspan (1999b), impaired social intelligence is central to the natural prototype of mental retardation that manifests itself in real-life situations, particularly in demanding interpersonal situations that are novel, ambiguous, or coercive.

The specific reasons why people with mental retardation so often fail to make effective decisions, however, are not yet well understood. Perhaps one barrier to reaching a full understanding of the decision-making processes of people with mental retardation has been that, until very recently, the theoretical focus in this body of literature has been almost exclusively cognitive. Recent efforts to explore the interplay of cognitive, motivational, and emotional factors in the decision making of people with mental retardation have been promising. The theoretical literature on decision making in people without mental retardation generally supports this broader perspective (see Hickson & Khemka, 1999b). In addition, researchers who have studied motivation in people with mental retardation have typically advocated a broader view. Zigler (1999), for example, admonished researchers

to look at the whole person with mental retardation by considering personality variables that include motivational and emotional
features.

In this chapter, the motivational aspects of decision making
in people with mental retardation are examined. Theoretical perspectives on motivation are considered followed by a discussion
of research on motivation and related personality factors in people with mental retardation. A general overview of theoretical perspectives and research on decision making is followed by a
focused look at the role of motivation in the interpersonal decision making of people with mental retardation. In the remainder
of the chapter, new directions for research and theory on motivation and decision making in mental retardation are explored in
light of a framework proposed to guide future research.

THEORETICAL
PERSPECTIVES ON MOTIVATION

Motivational factors are important determinants of decision-
making performance. In the context of decision making, motivation can affect whether a person chooses to engage in a
decision-making process at all as well as their selection of a goal
and of a means for attaining that goal. Traditional models of decision making have highlighted the motivational relevance of a person's self-perceptions of control in terms of his or her ability to
attain a particular goal and the extent to which he or she values
that goal.

The construct of control has a rich history in psychological
theory on human motivation. Examined within various theoretical frameworks, the emphasis has been on addressing perceptions of control from the perspective of personal expectancies or
behavior-outcome contingencies (see Bandura, 1977; Deci, 1975;
Rotter, 1966; Seligman, 1975). These theories contend that an
individual's personality, motivation, or expectancy beliefs can
influence cognitive processing, effort, and persistence in a given
situation or over time.

Other theorists have framed their work on motivation in
terms of individual goal selection and attainment of outcomes
that match valued goals or priorities (see Bandura, 1977; Deci &

Ryan, 1985; Ford, 1992; Higgins, 1997). The specific nature of a behavioral response is motivated by an individual's awareness of self-values and goals and the underlying need to reach valued goal conditions.

The remainder of this section includes a broad overview of prominent theories of motivation that focus on behavior-outcome contingencies that pertain to defining motivational processes in terms of future expectancies of attainability of desired outcomes. Next, theories are highlighted that focus on goal-related processes in motivation. Finally, Ford's (1992) broad-based motivational systems theory is considered along with the relevance of various theoretical constructs to interpersonal decision making.

Role of Perceptions of Control in Motivation

Rotter's (1966) social learning perspective posited that a person enters a situation with expectancies, based on past experience, regarding the probable outcomes of his or her behaviors. These expectancies for behavior-outcome contingencies are characterized in the construct of locus of control that has been researched widely in people with and without mental retardation. Locus of control refers to the generalized belief that one's outcomes are under the control (contingent upon) of one's own behavior (an internal locus of control orientation) versus the belief that outcomes are largely under the control of external factors such as luck, chance, or powerful others (an external locus of control orientation). A person with an internal locus of control orientation, therefore, views himself or herself as able to control consequences (hence attributing responsibility for outcomes to oneself) whereas a person with an external locus of control orientation views outcomes as primarily controlled by others (hence attributing responsibility for outcomes to factors other than oneself). It is implied that individuals with an internal locus of control orientation are able to see the contingency between their behavior and the outcome of a situation and, consequently, are likely to exert more effort and show greater persistence in the face of a challenging problem or decision than are individuals with an external locus of control orientation. Thus, locus of control allows one to predict whether a person is likely to engage in motivated, intentional action.

The theory of learned helplessness (Seligman, 1975) focuses on pervasive, causal interpretative beliefs (behavior-outcome expectancies) for negative events that reflect individual pessimism and demotivating patterns with negative affective consequences. Learned helplessness, defined as the perception of no control over outcomes (i.e., independence between behavior and outcomes), leads to attributions of failure to uncontrollable factors and decreased task perseverance following failure. The behavioral effects of learned helplessness (e.g., amotivation, passivity, disorganized action) are similar to those predicted by Rotter's (1966) social learning theory for individuals with external locus of control perceptions.

Attribution theories focus on people's causal analyses of, or attributions about, how events occur and influence future expectations, emotions, and performance (Fiske & Taylor, 1984). Through causal attributions, individuals explain their own and others' behaviors. Weiner (1979) presented a model of causal attributions in the context of achievement behavior suggesting that in an achievement situation, an individual searches for the cause of failure or success along three dimensions: locus (internal vs. external), stability (fixed vs. temporary), and controllability (controllable vs. uncontrollable). The most common and salient factors of achievement outcomes relate to individual ability, effort, luck, and task difficulty, where ability is considered to be an internal, uncontrollable, and fixed factor and effort is considered to be an external, controllable, and temporary factor (and therefore changeable). Generally, higher achievement is associated with giving oneself credit for success and attributing failure to a lack of effort or bad luck (Weiner, 1985). Individuals who acknowledge the importance of effort are more likely to engage in future tasks with higher motivation and more confidence. Attribution theories have provided the framework for altering individual attributions to make them more achievement-enhancing through attributional retraining that helps decrease learned helplessness (Dweck, 1975). Attribution of responsibility for outcomes is closely related to the locus of control construct.

Dweck (1991) proposed an attribution-based framework for studying the motivational processes of children. The framework is based on the premise that children operate from within an implicit theory of ability that determines their pursuit of goals in achievement situations. Children with an incremental theory view ability as a changeable and increasable and, therefore, controllable construct, whereas children with an entity theory view ability as a fixed and unchangeable and, therefore, uncontrollable construct. An incremental view of ability orients the individual toward self-development, high motivation, and a willingness to pursue challenges and persevere. An entity view of ability, on the other hand, is associated with self-judgment, low motivation, and a tendency to avoid challenges and to give up easily (Dweck & Leggett, 1988). An incremental theory of ability is reflected in a tendency to attribute failures to a lack of effort, on the assumption that when individuals believe that their performance is regulated by their own effort, they also believe that their performance and, hence abilities, can be increased through greater effort. An incremental theory seems akin to internal locus of control beliefs while an entity theory, like external locus of control beliefs, operates to discourage effort.

Self-efficacy theory (Bandura, 1977) focuses on situation-specific, individual expectancies or judgments of capabilities for effective action that help predict actual behavior. Bandura conceptualized control beliefs not as perceived responsibility for behavior as in the locus of control construct, but rather as an individual's perceived control over a given behavior in terms of self-efficacy or the subjective probability that one is capable of executing a certain course of action. Efficacy expectancies are regarded as prime motivators of human behavior and are linked to greater amounts and longer persistence of individual effort in the confrontation of obstacles and aversive experiences (Bandura, 1986). Self-efficacy beliefs have also been correlated with adaptive coping behavior (Bandura, Adams, & Meyer, 1977).

Rodin (1990) described the concept of desire for control as the extent to which people are motivated to want control (i.e., see themselves in control of the events in their lives). Measured along a continuum, a high desire for control is associated with the belief that outcomes are the result of personal action and not the action of others. A positive relationship between desire for control and achievement behavior is found with individuals having a high desire for control showing greater perseverance, maintaining higher aspiration levels, and responding with greater effort to difficult tasks, than with individuals with low desire for control. Burger and Cooper (1979) and Burger (1992) have also contended that there are persisting individual differences in motivation linked to people's motivational tendencies to control personal events in their lives. Individuals with a strong desire for control are more likely to take actions that reflect attempts to make their own decisions, instead of having decisions made for them, and to take actions that prevent any loss of their control.

Although diverse in terms of specific considerations and principles, a general position of the above theories is that individuals (conceptualized as agents) are motivated by specific perceptions of control, or personal agency beliefs, that determine how they approach and react to particular situations. Furthermore, the beliefs are a measure of a person's perceived potential (the expectancy) for control over his or her behaviors and do not represent the person's actual control over the behaviors. These beliefs play a critical role in decision making by determining whether a person who is faced with a coercive or manipulative interpersonal situation will be motivated to attempt an action to resist the manipulation.

Rotter (1966) indicated that individuals with an internal locus of control orientation would be more resistant to outside manipulation if they were aware of the manipulation as this would make them feel deprived of their ability to control the environment. Individuals with an external locus of control orientation, on the other hand, with their expectation that control would come from the outside, would be less resistant to any manipulation. Getter (1962), Pines and Julian (1972), Sherman (1984), and Strickland (1989) have supported Rotter's assertion in their studies. It is reasonable to conclude that individuals with an internal locus of control orientation, being more discriminating in which influences they accept, differ in their ways of handling social influence when compared to individuals with external perceptions of control.

An individual's self-awareness of his or her own capabilities and level of confidence, or personal agency beliefs, are critical to decision-making performance (Cacioppo & Petty, 1982; Fischhoff, 1975; Ford, 1992; Verplanken, 1993). Deci and Ryan (1987), Elms (1976), Janis (1974), Janis and Mann (1977), Lefcourt (1982),

Mann, Harmoni, and Power (1989), and Radford, Mann, Ohta, and Nakane (1993) emphasized the role of self-esteem, locus of control, self-efficacy, and other predispositional characteristics of the decision-maker in influencing decision-making competence and decision response styles.

Burnett, Mann, and Beswick (1989) and Radford et al. (1993) established a positive correlation between decisional self-esteem, defined as confidence and self-perception concerning the ability to make good decisions, and decisional vigilance response styles. Defensive avoidance, complacency, and hypervigilance response styles were found to be negatively correlated with decisional self-esteem and positively correlated with decisional stress. Mann, Harmoni, Power, and Beswick (1986) (cited in Mann et al., 1989) found a positive relationship between internality, greater decisional self-esteem, and higher performance on a decision-making recognition task for a group of adolescents 15–17 years old.

Ollendick, Greene, Francis, and Baum (1991) found externality to be related with impulsive decision making and distractibility. Studies by Deci and Ryan (1987) and Lent and Hackett (1987) have shown that perceived control can influence the type of educational and career choices an individual makes. Bandura and Wood (1988) indicated that individuals who believed strongly in their problem-solving capabilities performed more efficiently in complex decision-making situations. The importance of personality variables such as locus of control, self-attribution, and self-efficacy in decision-making performance has also been noted by Abery (1994).

Role of Goal-Related Processes in Motivation

In addition to the role of control beliefs, the role of goal-related processes in motivation has attracted considerable theoretical interest (Kuhl, 1986; Spaulding, 1994). Motivation plays a central role in determining which goal a person selects and how that person evaluates the possible consequences of a decision. Different desired goal-states motivate individuals to regulate themselves differently, leading to differences in both the emotional and the cognitive aspects of decision making.

The substantive content of a decision or the value of a decision outcome may determine the extent to which an individual will engage himself or herself in a decision-making activity (McGuire & McGuire, 1991; Simon 1985). Certain decisions may be of high personal relevance and interest to a decision-maker whereas others may be insignificant or of little interest. The motivation to engage in a decision-making event is derived from the value attached to goal attainability by the decision-maker. In addition, the literature provides considerable evidence that individuals' motivational beliefs (e.g., self-perceptions of control, efficacy expectations, goals, and purposes) influence decision-making engagement and performance.

Fishbein and Ajzen's (1975) theory of reasoned action and its extension, the theory of planned behavior (Ajzen & Madden, 1986), provide a conceptual framework for studying the effect of perceived behavioral control on the attainment of goals. The theory posits that an individual's intentions and expectations to pursue a particular goal are important motivational antecedents serving as direct predictors of a person's actual actions. Attitudes and beliefs about desired and expected outcomes and the perceived ease or difficulty of performing the goal-directed behaviors (the perceived behavioral control) determine intentions. Given favorable attitudes and sufficient pressures to perform a behavior, higher perceived behavioral control results in stronger intentions to achieve the goal.

Skinner, Chapman, and Baltes (1988) identified control beliefs that are useful in predicting certain actions and outcomes. Actions, or goal-intentional behaviors, are influenced by beliefs related to perceived control that involve understanding the relation among agents (individuals), means (or causes), and ends (or goal-related outcomes). Skinner et al. proposed a model of perceived control that comprises three distinct sets of beliefs: control beliefs are defined as individual expectancies about the ability to obtain desired outcomes; means-ends beliefs detail expectancies about the extent to which certain means or causes lead to desirable outcomes; and agency or capacity beliefs pertain to expectancies about the extent to which an individual possesses certain potential means for attaining outcomes. The capacity beliefs in this model are similar to Bandura's idea of self-efficacy beliefs as they pertain to whether an individual has or can acquire the means to perform certain behaviors.

Expectancy-value theories (e.g., Atkinson, 1957) view behavior as a function of individual expectancies of obtaining a particular outcome and the extent to which those outcomes are valued. Motivation for behavior is determined jointly by the outcome expectancies and the values. Individuals make likelihood judgments of attaining various goals in given situations, pursuing only those goals that seem valuable and attainable. Therefore, for an individual to be motivated to act, he or she must not only experience positive outcome expectancies but must also highly value the pursued outcome.

Self-determination theory (Deci & Ryan, 1985) has provided an impetus for thinking about the impact of motivation on individual actions and interactions as central to human agency. Based on Deci's (1975) theory of motivation, which helped clarify the roles of intrinsic and extrinsic motivation in an individual's capacity to effect changes in the environment, the self-determination theory was expanded to address the enduring motivational impact of individual experiences in shaping behavior and intentional action. According to Deci, extrinsic motivation is linked to performing behaviors to gain external rewards such as money and verbal praise. On the other hand, intrinsic motivation results in performing behaviors to satisfy internal sources of gratification related to satisfying curiosity or demonstrating that one is capable of exercising control. To achieve intrinsic motivation, decision-control (interpreted as the opportunity to make choices) and feelings of self-determination are central. Intrinsic motivation is seen as maintaining an individual's sense of choice over what happens and the ability to act on and adapt to environmental surroundings more competently.

Deci and Ryan (1985) described a continuum of self-determination involving three distinct personality orientations that result from differences in levels of intrinsic motivation among individuals: autonomy (the tendency to seek out opportunities to express self-determination and choice); control (the tendency to perform under external motivation or pressures); and impersonal (the tendency to believe that outcomes are not controllable). Individuals with an autonomous orientation tend to regulate choices based on self-awareness of needs and goals and are likely to be more internally motivated to achieve. At the other extreme, individuals with an impersonal orientation believe that choices are beyond intentional control and are likely to be amotivational or helpless. The theory also suggests that there is an inherently motivated developmental process whereby people build upon and refine their regulatory processes to integrate and internalize behaviors that allow them to be more self-determining than controlled.

Self-determination theory has generated a great deal of interest as it pertains to individuals with mental retardation. A number of related frameworks and assessment procedures have been developed to promote a better understanding of the components and organization of goal-related motivational patterns in individuals with mental retardation (see Abery, 1994; Mithaug, 1993; Wehmeyer, 1994b; 1998).

Higgins' (1997) *regulatory-focus theory* illustrates how individuals regulate themselves in decision-making situations. Individual motivational patterns, qualified by differences in goal content and goal setting, are described in terms of their component processes and behavioral consequences. Individuals pursue different decision outcomes, based on their differing motivational tendencies, seeking alternate goal states that may be either promotion-focused or prevention-focused. Promotion-focused motivational goals relate to accomplishment, advancement, nurturance, and growth. On the other hand, prevention-focused regulation is motivated by goals of avoiding danger and loss, maintaining safety, responsibility, and protection.

Mischel and Shoda (1995) highlighted personal goals and values as comprising important cognitive-affective units in the personality system. In proposing a *unified cognitive-affective personality system theory,* they identified different types of mediating processes (e.g., expectancies and beliefs, affect, goals, and self-regulatory plans) that are essential for activating behavior and accounting for individual variance in behavior across different situations. From a goal-orientation perspective, they suggested that goals influence the organization of the relationships among cognitive and affective units in the personality system that ultimately guides individual motivation of behavior over time. Individuals seek and respond to situations and outcomes guided by their personal goals and subjective values and organized by their self-regulatory plans and strategies.

The above theories continue to influence theory and research on motivation, most importantly through their consideration of goal concepts as a complex and integrated part of human motivation and behavior. Goal setting is hypothesized to serve an important cognitive function affecting motivation (Bandura, 1988; Locke & Latham, 1990; Schunk, 1991). In general, these theories identify a preferred or adaptive goal orientation as opposed to a less than optimal or maladaptive goal orientation for the pursuit and attainment of personal goals.

Motivational Systems Theory and Applications to Decision Making

The *motivational systems theory* (Ford, 1992) provides a comprehensive model for the study of motivation by integrating constructs from both perceptions of control and goal-orientation theories. Ford described motivation as the "organized patterning of an individual's personal goals, emotions, and personal agency beliefs" (p.78). These motivational elements represent anticipatory and evaluative psychological processes that help people prepare to act or get involved in activities in ways intended to produce desired outcomes. Personal goals represent thoughts about desired future states and outcomes and help regulate a person's activity to produce those desired states. Personal agency beliefs refer to motivational expectancies related to a person's capabilities, the skills, needed to attain goal-directed activities (capability beliefs) and to the responsiveness of a person's context or environment toward goal-attainment efforts (context beliefs). Emotional arousal processes reflecting different motivational influences serve the function of preparing a person to evaluate and handle complex behavioral demands tied to personally relevant events and consequences. Goals, personal agency beliefs, and emotions all work together in the process of decision making.

The broad overview of theories of motivation presented in the preceding sections provides a conceptual framework for understanding the issues involved in the definition and study of motivation in the context of decision making. Although the theories have explored motivation from a number of different per-spectives and in terms of a variety of constructs, they center on people's perception of and confidence in their ability to control and regulate important events in their lives. In addition, certain theories clarify the roles of goal identification and selection as important determinants of motivation to act.

Overall, the theories identify common characteristics of indi-viduals who are likely to display a poor motivational response to situations that pose challenges or risks. Many of these are charac-teristics frequently observed in people with mental retardation. In general, individuals with low personal agency beliefs (manifested as external locus of control perceptions, low self-efficacy beliefs, diminished perceived control, or an impersonal causality orienta-tion) experience low confidence in their ability, experience feel-ings of incompetence to obtain desired outcomes, demonstrate performance deficiencies, and behave in a helpless manner. On the other hand, individuals with high personal agency beliefs are likely to respond more adaptively to obstacles and failures, show resilient persistence, and be internally motivated to effect out-comes. Independent of personal agency beliefs, motivation is linked to the pursuit of valued and seemingly attainable goals. Interpreting motivational mechanisms in terms of personal agency beliefs and goal-directed behavior forms a theoretical basis for the study of the role of motivation in the decision making of people with mental retardation.

RESEARCH ON MOTIVATION AND RELATED PERSONALITY FACTORS IN PEOPLE WITH MENTAL RETARDATION

It is likely that perceptions of control and goal-related processes play pivotal roles in the decision-making performance of people with mental retardation, just as they do in people without mental retardation. Even when people with mental retardation can be shown to possess the cognitive skills and strategies needed for effective decision making, their decisions continue to reflect a variety of maladaptive patterns. These patterns include a failure to initiate action, a rigid reliance on past experience, and overre-liance on others in the decision-making situation (see Hickson &

Khemka, 1999b). The cognitive limitations associated with mental retardation cannot fully explain these patterns. An examination of existing research on motivational and personality factors suggests that some of these factors may be contributing to the decision-making difficulties of people with mental retardation.

Definitions of learned helplessness typically include at least two components, (1) a self-perception that an individual cannot exert control over a specific outcome and (2) evidence of deficits in response initiation and perseverance. The few existing studies involving people with mental retardation dealt primarily with performance deficits (Weisz, 1999). It was suggested that the development of helplessness may be fostered by high rates of failure feedback or attributions by others that lead them to tolerate low levels of performance in people with mental retardation (Weisz, 1999).

Weisz (1979) reported that children with mental retardation showed more evidence of helplessness on three performance measures than children without mental retardation, but only at mental age levels above 7.0. Weisz suggested that helplessness may be acquired gradually during development. In another study, Weisz (1981) found that after failure feedback, children with mental retardation declined in their use of effective strategies, while children without mental retardation did not show such a decline. The performance of the children with mental retardation was considered consistent with a learned helplessness interpretation. In addition, teachers rated children with mental retardation as more helpless than children without mental retardation on a teacher checklist. Gargiulo and O'Sullivan (1986) reported that children with mental retardation scored as more helpless than children without mental retardation on measures similar to those used by Weisz (1979, 1981).

Two additional studies involved comparisons between groups with and without mental retardation that were matched on chronological age rather than mental age. In 1985, Reynolds and Miller administered measures of both helplessness and depression to adolescents with and without mental retardation. They found that the adolescents with mental retardation obtained higher scores than the adolescents without mental retardation on both measures. Floor and Rosen (1975) also reported higher helplessness scores for individuals with mental retardation on several measures.

In a recent study, Palmer and Wehmeyer (1998) looked at the related construct of hopelessness in 10- to 19-year-old students with mental retardation, with learning disabilities, and without disabilities. Hopelessness was defined as "a negative expectation of oneself and the future" (Palmer & Wehmeyer, 1998, p. 130). In a study of children without disabilities, Kazdin, Rodgers, and Colbus (1986) reported that children with relatively high hopelessness scores were more depressed, had lower self-esteem, and received lower social behavior ratings by self and parents. Palmer and Wehmeyer (1998) found that students with mental retardation held less hopeful expectations for the future than students with learning disabilities and students without disabilities.

Learned helplessness among individuals with mental retardation has been linked to their exposure to repeated failures, to their inability to exercise control over outcomes, and to helplessness-inducing negative feedback that attributes their failure to uncontrollable factors. Zigler and Hodapp (1986) suggested that these factors lead individuals to distrust their own abilities and to seek outside help. It may be that self-perceptions of helplessness or hopelessness in people with mental retardation contribute to their tendency not to attempt a self-protective action in many decision-making situations where there is the potential for harm or danger.

Achenbach and Zigler (1963) focused on the discrepancy between the ideal self-image and the real self-image—differentiation increases with developmental level (Glick, 1999). It has been suggested that self-discrepancies may play a role in motivating behavior. Bandura (1990) proposed that people create challenging standards and then mobilize to attain their goals. When goal attainment reduces the discrepancy, they may set even higher standards. Similarly, according to Markus and Nurius (1986), positive possible selves give direction to desired future states (e.g., good job, love from family) and negative possible selves clarify what is to be avoided (e.g., unemployment, loneliness, and social rejection).

Much subsequent research has focused on self-esteem or self-worth. As emphasized in the work of Harter (1999) and her colleagues, self-esteem may be viewed as both a global construct and as many different domain-specific constructs, which can vary within an individual in terms of importance and self-perceived competence. Harter, Whitesell, and Junkin (1998) reported that normally achieving high school students expressed more positive feelings of self-worth than students with behavior disorders and learning disabilities in the domains of cognitive competence, likeability, athletic competence, job competence, and close friendship as well as on global self-worth. Harter et al. (1998) pointed out that it is essential to consider each student's importance ratings for these domains in planning interventions.

In a recent study, Khemka, Hickson, and Chatzistyli (1999) found significant differences between female adolescents with learning disabilities and mild mental retardation and those with moderate to severe mental retardation on only three of nine domains on the Harter Self-Perception Profile for Adolescents. The girls with mild disabilities reported higher self-esteem than did the girls with moderate to severe disabilities in the domains of physical appearance and job competence. Girls with moderate to severe disabilities reported higher self-esteem than did the girls with mild disabilities only for the domain of athletic competence, where scores were generally low for both groups. The two disability groups did not differ significantly on global self-worth.

The question of whether efforts should be made to increase self-esteem is somewhat controversial. Bandura (1997) has taken the position that self-esteem is not the construct to focus upon because it does not affect either personal goals or performance. Instead, Bandura has identified self-efficacy as a key variable with direct links to goals and performance. However, in a recent study, Yamusah (1998) reported that two effective methods for increasing self-esteem in multiple domains in adults with mental retardation were also associated with increases in both social and general self-efficacy, suggesting an extensive overlap between these constructs. Because both self-esteem and self-efficacy appear to be diminished in people with mental retardation, there may be more justification for interventions aimed at strengthening these characteristics in this population than in populations without disabilities. It is possible that low self-perceptions on these variables may discourage people with mental retardation from attempting to take action in challenging decision-making situations.

Mercer and Snell (1977), in their review of five studies that examined the locus of control orientations of individuals with mental retardation, found four of these studies (Fox, 1972; Gruen, Ottinger, & Ollendick, 1974; Reidel & Milgram, 1970; Shipe, 1971) to indicate that individuals with mental retardation are likely to be more externally oriented than their peers without mental retardation. Recently, Wehmeyer (1993b) found adolescents and adults with mental retardation to be more external when compared to their same-age peers with learning disabilities and to their nondisabled peers. Wehmeyer (1993b) also found external locus of control orientations as negatively impacting the career decision-making ability of adolescents with mental retardation.

Locus of control does not become more internal with age in populations with mental retardation as it does in populations without disabilities. Instead perceptions of adolescents and adults with mental retardation tend to remain largely external (Wehmeyer, 1993a, 1994c; Wehmeyer & Kelchner, 1996; Wehmeyer, Kelchner, & Richards, 1996; Wehmeyer & Palmer, 1997).

Wehmeyer (1994a) compared individuals with mental retardation in sheltered workshops with those in competitive settings and found individuals in sheltered workshops to have a higher external locus of control orientation than their counterparts in competitive, part-, or full-time employment. With competitive employment settings being associated with more internality in locus of control, the potential importance of greater opportunities for choice and control in shaping favorable perceptions of control orientation among individuals with mental retardation was established. Wehmeyer correlated internality with higher self-esteem, higher self-concept, and lower anxiety levels for individuals with mental retardation.

Wehmeyer and Palmer (1997) suggested several possible reasons for the external perceptions of control by people with mental retardation: (1) Interactions with nondisabled people in segregated environments have tended to foster dependency, limit choice and autonomy, and encourage overreliance on adults; (2) repeated failure experiences contribute to externality; and (3) people with mental retardation tend to become causal unrealists. They do not fully understand the relative contributions of effort, luck, and ability to positive outcomes and they tend to place more weight on external factors such as luck, chance, or fate.

Findings consistent with Wehmeyer and Palmer's (1997) hypotheses were reported by Koestner, Aube, Ruttner, and Breed (1995). They compared children with and without mental retardation on an attributional measure and found that children with mental retardation were less likely to attribute their failures to their own effort. Interpreting this result in light of Dweck's (1991) incremental theory, Koestner et al. (1995) concluded that children with mental retardation, in comparison to children without mental retardation, were significantly less likely to believe in an incremental theory of ability, i.e., to consider their performance or ability as malleable and improvable through their own effort.

These external perceptions of control may contribute to the difficulty faced by people with mental retardation in assessing the advisability of possible alternative courses of action in decision-making situations. Wehmeyer and Kelchner (1994) examined the role of perceptions of control in the interpersonal problem-solving performance of adolescents with mental retardation and found that a small (6–7%) but significant amount of the variability in the interpersonal problem-solving scores was accounted for by the personal control factors. Problem-solvers who generated a greater number of relevant solutions in a means-end problem-solving task held significantly higher perceptions of control (internal locus of control), self-esteem, and outcome expectancies. Wehmeyer and Kelchner concluded that the extent to which individuals believe in their ability to exercise control over the environment is predictive of their ability to function as efficient problem-solvers. Low perceptions of control over situations may limit a problem-solver's willingness to consider a wide range of alternative solutions as potentially attainable.

Outerdirectedness is indicated when a person in an unfamiliar situation chooses to imitate others or to use external cues or examples rather than attempting an independent solution to the problem. A body of research exists indicating that people with mental retardation are consistently more likely to be outerdirected than people without mental retardation (Bybee & Zigler,

1999). Turnure and Zigler (1964) suggested that a history of problem-solving failure may be a contributing cause of outerdirectedness. Alternatively, people with mental retardation may be less interested in the task than in sustaining contact with the other person (Zigler & Hodapp, 1986). Outerdirectedness in students with mental retardation has been found to increase after a difficult preceding task (Bybee & Zigler, 1992).

A related construct is low expectancy for success, commonly observed in people with mental retardation. This results in motivation to avoid failure rather than to achieve success (Cromwell, 1963; Bennett-Gates & Kreitler, 1999). A combination of outerdirectedness and low expectancy for success may contribute to the relatively high levels of other-dependent decision-making responses observed in people with mental retardation.

There is evidence that people with mental retardation exhibit both positive reaction tendencies, or a heightened desire for social reinforcement, and negative reaction tendencies, or a wariness or reluctance to interact with strangers. The former may be associated with social deprivation or neglect and the latter may be associated with abuse (Bennett-Gates & Zigler, 1999). These tendencies may come into play when people with mental retardation appear to place themselves at risk in order to please another person or to comply with that person's demands or expectations.

In addition to the studies described above, most of which have been focused on specific aspects of personality or motivation, there is an extensive literature in mental retardation pertaining to the role of motivation in achievement. Although most of this research and theory has not been applied directly to interpersonal decision making, some of the explanatory constructs may be useful in interpreting patterns of decision-making performance.

Borkowski and his colleagues (Borkowski, Carr, Rellinger, & Pressley, 1990; Carr, Borkowski, & Maxwell, 1991) have examined the interplay between the acquisition of cognitive and metacognitive strategies and a person's self-concept, perceptions of control, and attributional beliefs. Their studies provide empirical support for their metacognition theory, which predicts a bi-directional relationship between metacognition, or understanding about the efficacy of strategies, and positive self-esteem, internal locus of control, and a tendency to attribute success to effort, rather than to a stable characteristic such as ability. They point out that effort-based attributions must go hand in hand with knowing how to select and apply the specific strategies needed for success in a particular situation. Their recommendation that interventions include both strategy training and attribution training was supported by the results of a study designed to increase reading comprehension awareness and performance with underachieving students.

Another theoretical approach which has played a central role in the literature on motivation and achievement in people with mental retardation has been proposed and tested by Switzky and Haywood and their colleagues (Haywood & Switzky, 1985, 1986; Schultz & Switzky, 1990; Switzky & Schultz, 1988; Switzky, 1997a, 1997b, 1999). Much of their work has centered upon their working hypothesis that mental retardation involves a motivational self-system that interacts with cognitive and metacognitive factors to undermine learning efficiency (Switzky, 1997a). They invoke the construct of task-intrinsic motivation to describe the constellation of motivational characteristics that lead to efficient learning, a construct that has its roots in White's (1959) "effectance motivation" (to have an effect on the environment and master the challenges it presents). Also drawing upon Hunt's work (1963, 1971), Switzky has described intrinsic motivation as exploration "for the satisfaction of taking in and processing new information" (Switzky, 1999, p. 72). Task-intrinsic motivational factors include challenge, responsibility, creativity, learning opportunities, and achievement. People with mental retardation are characterized by a less efficient motivational pattern, labeled task-extrinsic motivation. Task-extrinsic motivational factors include external rewards, safety, comfort, and avoiding failure. It is well documented that people with mental retardation are more likely to be task-extrinsic than are people without mental retardation. These constructs constitute the core of motivational orientation theory (Haywood & Switzky, 1986; Switzky, 1997b). According to this theory,having an intrinsic-motivation orientation is associated with more effective learning than having an extrinsic-motivation orientation, incentives must be matched to the motivational orientations of individuals, and intrinsically motivated individuals may

4. MOTIVATION AND DECISION MAKING

have self-monitored reinforcement systems, making them less dependent on external reinforcement. These hypotheses have been associated with generally strong empirical support.

While the focus of most of the existing motivational theories in mental retardation has been upon achievement, the cognitive orientation theory developed by Kreitler and Kreitler (1988) was applied previously to a wide range of behaviors in populations without mental retardation, including achievement, smoking cessation, assertiveness, planning, and decision making. Because of its broad application, the cognitive orientation theory offers a framework for viewing motivational beliefs in a variety of contexts for individuals with mental retardation. Kreitler and Kreitler proposed their theory after noting the limitations of four earlier approaches to motivation in mental retardation to adequately account for individual differences: (1) the behavioral approach, (2) the personality-based approach, (3) the pychodynamic approach, and (4) the cognitive approach . The cognitive orientation theory is based on the premise that "cognitive contents guide behavior by orienting the person toward some behaviors and away from others" (p.92). The four-stage cognitive orientation theory tracks the processes that occur between input and behavior. The first stage, input identification, addresses the question "What is it?" The second stage, meaning generation, pertains to the question "What does it mean?" The third stage involves the activation of four types of beliefs, goal beliefs, self-beliefs, beliefs about norms and rules, and general beliefs. The four beliefs form a cognitive orientation cluster that orients behavior toward or away from a focal goal. The fourth stage, behavioral intent, addresses the question "What will I do and how will I do it?" This final stage consists of the behavior itself. In a series of studies using the Cognitive Orientation Questionnaire, Kreitler and Kreitler (1988) tested the ability of the four belief types to predict behavior in children with mental retardation. They found that measures of the four belief types did in fact predict a range of behaviors including rigidity, responsiveness to rewards, and performance after success and failure. Of particular interest is the finding that goal beliefs and beliefs about norms and rules played a more central role in the predictions of behavior by children with mental retardation than self-beliefs and general beliefs.

THEORETICAL PERSPECTIVES
ON DECISION MAKING

Important theoretical perspectives for decision-making research in mental retardation are provided by the extensive body of research and theory on decision making in people without mental retardation (see Hickson & Khemka, 1999b for a detailed review). A review of this literature reveals several prescriptive or reasoning theories (e.g., Newell & Simon, 1972; von Neumann & Morgenstern, 1944) that provide explanations of how decisions should be made or the types of formal decision rules that individuals could apply to maximize their decision-making competence. Descriptive theories or reasoned choice models (see Zey, 1992) outline the decision-making process or decision strategies that individuals adopt to arrive at reasoned choices in everyday real-life circumstances. These theories have been of most relevance to the study of interpersonal decision making in that they presume that decision-makers may not always apply specific decision rules to reach a decision and may instead rely on other less formal strategies, such as the use of heuristics, normative-affective factors, or motivational considerations.

A number of theorists have reflected on the contingent processes of motivation in explaining the role of motivation in person perception and social judgment behavior. Kruglanski (1996a, 1996b) has shown that motivation can affect cognition during information processing when a person constructs a knowledge representation of a particular situation. An individual's motivation for cognitive closure—the desire to gain definite knowledge or the need to avoid confusion or ambiguity—influences the amount and nature of information sought to construct the representation of the situation. An individual's motivation for cognitive closure exists on a continuum from a strong need for closure to a strong need to avoid closure (low need for closure). In decision-making situations, individuals with a high need for closure may engage in only cursory processing of available information in light of their motivation to act quickly, whereas individuals with a low need for immediate closure are likely to search more deeply for relevant information. In the event of wanting to avoid closure, an individual faces the cost of being unable to act or make decisions on an issue in a timely manner. On the other hand, a high need for closure may lead to motivations to act without seeking extensive information or generating fewer choice alternatives before making decisions. The need for closure is usually heightened in situations where individuals are faced with a time pressure to make judgments and lessened in situations where there is a high cost associated with making an error of judgment or with making a definite commitment, as in some interpersonal situations.

Kuhl (1986) has presented a taxonomy that emphasizes the interdependency of cognition, motivation, and emotion elements in decision making. According to Kuhl, cognition, emotion, and motivation each operate as a separate information processing subsystem performing unique functions in the process of decision making. The cognitive processes in decision making are involved in mediating the acquisition and representation of knowledge and information upon which decisions are made. The emotional processes are involved in evaluating the personal significance of information collected during decision making. The motivational processes are involved in the selection of goals relating to various alternative courses of action. At various stages of the decision-making process, the three components interact with each other in a variety of ways to determine final decision outcomes.

The importance of affective and emotional factors as determinants of individual decision-making performance is by now well established. Emotions serve as an important input in the process of behavioral choice and action and in determining the motivation for behavior. Mischel and Shoda (1995), Smith and Lazarus (1990), and Zajonc (1980) document that affects and emotions influence the processing of social information, influencing coping behavior and the pursuit of personal goals.

Etzioni (1988) has developed a normative-affective model of decision making that recognizes the importance of normative values and affect in decision making. According to his model, normative commitment (values) or affective involvement (emotions) governs the majority of choices or decisions that individuals make by influencing which information is considered and how it is processed and which options are considered and chosen. The degree to which normative-affective considerations as opposed to cognitive information processes drive decision making is represented by a continuum. Other theorists have emphasized the relevance of affective states or individual emotions such as passion, rage, and fervor in decision making. The effectiveness of decision making may decline in situations of high stress, anxiety, or emotion (Janis & Mann, 1977; Zey, 1992). According to Elster (1985), emotions play a negative role by overwhelming or subverting the rational mental processes during decision making. On the other hand, Maslow (1962) and Zajonc (1980) maintained that emotions serve a positive function in decision making. Other theorists have attributed a more neutral role to emotion, attributing to it the primary function of reordering processing priorities to adapt to changing situations (Clore, Schwarz, & Conway, 1994; Lazarus, 1991).

Individual perceptions of self-efficacy also affect emotional reactions to unfamiliar and potentially aversive situations (Bandura, 1982). Perceived coping inefficacy can trigger emotional arousal of fear and anxiety whereas feelings of controllability are likely to produce more adaptive emotions. Externality of control has been associated with several types of anxiety (Basgall & Snyder, 1988; Lefcourt, 1976; Ray & Katahn, 1968). Lefcourt (1982) identified perceived control as being an important moderator of personal stress, helping people cope better in stressful situations. Fiske and Taylor (1984) emphasized that the exercise of psychological control in aversive circumstances or stressful situations may be mediated by individual difference variables such as locus of control or preference for control.

DECISION MAKING
IN PEOPLE WITH MENTAL RETARDATION

Prior to our own interest in decision making, relatively little attention was focused on investigating personal and interpersonal decision making in individuals with mental retardation. The research that was available failed to provide a fully comprehensive picture of the decision-making capabilities of these individuals. However, the findings of the existing studies on decision-making processes, along with some related studies on problem solving, do suggest several serious shortcomings in the decision making of people with mental retardation. First, it is apparent that people with mental retardation often fail to apply any systematic decision-making process, but rather rely on a limited number of solutions drawn from their past experience that they apply to new situations in a rigid, inflexible manner. In addition, when people with mental retardation do attempt to apply a stepwise process, they tend to experience limited success at each stage of the process. For example, people with mental retardation tend to show incomplete comprehension of decision situations, they generate few alternative solutions, they may fail to anticipate the possible negative consequences of a course of action, and they often do not select an appropriate course of action (Castles & Glass, 1986; Healey & Masterpasqua, 1992; Jenkinson & Nelms, 1994; Smith, 1986; Tymchuk, Yokota, & Rahbar, 1990; Wehmeyer & Kelchner, 1994). (For a more detailed review of this literature, see Hickson & Khemka, 1999b.) Although these studies do serve to highlight decision making as an important area for continued investigation, their scope is limited by an emphasis on the role of cognition in decision making that overshadows the roles of the related processes of motivation and emotion. Furthermore, because few of the studies have involved direct comparisons of groups with and without mental retardation, little is known about the relative difficulty posed by various aspects of the decision-making process for people with mental retardation. Finally, the studies represent a wide range of decision-making and problem-solving tasks, making it difficult to compare studies and determine the relative difficulty of making decisions in various types of situations.

The approaches used to train individuals with mental retardation to handle interpersonal problems and decisions have been influenced heavily by the work of D'Zurilla and Goldfried (1971) and Spivack, Platt, and Shure (1976), who applied models highlighting the stepwise components of problem solving and decision making to improve the performance of children and adolescents without disabilities. Despite this influence, most training studies involving individuals with mental retardation have not addressed the complete constellation of components. (For a more detailed review of this literature, see Hickson & Khemka, 1999b.) Some studies have monitored the number of steps identified or applied, but more typically the studies have focused on a single step in the process, usually the generation of alternatives. This is not surprising, however, as most of the training studies have focused on problem-solving tasks, where the goal is predefined, rather than on decision-making tasks, where specification of a goal is part of the solution. Only two training studies employed actual decision-making tasks. In one study, Ross and Ross (1978) trained children with mental retardation to select the best of several alternative solutions to social environmental decision-making situations. In the other study, Tymchuk, Andron, and Rahbar (1988) used a multiple-baseline design to train nine mothers with mental retardation to identify and apply decision-making component steps to a set of child-care situations.

The remaining training studies focused on the generation of solutions to problem-solving situations where the goal was prespecified. Most of these studies used either a cognitive (Browning & Nave, 1993; Castles & Glass, 1986; Nezu, Nezu, & Arean, 1991; Ross & Ross, 1973, 1978) or behavioral (Martella, Marchand-Martella, & Agran, 1993; Park & Gaylord-Ross, 1989) approach to teach a stepwise process for generating alternative problem solutions. Even in a study by Vaughn, Ridley, and Cox (1983), which employed a broad-based social–cognitive training approach, the outcome focus was on the number of alternative solutions generated. Although these training studies were generally successful at teaching the participants to apply the steps to training problems, some of the studies suffered from methodological flaws such as small sample sizes and brief training periods. Generalization was limited and dependent variables generally failed to include measures of behavior in natural settings. Perhaps the greatest limitation of the training studies is that they typically failed to provide evidence that the quality of participants' solutions had improved. If training is to enable people with mental retardation to make better decisions in real-life community situations, many of which carry threats of danger, coercion, or abuse, then decision quality is of critical importance.

RESEARCH ON THE ROLE OF MOTIVATION IN THE INTERPERSONAL DECISION MAKING OF PEOPLE WITH MENTAL RETARDATION

The existing body of research pertaining to interpersonal decision making in people with mental retardation has yielded very little information on the impact of motivation on individual decision-making performance. The scope of this research has been limited by the previously noted emphasis on the role of cognition in decision making, with little attention to the related roles of motivation and emotion.

During the past several years, we have been involved in the systematic exploration of decision making by people with mental retardation in situations involving interpersonal conflict, coercion, and abuse. The studies summarized below address several issues that have not been fully investigated in past studies, specifically the comparison of people with and without mental retardation, the identification of predictors of decision-making performance, and the development of effective training approaches. In conducting these studies, we have expanded the focus beyond the cognitive aspects of decision making to include motivational and emotional factors that have been shown to be critical to performance on a variety of tasks in adolescents and adults with mental retardation and developmental disabilities (Abery, 1994; Kreitler & Kreitler, 1988; Wehmeyer & Kelchner, 1994). The intent of the studies was to examine concomitantly the relative contribution of cognitive and motivational determinants to decision-making performance.

A comparison of the decision-making skills of individuals with and without mental retardation was important in understanding the difficulty experienced by individuals with mental retardation in handling situations involving interpersonal conflict or danger. In an initial effort to apply a broader perspective to the study of interpersonal decision making, Hickson et al. (1998) conducted two studies that considered motivational and emotional, as well as cognitive, factors as possible sources of the decision-making difficulties of individuals with and without mental retardation. In the first study, male and female adults with mental retardation listened to vignettes depicting situations in which a protagonist was faced with a decision involving the possibility of interpersonal conflict, physical danger, or sexual assault. In the second study, adults without mental retardation received a paper-and-pencil version of the task. The vignettes each posed a conflict between a goal involving social or material gain (e.g., money) versus a goal involving a self-protective or socially responsible action to avoid a negative consequence (e.g., injury). Participants were asked what the protagonist should do and why.

Results of the two studies supported a broad-based conception of interpersonal decision making. Adults without mental retardation made vigilant decisions about 91% of the time, while adults with mental retardation made vigilant responses only 50% of the time. The group differences appeared to be related to both motivational and cognitive factors. Motivational differences between the two groups were reflected in different goal-selection patterns. The adults without mental retardation were somewhat more likely to recommend a negotiation approach that blended gain-oriented goals and safety- and responsibility-oriented goals and the adults with mental retardation were slightly more likely to recommend actions that involved seeking assistance. Results also indicated that women, both with and without mental retardation, produced considerably more vigilant responses than did men and were more likely to state possible negative consequences of failing to take vigilant action. These differences may have reflected higher levels of relevant past experience on the part of the women with some of the situations depicted in the vignettes, especially those involving a threat of sexual or physical assault. The findings of the two studies supported the importance of recognizing the roles of cognitive, motivational, and emotional factors in decision making as they relate to the experiences of women and men with mental retardation.

In interpersonal situations involving coercion or threats of abuse, self-system and personality variables are likely to be important cofactors in the way an individual assesses a risk situation and chooses an action that maximizes his or her self-protection and freedom. Low perceptions of control, poor self-esteem, and limited experience in choice and decision making can make individuals with mental retardation more vulnerable to abuse. There are some data to indicate that individuals with mental retardation hold more external locus of control orientations and lower self-efficacy feelings in comparison to individuals without mental retardation (Wehmeyer, 1993a). In a recent study, Jenkinson (1999) reported that young adults with intellectual disabilities who scored high on a measure of learned helplessness produced less appropriate decision responses to four vignettes depicting personal dilemmas than did young adults who scored low on the measure of learned helplessness.

In a study by Khemka and Hickson (1998) that compared 60 adults with and without mental retardation, equal numbers of females and males, on certain decisional behaviors and perceptions of control, adults with mental retardation were found to reflect relatively negative motivational patterns. In comparison to adults without mental retardation, adults with mental retardation reported greater externality in their locus of control orientation and lower self-efficacy beliefs. Adults with mental retardation also showed less adaptive decision behavior styles with high decisional stress and low decisional self-esteem. Significant relationships were noticed among perceptions of control and decision behavior scores for adults both with and without mental retardation. For instance, external locus of control orientation correlated positively with decisional stress ($r = .26$ / mr group; $r = .28$ / non mr group); self-efficacy correlated positively with decisional self-esteem ($r = .36$ / mr group; $r = .43$/ non mr group) and negatively with decisional stress ($r = -.28$ / mr group; $r = -.28$ / non mr group); decisional stress correlated negatively with decisional self-esteem ($r = -.48$ / mr group; $r = -.52$ / non mr group). In addition, a significant negative correlation was found between self-efficacy and external locus of control for adults without mental retardation ($r = -.36$).

Additional studies have further explored potentially important sources of interpersonal decision-making differences in individuals with and without mental retardation. Khemka, Hickson, and Kim (1998) compared women with and without mental retardation in their ability to suggest effective and independent prevention-focused decisions in response to simulated social interpersonal situations involving different types of abuse (sexual, physical, and verbal). In addition, differences between the two groups on perceptions of control (locus of control, self-efficacy) and decisional behaviors (decisional self-esteem, decisional stress, decisional vigilance) were explored. In this study, women with mental retardation provided far fewer independent prevention-focused decisions (40%), than did the women without mental retardation (62%) across all types of abusive situations. Furthermore, women with mental retardation, in comparison to women without mental retardation, held lower internal locus of control orientations and lower feelings of self-efficacy. Women without mental retardation also tended to have greater decisional self-esteem and higher decisional vigilance response styles.

In a related study, Khemka and Hickson (2000) investigated the ability of men and women with mental retardation to suggest prevention-focused decisions in response to simulated interpersonal situations of abuse. Decision-making responses across three types of abusive situations (physical, sexual, and psychological–verbal) were compared. Overall, participants suggested direct prevention-focused decisions aimed at resisting or stopping the abuse 45% of the time and other-dependent prevention-focused decisions, which consisted of reporting the abuse, 20% of the time. Prevention-focused decision making was higher in situations of physical abuse (59%) than in situations of sexual (51%) or psychological–verbal abuse (26%). In this study, men and women did not differ significantly in their decision-making performance, perhaps because comprehension differences between males and females (Hickson et al., 1998) were reduced by video presentation of the vignette situations. The findings did, however, demonstrate the sensitivity of decision making to situational factors. This suggests that situational and contextual variables impose differential demands that may play an important role in decision making.

Hickson and Khemka (1998) compared the performance of adult females and males with mental retardation on perceptions of control and decisional behaviors. Participants included 88 adults (44 females and 44 males) with mild and moderate mental retardation. Independent sample t-tests comparing females and males on locus of control, self-efficacy, decisional self-esteem, and decisional stress scores were performed. Female participants were significantly more external than the male participants on locus of control scores and held lower self-efficacy beliefs. Females also reported significantly more decisional stress than males, although no differences were noted on decisional self-esteem.

Two recent studies have focused on understanding the interplay of cognitive, motivational, and emotional factors as predictors of the interpersonal decision-making performance of individuals with mental retardation. Hickson and Khemka (1999b) examined the potential of several variables suggested by the theoretical and empirical literature to predict decision-making behaviors of individuals with mental retardation in response to different interpersonal situations, including those involving coercion or threat of abuse. Eighty-four adults with mild mental retardation, equal numbers of males and females, participated in this study. A stepwise multiple regression analysis was conducted with effective decision-making scores measured in response to simulated interpersonal situations as the criterion variable. The variables entered as potential predictors in this analysis included cognitive (IQ and social comprehension), motivational (self-efficacy and locus of control), emotional (perception of emotions and feelings), and personal experience (community independence and degree of residential independence) factors. The multiple regression analysis was completed in four steps, accounting for 39% of the variance. Four significant predictors that contributed to the proportion of variance accounted for (IQ, 16%; self-efficacy; 10%; community independence, 8%; and comprehension of emotions and feelings, 5%) spanned salient factors in the domains of cognition, motivation, emotion, and personal experience.

Hickson and Khemka (1999a) examined the potential of selected variables to predict the interpersonal decision-making performance of adolescent girls with mental retardation and developmental disabilities. The study included 101 girls attending various occupational and career development special education programs. Potential predictors were selected to represent the three basic processes of cognition, motivation, and emotion on the basis of previous theoretical and empirical work with this population. Sets of variables representing cognitive (knowledge of health and risk factors pertaining to birth control, knowledge of HIV, AIDS, etc.), motivational (locus of control, self-efficacy, self-determination, self-esteem, and decisional self-esteem), and emotional (decisional stress, and stress management) factors were entered as predictors in a hierarchical multiple regression analysis. Independent decision making measured in response to simulated interpersonal situations involving conflict or a threat of abuse was used as the criterion variable in the analysis. The results of the study showed that cognitive (19%), motivational (10%), and emotional variables (9%) all contributed significantly to the proportion of total variance (38%) accounted for. The findings suggest that although the cognitive factors contributed the most to the prediction of effective decision-making performance, motivational and emotional factors played a significant contributing role in decision making that was independent of cognitive factors. This conclusion supports the need to consider decision-making performance within a larger context encompassing cognitive and noncognitive variables.

Another important area of inquiry has been to examine the impact of different goal orientations on participants' decision-making preferences. In interpersonal situations, a number of desirable or conflicting personal and social goals can coexist and serve as additional influences on motivation. For example, interpersonal decision-making situations may involve alternative desirable goal states (e.g., gaining adult approval vs. pleasing a friend). In other interpersonal situations decision-makers may be presented with conflicting goals where individualistic goals (e.g., material or social gain) are pitted against more cooperative goals tied to moral or self-responsibility concerns (e.g., helping others or fulfilling family commitments). The decision-maker's preference for one goal state above another goal state contributes to the underlying motivational forces that influence the choice of decision actions.

Hickson and Khemka (2000) explored the nature of difficulties likely to be encountered by students with behavior and emotional disturbances in everyday interpersonal situations that pose potential conflicts between competing goals. Thirty-two adolescents (ages 12–14 years) were presented with a set of six vignettes, where each vignette described an interpersonal situation in which a protagonist is called upon to make a decision. In the vignettes, a conflict was set up between a possible promotion-focused goal involving social or material gain (e.g., pleasing a friend or getting a gift or money) versus a more prevention-focused goal involving a socially responsible action to avoid negative personal consequences (e.g., avoid getting into trouble or fulfilling school responsibilities). The vignettes were presented verbally and immediately after the presentation of each vignette the participants were asked to recommend what the protagonist should do in that situation. Responses were categorized as either reflecting negotiation between competing promotion-focused and prevention-focused goals or reflecting only the pursuit of prevention-focused goals. The study participants took into consideration both promotion-focused and prevention-focused goals while making their decisions 34% of the time, whereas they tended to adopt only a prevention-focused approach to decision making 59% of the time. The participants failed to suggest any decision or gave an irrelevant response to the vignette 7% of the time. The study was designed as a pilot study for future replication with additional participant groups, especially children and adolescents with mental retardation. In this study, we interpreted the motives of the participants as being reflected in the types of decisions recommended by them. For a more complete and accurate estimate of decision motives it would be important to ask the participants directly about their reasons for choosing particular courses of action.

In summary, our preliminary research studies on decision-making processes underscore the centrality and interdependence of cognition, motivation, and emotion in decision making. The studies provide empirical support for the importance of cognitive and noncognitive factors in predicting the interpersonal decision making of individuals with mental retardation. The research findings also highlight the limited ability of individuals with mental retardation to make independent and effective decisions in interpersonal situations of coercion and abuse, reinforcing the need for appropriate decision-making training. The need for training approaches that address both perceptions of control and goal-related motivational processes is supported.

With the growing awareness that decision-making and self-assertiveness skills are critical determinants of successful social adjustment and integration of individuals with mental retardation into community and work environments, there is an urgent need for effective training approaches for enhancing decision-making skills in individuals with mental retardation. The research on motivational components of decision making carries implications for designing interventions to influence individual motivational patterns. Interventions designed to promote adaptive motivational patterns might focus on assisting the decision-maker to adopt the particular personal agency beliefs about ability and control presumed to underlie adaptive motivational patterns or on altering existing patterns of personal goal preferences.

The applicability of a motivation-based training model was assessed in a study by Khemka (2000), where the aim of the training was to teach a decision-making strategy, to increase self-awareness of personal goals and values, and to induce resilient self-beliefs of decision-making efficacy in order to encourage increased exercise of control over decision-making outcomes. Khemka evaluated the effectiveness of a decision-making training approach incorporating motivational features in improving independent and vigilant handling of situations involving abuse by women with mild mental retardation. The study compared two training conditions with a control condition, (1) a traditional cognitive decision-making training approach providing instruction in the use of a cognitive decision-making strategy, and (2) an integrated cognitive and motivational decision-making training approach providing instruction in the use of a cognitive decision-making strategy with emphasis on increasing perceptions of control and goals clarification. A third condition consisted of no training. Thirty-six women with mild mental retardation were randomly assigned to one of the three conditions. Although both training approaches were effective relative to the control condition, the approach that addressed both cognitive and motivational aspects of decision making was superior to that addressing only the cognitive aspects of decision making. The superiority of the cognitive–motivational decision-making training approach was also reflected on a verbally presented generalization task that required the participants to respond to decision-making situations involving abuse from their own perspective (i.e., what they would do if they were ever in the situation themselves). In addition, participants showed higher internal locus of control perceptions after training, with improvements being more pronounced in the combined training condition. The findings of the study suggest that in order to improve the quality of decision responses, it is necessary to augment cognitive training with training that addresses the motivational aspects of decision making, including perceptions of control and goal selection.

Future efforts in decision-making training and research need to further explore the roles of the motivational and emotional components of decision making. Incorporating appropriate motivation-based interventions in decision-making training may help prevent the development of negative motivational systems, foster adaptive coping patterns, and enhance decision-making performance. The training must also emphasize independent goal orientation and evaluation. More research is needed on how best to produce changes in goal orientation and associated motivational patterns in producing more independent and effective decision responses across a range of situational contexts.

NEW DIRECTIONS IN MOTIVATION AND INTERPERSONAL DECISION MAKING IN MENTAL RETARDATION

The study of interpersonal decision making in individuals with mental retardation has been constrained by an emphasis on the cognitive aspects of decision making (Castles & Glass, 1986; Park & Gaylord-Ross, 1989; Ross & Ross, 1973, 1978; Tymchuk, et al., 1988). It is natural to assume that decision making is primarily a cognitive activity dependent on cognitive skills and strategies, such as generating alternative solutions and anticipating consequences. However, the lack of emphasis on motivational and emotional influences in decision making has resulted in only limited development of broad-based theory and research pertaining to individuals with mental retardation.

Recent studies are showing that cognitive abilities explain only a limited part of the variance in decision-making performance (Hickson & Khemka, 1999a, 1999b; Jenkinson, 1999). Evidence for the importance of perceptions of control over decision-making outcomes is gradually converging from diverse studies on decision making involving individuals with mental retardation. Hickson and Khemka (1999b) proposed a framework for the study of interpersonal decision-making processes from a broad perspective that includes motivational and emotional processes as well as cognitive processes as potentially important factors in decision making. In this chapter, we have expanded the Hickson and Khemka (1999b) framework to reflect upon motivational and emotional issues in decision making in greater detail. The new framework, shown in Fig. 4.1, is derived largely from recent empirical research investigating personal and interpersonal decision making in individuals with mental retardation (Hickson et al., 1998; Hickson & Khemka, 1999b; Khemka, 2000;

Khemka & Hickson, 2000). The framework is intended to encourage researchers to broaden their inquiry to include noncognitive factors such as motivational, emotional, and experiential factors, in addition to cognitive factors, in studying the decision making of individuals with mental retardation. It reflects the influence of a wide range of previous theoretical and empirical works discussed earlier in the chapter (e.g., Ford, 1992; Kuhl, 1986). In addition, the models of self-determination (e.g., Abery, 1994; Wehmeyer, 1996) and personal and social competence (Greenspan & Driscoll, 1997; Gumpel, 1994) that have emphasized the importance of decision-making skills in individuals with mental retardation form essential theoretical underpinnings of this framework.

FRAMEWORK FOR INTERPERSONAL
DECISION-MAKING RESEARCH

In the framework presented in Fig. 4.1, decision making is construed to be a multidimensional phenomenon that is shaped by the relative contributions of a number of factors, including cognitive and noncognitive (motivation and emotion) basic process variables. The three basic processes (cognition, motivation, and emotion) have been implicated in research as important contributors to the decision-making performance of individuals with mental retardation and to individual differences. Personal experience and situational context are variables that can potentially influence the operation of the three basic processes in decision making. The three basic processes, personal experience and situational context factors, and the four component steps of the decision-making process will be described in further detail.

The centrality of the role of cognition in interpersonal decision making is well established. Individual differences in decision making due to cognitive factors relate to the ability (or inability) to apply a systematic decision-making process. Application of a stepwise decision-making process requires the decision-maker to construct a cohesive representation of the decision-making situation, thereby drawing upon social knowledge and comprehension. The process also involves the cognitive appraisal of the situation as

FIG. 4.1.   *Framework for interpersonal decision-making research.*

BASIC PROCESSES			DECISION-MAKING COMPONENTS ▼
COGNITION	**MOTIVATION**	**EMOTION**	
• Social awareness and knowledge • Cognitive appraisal • Problem identification and representation	• Situational importance or goal relevance • Need for closure	• Personal significance of situation	┈┈➤ FRAMING
• Generation of options • Generalization of skills to novel situations	• Personal agency beliefs • Goal identification	• Time pressure or immediacy of decision • Emotion perception	──➤ ALTERNATIVES
• Estimation of contingency relationships between actions and consequences • Prediction of risks and benefits	• Environmental beliefs	• Sensitivity to consequences • Emotional coping strategies • Stress management strategies	──➤ CONSEQUENCES
• Weighing of costs and benefits of alternative options	• Goal priorities • Strength of promotion vs. prevention focus • Goal selection	• Emotional connection with past experiences • Sensation (thrill) seeking or risk avoidance tendencies	┈┈➤ ACTION

potentially harmful or potentially beneficial, the identification and definition of the decision problem, the generation of alternative solutions, the estimation of possible consequences of each of the alternatives, a comparison of their costs and benefits, and, finally, the selection of a course of action. The cognitive and self-regulatory processes in decision making also involve social perspective taking, risk perception, and the generalization and application of learned skills in novel decision-making situations.

The framework in Fig. 4.1 integrates different aspects of motivation as potential determinants of decision-making behavior. According to this view of the role of motivation in decision making, the motivational intent is assumed to be formed by perceptions of control that include personal agency beliefs and environmental beliefs (responsiveness of social environments to facilitate and support desirable decision-making opportunities and outcomes) and goal evaluation processes. The components of decision motivation are fundamentally interdependent and together define the expectancies a decision-maker has about whether he or she can make decisions that increase access to valued goals. The motivational beliefs are dependent on the person and circumstances involved.

Personal agency beliefs determine the expectancies of a decision-maker to effect positive outcomes in decision-making situations. Thus, believing that desired decision outcomes can be reached through individual effort and that outcomes are in one's control may motivate the decision-maker to pursue the decision-making activity. A low evaluation of one's personal capacity to control the environment creates a situation of perceived helplessness and may lead to defensive or avoidant decision-making strategies (e.g., shifting the responsibility of decision-making to someone else, accepting the status quo, or making hasty and impulsive decisions).

The psychological motivational processes underlying decision making are not unidirectional. The experience and outcomes of making a decision can affect the self-esteem of a decision-maker and thereby influence subsequent motivations to make decisions. A poor decision outcome can be threatening to the self, undermining one's confidence as a decision-maker, whereas a positive decision outcome can be motivationally enhancing in fostering one's sense of competence and control over a decision-making situation. The experience of being able to achieve desired outcomes and effect action is essential for motivated behavior (Deci & Ryan, 1991). Furthermore, individuals are likely to experience motivational inequalities if they perceive differences in competencies between themselves and others in a particular situation. In such instances, individuals may be quick to resign and give up their motivation and efforts to affect outcomes. Instead, they may be more likely to depend on others, be easily persuaded by others, and accept others' decisions. This may be especially true for individuals with mental retardation who have had a history of depending on others for their decision-making needs and who often have not had the requisite training and support needed to make decisions on their own in interpersonal situations. Research has shown that perceived inefficacy can lead to dependency on others and reduce chances for an individual to build the requisite skills needed for efficacious action (Bandura, 1982).

The characteristics of decision-making environments and opportunities can affect decision-makers' environmental beliefs in ways that might enhance or limit their motivational involvement in decision-making activities. Social environments that are responsive and supportive of independent and self-determined decision making are likely to contribute to favorable attitudes toward decision-making participation and performance. Conversely, social environments that foster dependency behaviors should eventually lead to negative self-evaluations and a sense of little control over the outcomes in one's life. Deci and Ryan (1991) emphasized the importance of autonomy supportive (vs. controlling) social contexts in promoting development of one's resources and adaptive self-regulation. Self-beliefs about coping capabilities for dealing with challenging or threatening environments are also known to regulate behavior involving risks (Bandura, 1988; Ozer & Bandura, 1990). The stronger the perceived coping self-efficacy, the less vulnerable people perceive themselves to be and the more discriminating they are in judging the riskiness of different situations. Therefore, a strong sense of self-efficacy creates a pattern of reduced perceived personal vulnerability to victimization and enhanced ability to distinguish between safe and risky situations. Conversely, low perceptions of efficacy lead to perceived vulnerability to victimization and a reduced tendency to attempt any self-protective action and a general inability to cope with potential risks.

Goals represent a primal orientation of motivation that drives a decision-maker's quality of engagement in a decision-making process. Decision goals represent motivation for decision-making performance in that they attach meaning to the alternative possibilities for decision actions and to the evaluation of consequences resulting from the different actions. In other words, the goals provide the criteria for evaluating and regulating a decision-making activity and they help identify and prioritize alternative options in the direction of desired states or outcomes. The value placed on particular goals when making a decision is determined by which goals are meaningful or relevant in a specific decision-making context as well as how personally important they are to the decision-maker. Ford (1992) has labeled these goal evaluative processes as goal relevance and goal importance, respectively. Goal evaluation also can be conceptualized as pertaining to the activities of goal identification and goal prioritization, as they operate to support goal selection, or the process of singling out the goal or goals that form the basis for the chosen course of action.

These goal-related processes serve to enhance an individual's perceptions of control. Without decision goals against which to evaluate decision alternatives or measure their consequences, decision-makers have little basis for judging the appropriateness or effectiveness of their decisions. Goal attainments provide indicators of making effective decisions, which helps in the verification of an individual's decision-making competence and adds to the experience of control and, therefore, to feelings of personal efficacy.

Emotions and affective values can influence the process of decision making in several ways. The need to engage oneself or remain indifferent to a particular decision is regulated by individual emotions. Decision-makers may experience different emotions (e.g., happiness or fright) in conjunction with their cognitive appraisals of decision-making situations. According to Lazarus (1991), most emotions involve interpersonal situations and depend upon the appraisal that there is "something to gain or lose" (p. 354). If there is no goal relevance, there is no possibility of an emotion (Lazarus, 1994). People may differ in their awareness of their emotional states and in their ability to perceive and identify specific emotions. Individual differences may also occur in the extent to which people are able to regulate their emotions or in the effectiveness of their strategies for coping with intense emotions or for handling stress.

Emotional reactions may be dependent on personal experience or on the personal relevance of the decision-making situation to the decision-maker. Interpersonal situations involving important consequences for the decision-maker are likely to be affect laden and generate a greater emotional reaction (Smith and Lazarus, 1990). The immediacy (under conditions of extreme stress or time pressure) of the need to make a decision and the decision-maker's sensitivity to the potential consequences of certain decision outcomes may intensify the emotional significance of certain decision-making situations. Emotions serve to enhance or limit the motivational involvement of a decision-maker, and in decision-making situations of high emotional engagement, emotions may also compel a decision-maker to undermine a cognitive decision-making process in favor of basing decisions entirely on emotional and affective considerations.

Personal experience can influence the operation of the basic processes and their relative contributions to the decision-making process. Personal experience is the avenue through which a decision-maker's personal background and relevant individual past experiences enter the decision-making process. Personal background encompasses personal characteristics such as age, gender, ethnicity, individual values, cultural norms and commitments, aspirations, and sensitivities to risk. Past experiences are likely to affect people's self-perceptions of personal efficacy and, more generally, their self-esteem. This may be especially true for individuals with mental retardation who are vulnerable to performance deficits and learned helplessness in their life histories. In addition, individuals with mental retardation may lack important decision-making experiences, especially with a wide range of independent choice and decision-making situations (Sands & Kozleski, 1994).

The framework takes into account the variability of an individual's decision-making behaviors across situations. Individual decision making and the relative contributions of cognition, motivation, and emotion can vary as a function of the specific situational context of the decision. The type and nature of a decision-making problem presents unique demands for the decision-maker, suggesting that it may be important to consider situational variables when studying decision making in individuals with mental retardation (Khemka & Hickson, 2000). Different types of situations present different demands for decision-making, thereby influencing an individual's coping abilities in such situations differentially. The type of decision and the accompany-

ing task demands and social expectations serve as situational fil-
ters that influence the extent to which an individual will engage
himself or herself in a decision-making process.

The framework also delineates the specific component steps
of the decision-making process (framing the problem, generating
alternatives, evaluating the consequences, and choosing an
action). The decision-making steps are enumerated to reflect a
generalized process of decision making, although the actual steps
followed by a decision-maker may vary from situation to situation. In certain situations, a decision-maker may even choose to
bypass the stepwise process and base decisions entirely on past
experiences or some strong predilection. At present, the framework presented in Fig. 4.1 shows the overall or cumulative impact
of key variables (basic processes, personal experience, and situational context factors) on the decision-making process. However,
future research is needed to monitor the differential effects of the
key variables on each of the components in the stepwise decision-
making process and to identify the direction and strength of such
relationships.

Figure 4.2 delineates some constituents of the four components of the decision-making process that emerged from our
review of the literature and from our own research as likely contributors to the decision-making difficulties experienced by individuals with mental retardation. Further research will be
necessary to clarify the actual importance of each of these factors
in various types of decision-making contexts.

CONCLUSIONS
AND FUTURE DIRECTIONS

Decision making is the evaluation and selection of an appropriate
course of action resulting in the attainment of relevant or desirable goals and consequences in specified decision-making environments. Effective decision making is defined as the ability to
independently make promotion-focused or prevention-oriented
decisions in one's best interest. Decision-making studies with
individuals with mental retardation (Hickson et al., 1998; Khemka
& Hickson, 2000; Khemka, 2000) reveal distinct decision response
patterns among these individuals characterized by an overre-

FIG. 4.2. *Constituents of the basic processes that may pose difficulties at the different stages of interpersonal decision making for individuals with mental retardation.*

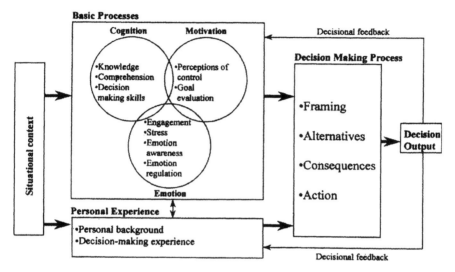

liance on other-dependent or avoidant decision making. Interpreting decision-making performance from Deci and Ryan's (1985) self-determination perspective, it is evident that any decision-making response that is initiated under pressure from others (compulsion), or coercion, lacks a sense of volition or choice and therefore does not represent self-determined behavior. Such behavior may still be intentional in the sense that the decision-maker chooses to go along with the external pressure at her or his own will, but as the choice is not truly independent of environmental influences it demonstrates controlled, not autonomous, decision making. The idea of personal agency with respect to decision-making outcomes thus refers to internally motivated and self-determined decision action.

Decision-making research in individuals with mental retardation has not fully dealt with the motivational and situational determinants of efficient decision-making performance. Recent studies (e.g., Hickson & Khemka, 1999b; Jenkinson, 1999; Khemka, 2000; Wehmeyer & Kelchner, 1994) have highlighted the importance of cognitive, personality, and situational factors in the interpersonal decision making of individuals with mental retardation, specifically in the context of interpersonal situations of coercion and abuse. The effective decision-maker approaches a decision-making situation in an active and goal-directed manner, not by reacting passively. From a motivational perspective, the decision-making process involves assessing alternative options and their potential consequences in light of one's personal agency beliefs, environmental expectations, and goals. In general, the recent research reflects an increased interest in and concern for motivational influences on decision making in individuals with mental retardation.

In light of a new impetus to achieve a broad-based understanding of decision making, the decision-making process is conceptualized as a system of interdependent cognitive, motivational, and emotional processes. Individuals may differ in how they encode a particular decision-making situation cognitively or in the way they react emotionally to a particular situation. Particular cognitions (thoughts) may interact with other cognitions derived from an individual's prior experiences and trigger, in response, different motivational or affective reactions. For effective decision making, an individual must not only have the knowledge and skills to generate optimal choices to produce the desired consequences, but also have the motivation to undertake and apply the decision-making process successfully toward goal attainment. Motivational and emotional processes determine how effectively an individual acquires and uses decision-making skills.

The underlying motivational processes in decision making are strongly influenced by the environmental or situational demands in various decision-making situations. The situational factors determine the affordability and likelihood that a person can access the required perceptions of control and select relevant personal goals in order to arrive at an effective decision. The organization of the decision-maker's cognitions and motivations reflects his or her experiences. A decision-maker's sense of competence is a function of whether he or she perceives himself or herself as successful at decision making or not, influenced greatly by his or her past decision-making experiences.

The relationship between decision-making behavior and the underlying processes is not necessarily one of direct correspondence, but is mediated by the interactions among the processes across different situations. The decision-making system is viewed as functioning as a whole, involving unique interconnections among the underlying processes. Recent research supports the view that cognitive processes interact with motivation and that decision responses are influenced by motivational variables such as individual beliefs, expectancies, and goal orientations. Future research is needed to understand the dynamic interplay of these relationships and how the decision-makers' resources (skills), goals, beliefs, and emotions combine to orchestrate the decision-making process. The ultimate goal of this research is to map the interrelationships among the basic processes that shape decision behavior so as to specify the precise requirements for effective interventions to reduce the decision-making vulnerabilities of people with mental retardation across a wide range of community situations.

Discrepancies between males and females in motivational patterns and decision-making behaviors as observed in several research studies suggest the need to further explore sex differences. A closer examination of other factors such as culture and verbal-communicative relationship styles as possible factors that may influence the perceptions and independent decision-making abilities of individuals with mental retardation is required. A number of definitional and methodological concerns exist in the study of motivational processes in interpersonal decision making. In our present conceptualization, we have chosen to view the basic processes of cognition, motivation, and emotion as interdependent, though individually represented constructs. However, further investigation of decision-making processes, especially as they are applied in real-life situations, might reveal a more moderate perspective on the distinctness of the basic processes. Decision making in specific situations may be so contextualized that it may be virtually impossible to clearly distinguish the underlying component processes without losing the significance or meaning of those processes. Such a perspective is being propounded by motivation theorists that argue for a contextualist view of socialization and the construction of knowledge (see Hickey, 1997).

REFERENCES

Abery, B. (1994). A conceptual framework for enhancing self-determination. In M. Hayden & B. Abery (Eds.), *Challenges for a service system in transition* (pp. 345–380). Baltimore, MD: Brookes.

Achenbach, T., & Zigler, E. (1963). Social competence and self-image disparity in psychiatric and non-psychiatric patients. *Journal of Abnormal and Social Psychology, 67*, 197–205.

Ajzen, I., & Madden, T. (1986). Prediction of goal-directed behavior: Attitudes, intentions, and perceived behavioral control. *Journal of Experimental Social Psychology, 22*, 453–474.

Atkinson, J. W. (1957). Motivational determinants of risk taking behavior. *Psychological Review, 64*, 359–372.

Bandura, A. (1977). Self-efficacy: Toward a unifying theory of behavioral change. *Psychological Review, 84*, 191–215.

Bandura, A. (1982). Self-efficacy mechanism in human agency. *American Psychologist, 37*(2), 122–147.

Bandura, A. (1986). *Social foundations of thought and action: A social cognitive theory.* Englewood Cliffs, NJ: Prentice-Hall.

Bandura, A. (1988). Self-efficacy conception of anxiety. *Anxiety Research, 1*, 77–98.

Bandura, A. (1990). Reflections on nonability determinants of competence. In J. Kollingian, Jr., & R. J. Sternberg (Eds.), *Competence considered: Perceptions of competence and incompetence across the lifespan* (pp. 315–362). New Haven, CT: Yale University Press.

Bandura, A. (1997). *Self-efficacy: The exercise of control.* New York: Freeman.

Bandura, A., Adams, N. E., & Meyer, J. (1977). Cognitive processes mediating behavioral change. *Journal of Personality and Social Psychology, 35*, 125–139.

Bandura, A., & Wood, R. (1989). Effect of perceived controllability and perfromance standards on self-regulation of complex decision-making. *Journal of Personality and Social Psychology, 56*, 805–814.

Basgall, J. A., & Snyder, C. R. (1988). Excuses in waiting: External locus of control and reactions to success-failure feedback. *Journal of Personality and Social Psychology, 54*(4), 656–662.

Bennett-Gates, D., & Kreitler, S. (1999). Expectancy of success in individuals with mental retardation. In. E. Zigler and D. Bennett-Gates (Eds.), *Personality development in individuals with mental retardation.* Cambridge, UK: Cambridge University Press.

Bennett-Gates, D., & Zigler, E. (1999). Motivation for social reinforcement: positive- and negative-reaction tendencies. In. E. Zigler and D. Bennett-Gates (Eds.), *Personality development in individuals with mental retardation.* Cambridge University Press.

Borkowski, J. G., Carr, M., Rellinger, E., & Pressley, M. (1990). Self-regulated cognition: Interdependence of metacognition, attributions, and self-esteem. In B.F. Jones & L. Idol (Eds.), *Dimensions of thinking and cognitive instruction.* (pp. 53–92). Hillsdale, NJ: Lawrence Erlbaum Associates.

Browning, P., & Nave, G. (1993). Teaching social problem-solving to learners with mild disabilities. *Education and Training in Mental Retardation and Developmental Disabilities, 28,* 309–317.

Burger, J. M. (1992). *Desire for control: Personality, social and clinical perspectives.* New York: Plenum Press.

Burger,J. M. & Cooper, H. M. (1979). The desirability of control. *Motivation and emotion, 3,* 381–393.

Burnett, P. C., Mann, L., & Beswick, G. (1989). Validation of the Flinders Decision Making Questionnaire in course decision-making. *Australian Psychologist, 24,* 285–292.

Bybee, J., & Zigler, E. (1992). Is outerdirectedness employed in a harmful or beneficial manner by students with and without mental retardation? *American Journal on Mental Retardation, 96*(5), 512–521.

Bybee, J., & Zigler, E. (1999). Outerdirectedness in individuals with and without mental retardation: a review. In. E. Zigler and D. Bennett-Gates (Eds.), *Personality development in individuals with mental retardation.* Cambridge, UK: Cambridge University Press.

Cacioppo, J. T., & Petty, R. E. (1982). The need for cognition. *Journal of Personality and Social Psychology, 42,* 116–131.

Carr, M., Borkowski, J. G., & Maxwell, S. E. (1991). Motivational components of underachievement. *Developmental Psychology, 27,* 108–118.

Castles, E. E., & Glass, C. R. (1986). Training in social and interpersonal problem-solving skills for mildly and moderately mentally retarded adults. *American Journal of Mental Deficiency, 91,* 35–42.

Clore, G. L., Schwarz, N., & Conway, M. (1994). Affective causes and consequences of social information processing. In R. S. Wyer & T. K. Srull (Eds.), *Handbook of social cognition* (Vol. 1, pp. 323–417). Hillsdale, NJ: Lawrence Erlbaum Associates.

Cromwell, R. (1963). A social learning approach to mental retardation. In N. R. Ellis (Ed.), *Handbook of mental deficiency.* New York: McGraw-Hill.

Deci, E. L. (1975). *Intrinsic motivation.* New York: Plenum Press.

Deci, E. L., & Ryan, R. M. (1985). The dynamics of self-determination in personality and development. In R. Schwarzer (Ed.), *Self-regulated cognitions in anxiety and motivation* (pp. 171–194). Hillsdale, NJ: Lawrence Erlbaum Associates.

Deci, E. L., & Ryan, R. M. (1987). *Intrinsic motivation and self-determination in human behavior.* New York: Plenum Press.

Deci, E. L., & Ryan, R. M. (1991). A motivational approach to self: Integration in personality. In R. Diensbier (Ed.), *Nebraska symposium on motivation: Vol. 38, Perspectives on motivation* (pp. 237–288). Lincoln: University of Nebraska Press.

Dweck, C. S. (1975). The role of expectations and attributions in the alleviation of learned helplessness. *Journal of Personality and Social Psychology, 31*(4), 674–685.

Dweck, C. S. (1991). Self theories and goals: Their role in motivation, personality, and development. In R. Dienstbar (Ed.), *Nebraska Symposium on Motivation* (pp. 199–235). Lincoln, NE: University of Nebraska Press.

Dweck, C. S., & Leggett, L. (1988). A social-cognitive approach to motivation and personality. *Psychological Review, 95,* 256–273.

D'Zurilla, T. J., & Goldfried, M R. (1971). Problem solving and behavior modification. *Journal of Abnormal Psychology, 78,* 107–126.

Elms, A. C. (1976). *Personality and politics.* New York: Harcourt Brace Jovanovich.

Elster, J. (1985). Sadder but wiser? Rationality and the emotions. *Social Science Information, 24,* 375–406.

Etzioni, A. (1988). Normative-affective factors: Toward a new decision-making model. *Journal of Economic-Psychology, 9,* 125–150.

Fischbein, M., & Ajzen, I. (1975). *Belief, attitude, intention, and behavior: An introduction to theory and research.* Reading, MA: Addison-Wesley.

Fischhoff, B. (1975). Hindsight = foresight: The effect of outcome knowledge on judgement under uncertainty. *Journal of Experimental Psychology: Human Perception and Performance, 1,* 288–299.

Fiske, S. T., & Taylor, S. E. (1984). *Social cognition.* Reading, MA: Addison-Wesley.

Floor, L., & Rosen, M. (1975). Investigating the phenomenon of helplessness in mentally retarded adults. *American Journal of Mental Deficiency, 79*(5), 565–572.

Ford, M.E. (1992). *Motivating humans: Goals, emotions, and personal agency beliefs.* Newbury Park, CA: Sage.

Fox, P. B. (1972). Locus of control and self-concept in mildly retarded adolescents. *Dissertation Abstracts, 33,* 2807B.

Gargiulo, R. M., & O'Sullivan, P. S. (1986). Mildly mentally retarded and non-retarded children's learned helplessness. *American Journal of Mental Deficiency, 91,* 203–206.

Getter, H. (1962). *Variables affecting the value of reinforcement in verbal conditioning.* Unpublished doctoral dissertation, Ohio State University.

Glick, M. (1999). Developmental and experiential variables in the self-images of people with mild mental retardation. In. E. Zigler and D. Bennett-Gates (Eds.), *Personality development in individuals with mental retardation.* Cambridge, UK: Cambridge University Press.

Greenspan, S. (1996). There is more to intelligence than IQ. In D. S. Connery (Ed.), *Convicting the innocent* (pp. 136–151). Cambridge, MA: Brookline Books.

Greenspan, S. (1999a). A contextualist perspective on adaptive behaviour. In R. L. Schalock (Ed.), *Adaptive behavior and its measurement: Implications for the field of mental retardation* (pp. 61–80). Washington, DC: American Association on Mental Retardation.

Greenspan, S. (1999b). What is meant by mental retardation? *International Review of Psychiatry, 11,* 6–18.

Greenspan, S., & Driscoll, J. (1997). The role of intelligence in a broad model of personal competence. In P. P. Flanagan, J. L. Genshaft, & P. L. Harrison (Eds.), *Contemporary intellectual assessment: Theories, tests, and issues.* New York: Guilford.

Gruen, G., Ottinger, D., & Ollendick, T. (1974). Probability learning in retarded children with differing histories of success and failure in school. *American Journal of Mental Deficiency, 79,* 417–423.

Gumpel, T. (1994). Social competence and social skills training for persons with mental retardation: An expansion of a behavioral paradigm. *Education and Training in Mental Retardation and Developmental Disabilities, 29,* 194–201.

Harter, S. (1999). *The construction of the self, a developmental perspective.* New York: Guilford.

Harter, S., Whitesell, N. R., & Junkin, L. J. (1998). Similarities and differences in domain-specific and global self-evaluations of learning-disabled, behaviorally-disordered, an normally-achieving adolescents. *American Educational Research Journal, 35,* 653–680.

Haywood, H. C., & Switzky, H. N. (1985). Work response of mildly mentally retarded adults to self-versus external regulation as a function of motivational orientation. *American Journal of Mental Deficiency, 90,* 151–159.

Haywood, H. C., & Switzky, H. N. (1986). Intrinsic motivation and behavior effectiveness in retarded persons. In N. R. Ellis & N. W. Bray (Eds.), *International review of research in mental retardation* (Vol. 14). Orlando, FL: Academic Press.

Healey, K. N., & Masterpasqua, F. (1992). Interpersonal cognitive problem-solving among children with mild mental retardation. *American Journal on Mental Retardation, 96,* 367–372.

Hickey, D.T. (1997). Motivation and contemporary socio-constructivist instructional perspectives. *Educational Psychologist, 32*(3), 175–193.

Hickson, L., Golden, H., Khemka, I., Urv, T., & Yamusah, S. (1998). A closer look at interpersonal decision making in adults with and without mental retardation. *American Journal on Mental Retardation, 103*(3), 209–224.

Hickson, L., & Khemka, I. (1998). *Examining social interpersonal decision-making skills of adults with mental retardation: Implications for training.* Paper presented at the Gatlinburg Conference on Research and Theory in Mental Retardation and Developmental Disabilities, Charleston, SC.

Hickson, L., & Khemka, I. (1999a). *Applicability of a decision-making framework for adolescents with developmental disabilities in interpersonal situations.* Paper presented at the 32nd Gatlinburg Conference on Research and Theory in Mental Retardation and Developmental Disabilities, Charleston, SC.

Hickson, L., & Khemka, I. (1999b). Decision Making and Mental Retardation. In L. M. Glidden (Ed.), *International review of research in mental retardation* (Vol 22). San Diego: Academic Press.

Hickson, L., & Khemka, I. (2000). *Integration of arts in schools for students with disabilities: Challenges and success.* Paper to be presented at the CEC Annual Convention, Vancouver, BC.

Higgins, T., (1997). Beyond pleasure and pain. *American Psychologist, 52*(12), 1280–1300.

Hunt, J. McV. (1963). Motivation inherent in information processing and action. In O.J. Harvey (Ed.), *Motivation and social interaction: cognitive determinants* (pp.35–94). New York: Ronald.

Hunt, J. McV. (1971). Toward a history of intrinsic motivation. In H.I. Day, D. E. Berlyne, & D. E. Hunt (Eds.), *Intrinsic motivation: A new direction in education* (pp. 1–32). Toronto: Holt.

Janis, I. L. (1974). Vigilance and decision-making in personal crises. In D. A. Hamburg & C. V. Coelho (Eds.), *Coping and adaptation*. New York: Academic Press.

Janis, I. L., & Mann, L. (1977). *Decision making: A psychological analysis of conflict, choice and commitment*. New York: The Free Press.

Jenkinson, J., & Nelms, R. (1994). Patterns of decision-making behaviour by people with intellectual disability: An exploratory study. *Australia and New Zealand Journal of Developmental Disabilities, 19*, 99–109.

Jenkinson, J. C. (1999). Factors affecting decision-making by young adults with intellectual disabilities. *American Journal on Mental Retardation, 104*, 320–329.

Kazdin, A. E., Rodgers, A., & Colbus, D. (1986). The hopelessness scale for children: psychometric characteristics and concurrent validity. *Journal of Consulting and Clinical Psychology, 54*, 241–245.

Khemka, I. (2000). Increasing independent decision-making skills of women with mental retardation in simulated interpersonal situations of abuse. *American Journal on Mental Retardation, 105*, 387–401.

Khemka, I., & Hickson, L. (1998). *Individuals with mental retardation handling interpersonal situations involving abuse: Implications for prevention*. Paper presented at the Annual Convention of the Council for Exceptional Children, Minneapolis, MN.

Khemka, I., & Hickson, L. (2000). Decision-making by adults with mental retardation in simulated situations of abuse. *Mental Retardation, 38*, 15–26.

Khemka, I., Hickson, L., & Chatzistyli, K. (1999). *An evaluation of a school-based substance abuse prevention program for female adolescents with developmental disabilities*. Paper presented at AAMR 123rd Annual Meeting, New Orleans, LA.

Khemka, I., Hickson, L., & Kim, C. (1998). *Effective decision making in social interpersonal situations involving abuse: Comparisons between women with and without mental retardation*. Paper presented at the Annual Convention of the American Association on Mental Retardation, San Diego, CA.

Koestner, R., Aube, J., Ruttner, J., & Breed (1995). Theories of ability and the pursuit of challenge among adolescents with mild mental retardation. *Journal of Intellectual Disability Research, 39*, 57–65.

Kreitler, S., & Kreitler, H. (1988). The cognitive approach to motivation in retarded individuals. In N. R. Ellis & N. W. Bray (Eds.), *International review of research in mental retardation* (Vol. 15). Orlando, FL: Academic Press.

Kruglanski, A. W. (1996a). A motivated gatekeeper of our minds: Need-for-closure effects on interpersonal and group processes. In R.M. Sorrentino & E. T. Higgins (Eds.), *Handbook of motivation and cognition* (Vol. 3). New York: Guilford.

Kruglanski, A. W. (1996b). Motivated social cognition: Need for closure effects on memory and judgment. *Journal of Experimental Social Psychology, 32,* 254–270.

Kuhl, J. (1986). Motivation and information processing: A New look at decision making, dynamic change, and action control. In R. M. Screntino & E. Tony Higgins (Eds.), *Handbook of motivation & cognition.* New York: Guilford.

Lazarus, R. (1994). Universal antecedents of the emotions. In P. Ekman & R. J. Davidson (Eds.), *The nature of emotion* (pp. 163–171). New York: Oxford University Press.

Lazarus, R. S. (1991). *Emotion and adaptation.* New York: Oxford.

Lefcourt, H. M. (1976). *Locus of control: Current trends in theory and research.* Hillsdale, NJ: Lawrence Erlbaum Associates.

Lefcourt, H. M. (1982). *Locus of control: Current trends in theory and research* (2nd ed.). Hillsdale, NJ: Lawrence Erlbaum Associates.

Lefkowitz, B. (1997). *Our guys: The Glen Ridge rape and the secret life of the perfect suburb.* Berkeley, CA: University of California Press.

Lent, R. W., & Hackett, G. (1987). Career self-efficacy: Empirical status and future directions. *Journal of Vocational Behavior, 30,* 347–382.

Locke, B. A., & Latham, G. P. (Eds.). (1990). *A theory of goal setting and task performance.* Englewood, NJ: Prentice-Hall.

Mann, L., Harmoni, R., & Power, C. (1989). Adolescent decision-making: The development of competence. *Journal of Adolescence, 12,* 265–278.

Martella, R. C., Marchand-Martella, N. E., & Agran, M. (1993). Using a problem-solving strategy to teach adaptability skills to individuals with mental retardation. *Journal of Rehabilitation, 59,* 55–60.

Markus, H., & Nurius, P. (1986). Possible selves. *American Psychologist, 41,* 954–969.

Maslow, A. H. (1962). *Toward a psychology of being.* Princeton, NJ: Nostrand.

McGuire, W. J., & McGuire, C. V. (1991). The content, structure, and operation of thought systems. In R. S. Wyer, & T. K. Srull (Eds.), *Advances in Social Cognition* (Vol. IV). Hillsdale, NJ: Lawrence Erlbaum Associates.

Mercer, C. D., & Snell, M. E. (1977). *Learning theory research in mental retardation: Implications for teaching.* Columbus, OH: Charles E. Merrill.

Mischel, W., & Shoda, Y. (1995). A cognitive-affective system theory of personality: Reconceptualizing situations, dispositions, dynamics, and invariance in personality structure. *Psychological Review, 102*(2), 246–268.

Mithaug, D. E. (1993). *Self-regulation theory. How optimal adjustment maximizes gain.* Westport, CT: Praeger.

Newell, A., & Simon, H. A. (1972). *Human problem solving.* Englewood Cliffs, NJ: Prentice-Hall.

Nezu, C. M., Nezu, A. M., & Arean, P. (1991). Assertiveness and problem-solving training for mildly mentally retarded persons with dual diagnosis. *Research in Developmental Disabilities, 12,* 371–386.

Ollendick, T. H., Greene, R. W., Francis, G., & Baum, C. G. (1991). Sociometric status: Its stability and validity among neglected, rejected and popular children. *Journal of Child Psychology and Psychiatry and Allied Disciplines, 32,* 525–534.

Ozer, E. M., & Bandura, A. (1990). Mechanisms governing empowering effects: A self-efficacy analysis. *Journal of Personality & Social Psychology, 58,* 472–486.

Palmer, S. B. & Wehmeyer, M. L. (1998). Students' expectations of the future: Hopelessness as a barrier to self-determination. *Mental Retardation, 36*(2), 128–136.

Park, H. S., & Gaylord-Ross, R. (1989). A problem-solving approach to social skills training in employment settings with mentally retarded youth. *Journal of Applied Behavior Analysis, 22,* 373–380.

Pines, H. A., & Julian, J. W. (1972). Effects of task and social demands on locus of control differences in information processing. *Journal of Personality, 40,* 407–416.

Radford, M. H., Mann, L., Ohta, Y., & Nakane, Y. (1993). Differences between Australian and Japanese students in decisional self-esteem, decisional stress, and coping styles. *Journal of Cross-Cultural Psychology, 24,* 284–297.

Ray, W., & Katahn, M. (1968). Relaxation of anxiety to locus-of-control. *Psychological Reports, 3,* 1196.

Reidel, W. W., & Milgram, N. A. (1970). Level of aspiration, locus of control and achievement in retardates and normal children. *Psychological Reports, 27,* 551–557.

Reynolds, W.M., & Miller, K.L. (1985). Depression and learned helplessness in mentally retarded and nonmentally retarded adolescents:

An initial investigation. *Applied Research in Mental Retardation, 6,* 295–306.

Ross, D. M., & Ross, S. A. (1973). Cognitive training for the EMR child: Situational problem solving and planning. *American Journal of Mental Deficiency, 78,* 20–26.

Ross, D. M., & Ross, S. A. (1978). Cognitive training for EMR childres: Choosing the best alternative. *American Journal of Mental Deficiency, 82,* 598–601.

Rotter, J. B. (Ed.). (1966). Generalized expectancies for internal versus external control of reinforcement. *Psychological Monographs, 80*(10), 1–28.

Sands, D. J., & Kozleski, E. B. (1994). Quality of life differences between adults with and without disabilities. *Education and Training in Mental Retardation, 29,* 90–101.

Schultz, G. F., & Switzky, H. N. (1990). The development of intrinsic motivation in students with learning problems: Suggestions for more effective instructional practice. *Preventing School Failure, 34,* 14–20.

Schunk, D. H. (1991). Self-efficacy and academic motivation. *Educational Psychologist, 26*(3 & 4), 207–231.

Seligman, M. E. (1975). *Helplessness: On depression, development and death.* San Francisco: Freeman.

Sherman, L. W. (1984). Development of children's perceptions of internal locus of control: A cross-sectional and longitudinal analysis. *Applied Research in Mental Retardation, 6,* 307–317.

Shipe, D. (1971). Impulsivity and locus of control as predictors of achievement and adjustment in mildly retarded and borderline youth. *American Journal of Mental Deficiency, 76,* 12–22.

Simon, H. A. (1985). Human nature in politics: The dialogue of psychology with political science. *American Political Science Review, 79,* 293–304.

Skinner, E.A., Chapman, M., & Baltes, P.B. (1988). Control, means-ends, and agency beliefs: A New conceptualization and its measurement during childhood. *Journal of Personality and Social Psychology, 54*(1), 117–133.

Smith, C. A., & Lazarus, R. S. (1990). Emotion and adaptation. In L. A. Pervin (Ed.), *Handbook of Personality: Theory and Research* (pp. 609–637). New York: Guilford.

Smith, D. C. (1986). Interpersonal problem-solving skills of retarded and nonretarded children. *Applied Research in Mental Retardation, 7,* 431–442.

Spaulding, W. D. (1994). Introduction. In W. D. Spaulding (Ed.), *Integrative views of motivation, cognition, and emotion, Vol. 41 of the Nebraska Symposium on Motivation* (pp. ix-xii). Lincoln, NE: University of Nebraska Press.

Spivack, G., Platt, J. J., & Shure, M. B. (1976). *The problem-solving approach to adjustment.* San Francisco: Jossey-Bass.

Strickland, B. (1989). Internal-external control expectancies: From contingency to creativity. *American Psychologist, 44*(1), 1–12.

Switzky, H. N. (1997a). Individual differences in personality and motivational systems in persons with mental retardation. In W. W. Maclean, Jr. (Ed.), *Ellis handbook of mental deficiency, psychological theory and research* (3rd ed., pp. 343–377). Mahwah, NJ: Lawrence Erlbaum Associates.

Switzky, H. N. (1997b). Mental retardation and the neglected construct of motivation. *Education and Training in Mental Retardation and Developmental Disabilities, 32*(3), 194–196.

Switzky, H. (1999). Intrinsic motivation and motivational self-system processes in persons with mental retardation. In E. Zigler & D. Bennett-Gates (Eds.), *Personality development in individuals with mental retardation* (pp. 70–106). New York: Cambridge University Press.

Switzky, H. N., & Schultz, G. F. (1988). Intrinsic motivation and learning performance: Implications for individual education programming for learners with mild handicaps. *RASE, 9*(4), 7–14.

Turnure, J. E., & Zigler, E. (1964). Outer-directedness in the problem-solving of normal and retarded children. *Journal of Abnormal and Social Psychology, 69,* 427–436.

Tymchuk, A, J., Andron, L., & Rahbar, B. (1988). Effective decision-making/problem-solving training with mothers who have mental retardation. *American Journal on Mental Retardation, 92,* 510–516.

Tymchuk, A, J., Yokota, A., & Rahbar, B. (1990). Decision-making abilities of mothers with mental retardation. *Research in Developmental Disabilities, 11,* 97–109.

Vaughn, S. R., Ridley, C. A., & Cox, J. (1983). Evaluating the efficacy of an interpersonal training program with children who are mentally retarded. *Education and Training of the Mentally Retarded, 18,* 191–206.

Verplanken, B. (1993). Need for cognition and external information search: Responses to time pressure during decision-making. *Journal of Research in Personality, 27,* 238–252.

Von Neumann, J., & Morgenstern, O. (1944). *Theory of Games and Economic Behavior*. Princeton, NJ: Princeton University Press.

Wehmeyer, M. L. (1993a). Factor structure and construct validity of a locus of control scale with individuals with mental retardation. *Educational and Psychological Measurement, 53*, 1055–1066.

Wehmeyer, M. L. (1993b). Perceptual and psychological factors in career decision-making of adolescents with and without cognitive disabilities. *Career Development of Exceptional Individuals, 16*, 135–146.

Wehmeyer, M. L. (1994a). Employment status and perceptions of control of adults with cognitive and developmental disabilities. *Research in Developmental Disabilities, 15*(2), 119–131.

Wehmeyer, M. L. (1994b). Perceptions of self-determination and psychological empowerment of adolescents with mental retardation. *Education and Training in Mental Retardation and Developmental Disabilities, 29*(1), 9–21.

Wehmeyer, M. L. (1994c). Reliability and acquiescence in the measurement of locus of control with adolescents and adults with mental retardation. *Psychological Reports, 75*, 527–537.

Wehmeyer, M. L. (1996). Self-determination as an educational outcome. In D. J. Sands & M. L. Wehmeyer (Eds.), *Self-determination across the life span*. Baltimore: Brookes.

Wehmeyer, M. L. (1998). Self-determination and individuals with significant disabilities: examining meanings and misinterpretations. *The Association for Persons with Severe Handicaps, 23*(1), 5–16.

Wehmeyer, M. L., & Kelchner, K. (1994). Interpersonal cognitive problem-solving skills of individuals with mental retardation. *Education and Training in Mental Retardation and Developmental Disabilities, 29*, 265–278.

Wehmeyer, M. L., & Kelchner, K. (1996). Perceptions of classroom environment, locus of control and academic attributions of adolescents with and without cognitive disabilities. *Career Development for Exceptional Individuals, 19*, 15–29.

Wehmeyer, M. L., Kelchner, K., & Richards, S. (1996). Essential characteristics of self—determined behavior of individuals with mental retardation. *American Journal on Mental Retardation, 100*, 632–642.

Wehmeyer, M. L. & Palmer, S. B. (1997). Perceptions of control of students with and without cognitive disabilities. *Psychological Reports, 81*, 195–206.

Weiner, B. (1979). A theory of motivation for some classroom experiences. *Journal of Educational Psychology, 71,* 3–25.

Weiner, B. (1985). *Human motivation.* New York: Springer-Verlag.

Weisz, J. R. (1979). Perceived control and learned helplessness among mentally retarded and nonretarded children: A developmental analysis. *Developmental Psychology, 15*(3), 311–319.

Weisz, J. R. (1981). Learned helplessness in black and white children identified by their schools as retarded and nonretarded: Performance deterioration in response to failure. *Developmental Psychology, 17,* 499–508.

Weisz, J. R. (1999). Cognitive performance and learned helplessness in mentally retarded persons. In. E. Zigler and D. Bennett-Gates (Eds.), *Personality development in individuals with mental retardation.* Cambridge, UK: Cambridge University Press.

White, R. W. (1959). Motivation reconsidered: The concept of competence. *Psychological Review, 66,* 297–333.

Yamusah, S. (1998). *An investigation of the relative affectiveness of the composite approach and the phenomenological method for enhancing self-esteem in adults with mental retardation.* Doctoral Dissertation, Teachers College, Columbia University, New York.

Zajonc, R. B. (1980). Feeling and thinking: Preferences need no inferences. *American Psychologist, 35,* 151–175.

Zey, M. (Ed.). (1992). *Decision-making: Alternatives to rational choice models.* Newbury Park, CA: Sage.

Zigler, E. (1999). The individual with mental retardation as a whole person. In. E. Zigler and D. Bennett-Gates (Eds.), *Personality development in individuals with mental retardation.* Cambridge, UK: Cambridge University Press.

Zigler, E., & Hodapp, R. M. (1986). *Understanding mental retardation* (pp. 115–135). Cambridge, UK: Cambridge University Press.

5

Etiology and Personality Motivation: Direct and Indirect Effects

Robert M. Hodapp

UCLA Graduate School of Education & Information Studies

Although all sciences have progressed over the past few decades, the most striking advances have arguably occurred in genetics. Among the changes that took place during his 7–year tenure as editor of *American Journal of Human Genetics*, Charles Epstein (1996) highlighted:

- Continuing success of the Human Genome Project;
- Discovery of triplet repeat diseases;
- First uses of gene therapy;
- Discovery of microdeletion syndromes;
- Mouse models for many genetic disorders; and
- New methods for prenatal screening and diagnosis.

As this list indicates, most advances involve identifying and understanding the normal and abnormal workings of numerous genes on virtually every human chromosome. Within mental retardation, genetic discoveries include identifying approximately 750 different genetic disorders associated with mental retardation (Opitz, 1996). For many of these disorders, geneticists and other biomedical workers have identified physical features and associated health or medical problems: Witness, for example, the recent criteria that allow pediatricians to diagnose children with Prader-Willi syndrome (Holm et al., 1993). Although certain aspects of behavior are sometimes included within these criteria (e.g., hyperphagia in Prader-Willi), most such screening instruments highlight the child's height, weight, facial features, and specialized medical issues.

However, in most phenotypic work to date, researchers have paid only sporadic attention to so-called behavioral phenotypes of different genetic disorders. Even when they have been discussed, such behaviors have been described only grossly. Thus, early behavioral work on fragile X syndrome characterized the language of these males as "sing-songy" (see Dykens, Hodapp, & Leckman, 1994, for a review), and early work on Williams syndrome considered these children as "friendly and outgoing." In short, at the same time as the new genetics has revolutionized the identification and medical management of many of the 750 different genetic disorders of mental retardation, knowledge about behavior has lagged far behind. Before discussing the link between genetic disorders and personality-motivational functioning, then, it is important to first discuss the state of the art concerning the behaviors of various genetic disorders of mental retardation.

BEHAVIORAL
EFFECTS OF GENETIC DISORDERS

Researchers are considerably deficient in understanding the behaviors of different genetic disorders for three reasons. First, the sheer number of different genetic disorders of mental retardation—approximately 750 (and growing)—makes it difficult to study each in depth. Many of these disorders are also relatively rare, making in-depth behavioral studies difficult without cross-center collaborations. Ironically, such cross-center collaborations—so common within genetics and other biomedical fields—remain uncommon for most social scientists studying behavior in individuals with mental retardation.

A second, and probably more important, reason concerns the social structure of behavioral research in mental retardation. Here we refer to the two cultures of behavioral work in mental retardation, the division between social scientists and biomedical workers. Although this phenomenon is detailed elsewhere (Hodapp & Dykens, 1994), the basic point is that behavioral work in mental retardation is carried out by two, rarely overlapping groups of workers. The first group includes clinical, behavioral, information-processing, social, and developmental psychologists, special educators, and social workers. This group is expert in the measurement of behavior and in the various theoretical perspectives used throughout the social sciences to understand complex human behavior. Unfortunately, most members of this group have little understanding or appreciation of genetics and genetic etiology. Historically, most social scientists have routinely grouped together individuals with different genetic disorders based on their level of impairment. We thus see studies of persons with mild, moderate, severe, and profound mental retardation, but whose cause of mental retardation varies from individual to individual. Such mixed-group studies constitute as many as 80 to 90% of behavioral studies in journals such as the *American Journal on Mental Retardation, Research in Developmental Disabilities,* and *Mental Retardation* (Dykens, 1996).

The other culture includes geneticists, pediatricians, psychiatrists, and other biomedically oriented personnel. These workers know well the different genetic etiologies, their physical features, and their medical needs. Their studies examine the behavior of groups of individuals with one specific etiology (e.g., fragile X syndrome) or compare individuals with one etiology (fragile X syndrome) to those with another etiology (Down syndrome). Unfortunately, these biomedical workers are less well-trained in behavioral assessment and explanation. In essence, then, behavioral work in mental retardation features two distinct, rarely interacting sets of workers. As a result, there are few in-depth behavioral studies on most of the 750 different genetic disorders of mental retardation.

The third important reason for the lack of behavioral work concerns varying definitions of the term *behavioral phenotype.* Although a small but growing set of primarily American and

British researchers has become interested in the specific behaviors of different genetic disorders, these researchers have disagreed about what behavioral phenotypes are and how they should be studied. Some feel that the term should be restricted to a behavior that is unique to one specific syndrome and that occurs in almost all persons with that syndrome (Flynt & Yule, 1994); others hold the view that a behavioral phenotype need not be unique to only one syndrome nor occur in every person with that syndrome (Rosen, 1993).

For my purposes, I employ a definition closer to the latter position, a definition that describes behavioral phenotypes in more probabilistic terms. According to Dykens (1995), a behavioral phenotype "may best be described as the heightened probability or likelihood that people with a given syndrome will exhibit certain behavioral or developmental sequelae relative to those without the syndrome" (p. 523; see also Dykens, chap. 6, this volume).

Three aspects of this definition are noteworthy.

1. Not every person with a specific genetic disorder will show that disorder's characteristic behavior. This first aspect emphasizes the probabilistic nature of the behavioral outcomes of specific genetic disorders of mental retardation. Although researchers sometimes think of different genetic disorders as dictating that all children or adults show particular behaviors, genetic disorders are more precisely thought of as predisposers of particular behaviors. Not every child with Prader-Willi syndrome will show hyperphagia, nor will every child with Williams syndrome show high-level verbal abilities or hypersociability nor every male with fragile X syndrome show gaze aversion. Granted, in each disorder, most individuals will show the syndrome's characteristic behaviors, but exceptions do occur.

    Furthermore, understanding within-syndrome variability constitutes one of the most interesting aspects of syndrome-specific research. In Prader-Willi syndrome, for example, it may be the case that the syndrome's two variants—paternal deletion (a deletion on the paternally inherited chromosome 15) and maternal disomy (two chromosome 15s from the mother)—show subtle behavioral differences in terms of both IQ and proneness to certain maladaptive behaviors (Dykens, Cassidy, & King, 1999). In the same way, certain environmental or other input may dampen or exacerbate particular behaviors in different genetic etiologies. Just as genetic history predisposes—but does not determine—one to develop, say, high blood pressure, so too do genetic disorders predispose—but not determine—an individual to develop particular behaviors.

2.   A single behavior may be characteristic of a genetic disorder but be either unique or shared with one or more additional genetic disorders. In certain definitions of behavioral phenotype, researchers have considered that a particular genetic disorder shows a phenotype only when one or more behaviors are unique to one syndrome. And indeed, such examples do occur. Note, for example, hyperphagia in Prader-Willi syndrome, extreme self-mutilation in Lesch-Nyan syndrome, putting objects into bodily orifices and self-hugging in Smith-Magenis syndrome, and the cat-like cry in cri-du-chat syndrome. Each constitutes behaviors that, at least at the moment, appear unique to only one syndrome.

For most behaviors, however, two or more genetic disorders share certain characteristic behaviors. For example, hyperactivity seems to be common in males with fragile X syndrome (Dykens et al., 1994), as well as in children with Williams syndrome (Udwin, Yule, & Martin, 1987). Hyperactivity can thus be considered characteristic of both disorders: compared to a representative sample of persons with mental retardation—or even compared to individuals with certain other etiologies (e.g., Prader-Willi syndrome, Down syndrome)—hyperactivity is much more common in both fragile X and Williams syndromes. At the same time, however, hyperactivity is unique to neither.

Behaviors that characterize a specific mental retardation syndrome can therefore be considered as either totally or partially specific to a single etiology (Hodapp, 1997). Total specificity sometimes occurs, but the more common occurrence is partial specificity, the case in which two or more etiological groups show a particular behavior either much more often than the population with mental retardation in general or much more often compared to other etiological groups. In addition to being more common, partial specificity is also interesting in that it begins to illustrate the common pathways to various behavioral outcomes. Such pathways should eventually reveal the genetic, biochemical, embryological, neurological, or other mechanisms by which certain behaviors come about.

3. Genetic disorders lead to both direct and indirect behavioral effects. A final issue concerns the nature of the effects of genetic disorders on behavior. Until now, direct effects have been discussed, that is, those effects of a specific genetic disorder on the behavior(s) of individuals with that disorder. Thus, through a long and yet-to-be-determined chain of events, the (Prader-Willi) deletion on chromosome 15 predisposes the individual to hyperphagia, just as the triplet repeats involved in fragile X syndrome and the deletion on chromosome 7 involved in Williams syndrome predispose individuals toward hyperactivity. In short, only the direct effects of a genetic disorder on one or more of the individual's behaviors have been examined.

But there is another sense by which genetic disorders show their effects, and this sense might be called a genetic disorder's *indirect effects* (Hodapp, 1997). Indirect effects can best be understood by employing several ideas common to the study of typically developing children from the late 1960s on (Hodapp, 1999). In short, just as parents influence their children, socializing them every day to become increasingly adult-like over time, so too do children affect their parents. This view, called interactionism, was developed by Richard Bell (1968) and led to a host of studies of mother-child, father-child, sibling-sibling, and peer-peer interactions beginning in the early 1970s. Partly because interactionism was a response to the reigning paradigm of socialization—by which parents affect children—most interactional work reversed the direction of effects. Researchers tried to understand the ways in which the child's behaviors or personal characteristics (e.g., the child's gender or age) elicit changes in the behaviors of a mother, father, sibling, or peer.

This perspective of children affecting adults can also be applied to children with different genetic disorders. If children with a specific genetic disorder are more likely to show particular behaviors, parents too may react in particular ways. In essence, a link may run from genetic disorder, to higher likelihood or predisposition to one or more behaviors, to specific parental reactions and behaviors.

This chapter applies to the personality-motivational field the ideas of behavioral phenotypes as heightened predispositions toward particular behaviors and as having effects that can be either partially or totally specific. Most important, this chapter considers the effects of genetic mental retardation disorders as being both direct and indirect and begins to spell out a model highlighting both direct and indirect effects for the study of personality and motivational functioning in individuals with mental retardation.

DIRECT EFFECTS ON PERSONALITY-MOTIVATIONAL FUNCTIONING: THE EXAMPLE OF DOWN SYNDROME

Because the direct effects of genetic disorders on personality are considered in more depth elsewhere in this volume (Dykens, chap. 5), they are only mentioned here only briefly. Specifically, we use as an example the case of Down syndrome. The Down syndrome example will then be continued when considering the indirect effects of genetic disorders on personality-motivational functioning.

Down Syndrome: Issues Concerning a Behavioral Phenotype

As the most commonly occurring and well-known type of mental retardation, Down syndrome has taken on an interesting status for researchers studying behavior in individuals with mental retardation. Almost alone among the 750 different genetic disorders of mental retardation, Down syndrome has a rich history of sophisticated behavioral work. In one survey, almost half (46%) of all etiology-based behavioral studies in the principal journals in the area of mental retardation focused on Down syndrome

(Hodapp, 1996). In addition, Down syndrome often serves as the control or contrast group for researchers examining autism or even other genetic forms of mental retardation (e.g., Williams syndrome). To both the public and professionals alike, Down syndrome has become the prototypical mental retardation syndrome, considered a stand-in for the population with mental retardation in general.

In contrast, recent studies question just how typical Down syndrome really is. Compared to others with mental retardation, groups with Down syndrome differ physically, medically, and behaviorally. Physically, these individuals more often show epicanthal folds, transverse palmer creases, and other physical sequelae (Pueschel, 1990). Medically, virtually all persons over age 40 show the plaques and tangles characteristic of Alzheimer's disease, although these plaques and tangles may differ slightly from the usual Alzheimer's presentation, and dementia may not occur until many years after plaques and tangles first appear (Wisniewski, Kida, & Brown, 1996).

But the most interesting phenotypic differences may concern various aspects of behavior. For example, groups with Down syndrome seem more likely than other groups with mental retardation to show increased abilities in visual over auditory processing (Hodapp, Evans, & Gray, 1999; Pueschel, Gallagher, Zartler, & Pezzullo, 1987). This finding was recently used to support the teaching of early literacy skills to these children (Buckley, Bird, & Byrne, 1996). In addition, compared to their overall cognitive levels, children with Down syndrome show particularly poor grammatical abilities (Fowler, 1990), and their receptive language abilities clearly outpace their expressive language skills, particularly past the toddler years (Miller, 1992). Although not every person with Down syndrome necessarily shows these physical, medical, or behavioral characteristics, all seem more common in Down syndrome than in the mental retardation population in general.

Personality-Motivational Functioning

Moving to personality-motivational functioning, one can again see the possibility of differences when comparing individuals with Down syndrome to groups with heterogeneous causes for their retardation. Indeed, the possibility of a distinct Down syndrome personality was first suggested by Langdon Down (1866), who noted that "They have considerable power of imitation, even bordering on being mimics. They are humorous, and a lively sense of the ridiculous often colours their mimicry" (Dunn, 1991, p. 828). Although investigators over the years have varied somewhat in how they characterize these individuals, most writers have considered persons with Down syndrome as sociable, friendly, and good-natured (Gibson, 1978).

Before describing research directly related to this issue, it is important to realize that the presence of a Down syndrome personality—or even of a specific behavioral phenotype for Down syndrome—remains controversial (see Fidler & Hodapp, 1998; Gelb, 1997). Many families and researchers associated with the syndrome feel that the possible presence of such a Down syndrome personality denigrates individuals with the syndrome. As mentioned previously, though, it is important to note that behavioral phenotypes involve probabilistic statements (Dykens, 1995). In the studies below, any evidence of differences between Down syndrome and other groups with retardation involves a group difference: Not all members of Down syndrome need share any of the syndrome's characteristic behaviors.

Given these caveats, we can now examine sociability, one aspect of personality functioning that has received research attention (Kasari & Hodapp, 1996). Specifically, young children with Down syndrome look longer to faces than to objects or other events (Kasari, Freeman, Mundy, & Sigman, 1995)—they seem to have an interest in and fascination for people not seen in children with other types of mental retardation. In addition, these children have more positive affect (as reported by parents) than do children with autism or with mental retardation of unknown etiology (Capps, Kasari, Yirmiya, & Sigman, 1993).

Most intriguing, however, may be the reactions of children with Down syndrome as they try to solve difficult tasks. Consider Pitcairn and Wishart's (1994) study that compared children with Down syndrome, mental-age-matched nonretarded children, and mental-age-matched children with mixed etiologies of mental retardation. All three groups were administered a series of impossible tasks, such as putting a round peg into a square hole. In contrast to the other two groups, children with Down syndrome "exploited their social skills, producing a variety of distracting behaviors that focused attention (their own and that of the experimenter) away from the task at hand" (p. 489). Pitcairn and Wishart (1994) referred to these displays as party tricks and suggest that these children appear to be attempting to charm their way out of a difficult situation. Kasari and Freeman (in press) gave similar puzzle tasks to 5-to 12-year-old children with Down syndrome, mental age-matched typically developing children, and mental-age-matched children with nonspecific mental retardation. Even such older children with Down syndrome more often looked to adults and asked for help and took longer to complete the task. During both the toddler and the school-age years, then, children with Down syndrome use their social skills to avoid performing difficult tasks.

In addition to research examining issues of sociability, several studies have directly examined the personalities of children with Down syndrome. For example, Wishart and Johnston (1990) asked parents, teachers, and students to rate children's personalities along 23 items specifically chosen to tap into the stereotypical personality of persons with Down syndrome. According to its authors, the study's findings debunk the myth of a stereotypical Down syndrome personality, as adults with more (versus less) experience with children with the disorder rated items lower. Mothers, too, scored relatively lower when asked to report on a typical child with Down syndrome. However, mothers scored exceptionally high when asked to rate the personality of their own child with Down syndrome. On a scale ranging from 23 (1, or lowest, on every item of the Down syndrome personality) to 115 (5, or highest, on every item), mothers of children with Down syndrome averaged 97 points (or 4.22 points per item). Such scores were higher than scores for all other groups. Strangely, then, while teachers and students may not think that persons with Down syndrome show a particular personality—and mothers do not when considering children with Down syndrome in general—mothers highly endorse many elements of this personality when rating their own children with Down syndrome.

INDIRECT EFFECTS
ON PERSONALITY-MOTIVATIONAL
FUNCTIONING

Given that different genetic disorders show particular behavioral predispositions, it may be possible that such behavioral effects in turn influence individuals in the child's surrounding environments. Although there is less support for such indirect effects than for genetic disorders' direct effects, some early findings are suggestive. Continuing the example of Down syndrome, this section first describes studies of three of the surrounding environments of children with Down syndrome—parents, families, and siblings—and then discusses possible reasons for any differences found.

Indirect Effects of Down Syndrome on Parents, Families, and Siblings

In overviewing the possible indirect effects of Down syndrome, we begin with the views of parents. In addition to parents' perceptions that their own children do, in fact, conform to a particular Down syndrome personality, recent studies also show such parental views in interview form. In a series of interviews, Hornby (1995) noted that, among fathers of 7- to 14-year-old children with Down syndrome, a full 46% commented on their children's cheerful personalities (this was fathers' most common spontaneous comment). In addition, nearly one third of fathers referred to their children as being lovable, and nearly one fourth described their children as sociable or friendly. Similarly, in Carr's (1995) 20-year longitudinal study, over half of the children with Down syndrome were described as "affectionate," "lovable," "nice," and "gets on well with people"—these percentages were similar to same-aged nonretarded peers. Although neither study compared parental perceptions of children with Down syndrome to parental perceptions of children with mixed (or other) etiologies, they do show that parents react positively to their children's perceived pleasant personalities.

Families, too, react positively to their children with Down syndrome. Here the research compares families of children with

Down syndrome to families of children with mental retardation in general or with other disabilities (e.g., autism or emotional disorder). In almost every case, families of children with Down syndrome show lower levels of stress and better coping than families of same-aged children with other disorders. To give but a few examples, when compared with children with autism and children with unidentified mental retardation, parents of children with Down syndrome exhibit significantly lower amounts of stress (Holroyd & MacArthur, 1976; Kasari & Sigman, 1997; Sanders & Morgan, 1997; Seltzer, Krauss, & Tsunematsu, 1993). In a study that classified families of children with mental retardation into varying types, a full 66% of the *cohesive-harmonious* families—the most intact family type—were comprised of families of children with Down syndrome (Mink, Nihira, & Myers, 1983). Compared to mothers of children with other disabilities, mothers of children with Down syndrome even report experiencing greater support from friends and the greater community (Erikson & Upshure, 1989).

This advantage to families of children with Down syndrome occurs across a range of ages and relative to a variety of contrast groups. The above-mentioned studies, for example, examined families of persons with mental retardation who ranged from below 2 years (Erikson & Upshure, 1989) up through 25 years of age (Seltzer et al., 1993). In addition, some studies compared individuals with Down syndrome to other groups with retardation and some to groups of children with autism. In one study (Thomas & Olsen, 1993), researchers began by considering families of adolescents with Down syndrome as *problem families,* akin to two groups of families of adolescents with emotional disturbance. As the study progressed, however, these researchers—finding no group differences—combined their "normal" and Down syndrome families into a single control group, concluding that families of children with Down syndrome were not really problem families after all. Although an occasional study does not find the Down syndrome advantage (e.g., Cahill & Glidden, 1996), in most studies families of individuals with Down syndrome cope better than families of children and adults with other disabilities.

This Down syndrome advantage may even extend to siblings. In two large-scale studies, siblings were found to have few interpersonal problems with their brothers or sisters with Down syndrome (Carr, 1995; Byrne, Cunningham, & Sloper, 1988). Comparing quarrels in sibling dyads when the index child (Down syndrome vs. typically developing) was 11 years of age, Carr (1995) found that 37% of the Down syndrome siblings had no quarrels and 44% had some quarrels; these compare to 18% with no quarrels and 54% with some quarrels among control siblings. As Carr (1995) noted, "The picture is then of quite harmonious relationships between the young people with Down's syndrome and their sibs" (p. 122).

So too may siblings of children with Down syndrome cope better than siblings of children with other etiologies of mental retardation. In a recently completed study, we compared older siblings of children with Down syndrome to age- and gender-matched siblings of children with 5p- syndrome (Wijma & Hodapp, 2001). As expected, older siblings of children with 5p- syndrome displayed more concerns in a variety of areas. These siblings showed more interpersonal concerns, involving higher endorsements of such items as "I don't want to bother my parents with my worries" and "I wish that my parents would spend less time with my brother/sister." Compared to same-aged older siblings of children with Down syndrome, siblings of children with 5p- also showed more concerns about intrapersonal issues such as "I feel sad about my brother's/sister's disability" or "I wish that there were something that I could do about my brother's/sister's disability." Just as parents and families seem affected differently by children with different types of mental retardation, so too are these children's older siblings affected differently than older siblings of children with 5p-syndrome.

Mechanisms by Which Indirect Effects Operate

Until now, we have discussed indirect effects without regard to why such differences occur. Why is it that parents, families, and siblings seem less adversely affected when the child with disabilities has Down syndrome versus some other mental retardation (or other) disorder?

Although there are presently no clear answers to this question, many possibilities exist. One possibility might involve characteristics associated with Down syndrome. For example, mothers of children with Down syndrome are, as a group, older than mothers of children with other types of mental retardation (Cahill & Glidden, 1996). As older parents, these mothers might also be expected to have more children, more experience with the parenting role, and more maturity.

Another possible mechanism concerns the many active parent groups in Down syndrome. Although parents of children with many etiologies form national and local organizations, groups are probably more numerous and more active in Down syndrome. Such organizations allow parents the opportunity to befriend and confide in others who share the difficult changes that parenting a child with Down syndrome brings about for the family, for the couple, and for schooling and other social services (Hodapp, 1995). In addition, as noted above, Down syndrome is by far the best-known and accepted mental retardation disorder among the general public.

Although differences in mothers and in surrounding environments may partially account for the Down syndrome difference, aspects of the child are probably most important. In considering the reactions to children with Down syndrome, three specific characteristics stand out: (1) sociability and possibly pleasant personality; (2) lack of psychopathology; and (3) appearance.

1.   Sociability and personality. As the old song says: "When you're smiling, the whole world smiles with you." Each of us, it seems, reacts positively to pleasant, people-oriented people, and Down syndrome may indeed predispose children to pleasant, people-oriented personalities. Consider only the most straightforward of sociable behaviors, that children with Down syndrome look longer to the faces of others than to objects or other events (Kasari et al., 1995). While eye contact is an obvious social skill, it is not a trivial one. Indeed, children with certain disorders find it difficult to even look to others and make eye contact. Children with autism (Kasari & Bauminger, 1998) and boys with fragile X syndrome (Dykens et al., 1994) rarely directly gaze toward others. Whatever the reasons for this lack of eye contact (uninterest in others or

extreme social anxiety), this behavior makes interactions difficult. In short, most adults find it difficult to interact with children who look away.

2. Lack of psychopathology. Another interesting feature of Down syndrome is a general lack of psychopathology. Although not always found, most studies find relatively low levels of psychopathology in children with Down syndrome. Although percentages of children with Down syndrome who have psychiatric disturbance range from 15 to 38% (Hodapp, 1996), such percentages are generally lower than those found in same-aged children with mixed etiologies (Dykens, 1996; Dykens & Kasari, 1997).

Furthermore, those maladaptive behaviors that do exist most often involve problems centering on conduct, attentional, and generally disruptive behaviors (Gath & Gumley, 1986; Meyers & Pueschel, 1991). Although such problems can be difficult, fewer children with Down syndrome display more severe psychiatric problems—particularly autism or severe psychoses (Dykens & Volkmar, 1997). In short, while psychiatric disorders exist in children with Down syndrome, these disorders may occur in lower percentages and, in general, involve less severe types of psychopathology.

Conversely, high levels of maladaptive behavior and psychopathology seem to relate to increased levels of family stress. Correlating symptoms on Achenbach's Child Behavior Checklist (CBCL) with various measures of parental stress, we have found that children displaying more behavior problems have families with more overall stress, more parent and family problems, and more parental pessimism. This connection has now been found within three different etiological groups: Prader-Willi syndrome (Hodapp, Dykens, & Masino, 1997), 5p- (or cri-du-chat) syndrome (Hodapp, Wijma, & Masino, 1997), and Smith-Magenis syndrome (Hodapp, Fidler, & Smith, 1998). In each group, levels of child psychopathology constituted the best predictor of parent and family stress, better than the child's age, sex, degree of intellectual impairment, family support, or any other predictor measured.

3. Appearance. Although J. Langdon Down was the first to note the "mongoloid" facial characteristics of children with Down

syndrome, the child's facial appearance—or, more specifically, its effects on others—has yet to be examined in depth.
When considering the reactions of others, an important
aspect of a person's face may be the degree to which a face
seems immature or babylike. Zebrowitz (1997) recently
described uniform adult reactions when interacting with
infants. These behaviors include the extended mutual gaze
between adults and babies and an eyebrow flash in adults,
such that adults come eyeball-to-eyeball with a baby on a first
encounter. Zebrowitz attributes these warm, familiar reactions to the ability of infants to disarm adults. In effect, the
infant's appearance communicates to the adult that the baby
is developmentally immature and is dependent on the adult
for survival.

   Given its probable evolutionary importance, such "babyface reactions" may be "overgeneralized to individuals whose appearance merely resembles" a baby in some way (Zebrowitz, 1997, p.
56). When this overresponsiveness is manifested in reactions to
adults who retain babylike facial proportions, Zebrowitz terms
this the *babyface overgeneralization*. Across numerous studies, ob-
servers attribute higher ratings of warmth, weakness, and naiveté
to pictures of adult faces with babylike features (Berry &
McArthur, 1985, 1986; Zebrowitz & Montepare, 1992;
Zebrowitz, Olson, & Hoffman, 1993). These features lead others
to perceive individuals as dependent and to foster warm, protective responses.
   What characterizes a babyfaced appearance? From Zebrowitz's
studies, faces considered babylike (and which elicit protective responses) include those that have larger eyes relative to the face; a
small, concave nose with a sunken bridge; redder lips that are proportionately smaller than adults'; larger forehead and shorter
chin, resulting in lower vertical placement of features on the face;
and fuller cheeks and rounder chin, resulting in a rounder face
(Berry & McArthur, 1986). Although a face with all features will
be rated as most immature, the effect is still found for varying
combinations of individual features (Zebrowitz, 1997).

Individuals with Down syndrome have many of these baby-like facial features. Compared to age- and sex-matched typically developing children, Allanson, O'Hara, Farkas, and Nair (1993) found that Down syndrome faces characteristically show striking negative nasal protrusion (similar to Zebrowitz's sunken bridge), reduced ear length (i.e., smaller features), reduced mouth width (i.e., smaller mouth), head length shorter than width (i.e., rounder face), and lower facial width (i.e., lower placement of features on the face).

These results suggest that individuals with Down syndrome have babyface features and, as a result, are included in the babyface overgeneralization. Consequently they may be eliciting more protective and positive reactions from others, as do their typically developing babyfaced peers.

In Fidler and Hodapp (1999), adults were shown to react to these faces as they would to younger children. The study involved showing college undergraduates three sets of faces: one of children with Down syndrome, one of children with 5p- syndrome (who generally have longer, more adult-like faces), and one of typically developing children. Each set consisted of one 8-year-old, one 10-year-old, and one 12-year-old. Respondents considered the Down syndrome faces as younger, more dependent, and more in need of help and assistance. In a second portion of this study, we examined whether the babyface overgeneralization holds within the Down syndrome group. We asked respondents to rate pictures of twelve 10-year-old children with Down syndrome, but whose faces were either higher or lower on their objectively measured degrees of babyfaceness. Again, more babyfaced children were considered to be warmer, more honest, naïve, and dependent.

Taken together, children with Down syndrome show the workings of both direct and indirect effects on personality and motivational functioning. Although findings remain controversial, it does appear that these children tend to have pleasant personalities, engage in frequent, socially oriented behaviors, and have less psychopathology (especially the most severe psychopathologies). Children with Down syndrome may also have facial characteristics that are more babylike than same-aged retarded and typically developing peers. These more direct effects, in turn, seem to engender more loving, less stressful reactions from parents, families, and peers and more protective, nurturant reactions from surrounding adults.

TOWARD AN INTERACTIONAL-
TRANSACTIONAL VIEW OF PERSONALITY
AND MOTIVATION
IN DIFFERENT ETIOLOGICAL GROUPS

Findings of direct and indirect genetic disorders of mental retardation shed a new, unexpected light on personality and motivation in individuals with mental retardation. For the most part, such personality-motivational work has focused on only one corollary of mental retardation: that individuals with mental retardation fail more often. To date, studies have involved such issues as learned helplessness (Weisz, 1981), decreased expectancy of success (Gruen, Ottinger, & Ollendick, 1974; Zigler, 1971), and outerdirectedness, the ways in which persons with mental retardation look toward others for solutions to difficult problems (Bybee & Zigler, 1998).

But less efficient intellectual abilities are not the sole direct effect of different genetic etiologies of mental retardation. As the Down syndrome example shows, persons with different genetic disorders of mental retardation oftentimes show distinct social abilities and personality styles. Though not every person with Down syndrome is the same, as a group persons with Down syndrome seem more social, more interested in people, and, possibly, more pleasant and outgoing.

Consequently, individuals with Down syndrome receive different interactions from those in their surrounding environments. The perception of most individuals with Down syndrome as more personable and person-oriented leads, in turn, to parents who remark on the pleasant, cheerful personalities of their children.

In considering direct and indirect effects of genetic disorders, the mental retardation field may have too narrowly focused its examinations of personality and motivation. In effect, a more interactional, even transactional, view seems needed. This more interactional-transactional perspective goes beyond the view that personalities and motivational structures are the result of failures or that failure constitutes mental retardation's sole critical component. An interactional-transactional view emphasizes the need to consider both direct and indirect effects of genetic mental retardation disorders. Just as different genetic disorders predispose persons with that disorder to different personality styles and other personal characteristics, these characteristics become exacerbated or lessened by each child's interactions with the surrounding interpersonal environment. These ongoing reactions, in turn, serve to either reinforce or negate already-existing personality and motivational characteristics.

Although most researchers would consider an interactional-transactional analysis as amenable to personality-motivational work in mental retardation, the larger, more interesting questions remain unanswered. Indeed, when considering personality-motivational functioning, the important questions involve not whether transactional relations occur, but how.

To pose only the most basic of questions, how, exactly, does the child's personality or motivational style interact with surrounding adults? Which specific behaviors does a cheerful, person-oriented personality elicit from surrounding adults? In Down syndrome, are parental behaviors even elicited most by the child's behavior, or equally (or more) by the child's facial appearance or by the helpful effects of parent groups or society's acceptance of this one syndrome?

In the same way, how do such adult-child interactions and transactions change over the child's development? Consider, for example, the finding that Prader-Willi syndrome is a two-stage disorder (Dykens & Cassidy, 1996), with infants and young toddlers oftentimes showing failure-to-thrive and the hyperphagia and other food-related behaviors only beginning later in the preschool period. How do families react to the shift from worrying that their toddler might fail to thrive at one age, only to be worried about the child's weight ballooning out of control only a year or two later? Similar changes in child behaviors with development may characterize the language abilities of Williams syndrome (which may not be as advanced early on) and Down syndrome (which may show dampened affect in infancy but not at later ages). In short, a more dynamic, transactional sense of child-adult interaction is necessary when considering the interactive aspects of personality and motivation in different genetic disorders of mental retardation.

In yet another set of questions, adult-child interactions and transactions may occur differently to different people in the child's surrounding environments. When confronted with the child with Down syndrome's social party pieces, are teachers as charmed as parents? How do such behaviors affect peers or siblings? Again, no answers to these questions currently exist.

Ultimately, genetic etiologies' direct and indirect effects matter for both theory and practice. Theoretically, such insights tell researchers more about mental retardation and the interplay of specific types of mental retardation and the child's surrounding environments. On a more practical level, such studies inform intervention efforts. If indeed children with different types of mental retardation differ in their personalities, learning styles, or cognitive, linguistic, or adaptive strengths and weaknesses, then specific, tailored interventions become possible (Hodapp & Fidler, 1999). Families, peers, and siblings can be counseled about behaviors and characteristics typical of different etiologies, and interventions can be developed for these individuals as well.

In essence, by examining both direct and indirect effects of genetic disorders, we broaden the study of personality and motivational functioning in children with mental retardation and their families. As this review shows, we currently have more questions than answers. But, then again, in looking at the geneticist Charles Epstein's review of genetic progress over the past decade, that field as well had more questions than answers only a short time ago. Although it is unlikely that the field of personality motivation will progress as quickly or on as many fronts as the study of human genetics, researchers can look forward to many exciting discoveries in the years ahead. Such discoveries, in turn, can provide more information about personality-motivational functioning, as well as point the way to new, more targeted, programs of intervention.

ACKNOWLEDGMENT

I thank Elisabeth Dykens for her helpful comments on earlier drafts of this chapter.

REFERENCES

Allanson, J. E., O'Hara, P., Farkas, L. G., & Nair, R. C. (1993). Anthropometric craniofacial pattern profiles in Down syndrome. *American Journal of Medical Genetics, 47*(5), 748–752.

Bell, R. Q. (1968). A reinterpretation of direction of effects in studies of socialization. *Psychological Bulletin, 75,* 81–95.

Berry, D. S., McArthur, L. Z. (1985). Some components and consequences of a babyface. *Journal of Personality and Social Psychology, 48*(2), 312–323.

Berry, D. S., McArthur, L. Z. (1986). Perceiving character in faces: The impact of age-related craniofacial changes on social perception. *Psychological Bulletin, 100,* 3–18.

Buckley, S., Bird, G., & Byrne, A. (1996). The practical and theoretical significance of teaching literacy skills to children with Down's syndrome. In J.A. Rondal, J. Perera, L. Nadel, & A. Comblain (Eds.), *Down's syndrome: Psychological, psychobiological, and socio-educational perspectives* (pp. 119–128). London: Whurr.

Bybee, J. A., & Zigler, E. (1998). Outerdirectedness and emotional development in children with mental retardation. In J. A. Burack, R. M. Hodapp, & E. Zigler (Eds.), *Handbook of mental retardation and development* (pp. 434–461). Cambridge, UK: Cambridge University Press.

Byrne, E. A., Cunningham, C. C., & Sloper, P. (1988). *Families and their children with Down's syndrome.* London: Routledge.

Cahill, B. M., & Glidden, L. M. (1996). Influence of child diagnosis on family and parent functioning: Down syndrome versus other disabilities. *American Journal on Mental Retardation, 101,* 149–160.

Capps, L., Kasari, C., Yirmiya, N., & Sigman, M. (1993). Parental perception of emotional expressiveness in children with autism. *Journal of Consulting and Clinical Psychology, 61,* 475–484.

Carr, J. (1995). *Down's syndrome: Children growing up.* Cambridge, UK: Cambridge University Press.

Down, J. L. (1866). Observations on an ethnic classification of idiots. *London Hospital Reports, 3,* 259–262.

Dunn, P. M. (1991). Dr. Langdon Down (1828–1896) and "mongolism." *Archives of Disease in Childhood, 66,* 827–828.

Dykens, E. M. (1995). Measuring behavioral phenotypes: Provocations from the "new genetics." *American Journal on Mental Retardation, 99,* 522–532.

Dykens, E. M. (1996). DNA meets DSM: Genetic syndromes' growing importance in dual diagnosis. *Mental Retardation, 34,* 125–127.

Dykens, E. M. (this volume). Personality and psychopathology: New insights from genetic syndromes.

Dykens, E. M., & Cassidy, S. B. (1996). Prader-Willi syndrome: Genetic, behavioral, and treatment issues. *Child and Adolescent Clinics of North America, 5,* 913–928.

Dykens, E. M., Cassidy, S. B., & King, B. H. (1999). Maladaptive behavior differences in Prader-Willi syndrome associated with paternal deletion versus maternal uniparental disomy. *American Journal on Mental Retardation, 104,* 67–77.

Dykens, E. M., Hodapp, R. M., & Leckman, J. F. (1994). *Behavior and development in fragile X syndrome.* In (A. E. Kazdin, Series Ed.), *Sage Series on Developmental Clinical Psychology and Psychiatry* (Vol. 28). Newbury Park, CA: Sage Publications.

Dykens, E. M., & Kasari, C. (1997). Maladaptive behavior in children with Prader-Willi syndrome, Down syndrome, and non-specific mental retardation. *American Journal on Mental Retardation, 102,* 228–237.

Dykens, E. M., & Volkmar, F. R. (1997). Medical conditions associated with autism. In D.J. Cohen & F. R. Volkmar (Eds.), *Handbook of autism and pervasive developmental disorders* (2nd ed., pp. 388–407). New York: John Wiley.

Epstein, C. J. (1996). ASHG Presidential Address: Toward the 21st century. *American Journal of Human Genetics, 60,* 1–9.

Erikson, M., & Upshure, C. C. (1989). Caretaking burden and social support: Comparison of mothers of infants with and without disabillities. *American Journal on Mental Retardation, 94,* 250–258.

Fidler, D. J., & Hodapp, R. M. (1998). The importance of typologies for science and service in mental retardation. *Mental Retardation, 36,* 489–495.

Fidler, D. J., & Hodapp, R. M. (1999). Craniofacial maturity and perceived personality in children with Down syndrome. *American Journal on Mental Retardation, 104,* 410–421.

Flynt, J., & Yule, W. (1994). Behavioural phenotypes. In M. Rutter, E. Taylor, & L. Hersov (Eds.), *Child and adolescent psychiatry: Modern approaches* (3rd ed., pp. 666–687). London: Blackwell Scientific.

Fowler, A. (1990). Language abilities in children with Down syndrome: Evidence for a specific syntactic delay. In D. Cicchetti & M. Beeghly

(Eds.), *Children with Down syndrome: A developmental approach* (pp. 302–328). New York: Cambridge University Press.

Gath, A., & Gumley, D. (1986). Behaviour problems in retarded children with special reference to Down's syndrome. *British Journal of Psychiatry, 149,* 156–161.

Gelb, S. A. (1997). The problem of typological thinking in mental retardation. *Mental Retardation, 35,* 448–457.

Gibson, D. (1978). *Down's syndrome: The psychology of mongolism.* Cambridge, UK: Cambridge University Press.

Gruen, G., Ottinger, D., & Ollendick, T. (1974). Probability learning in retarded children with different histories of success and failure in school. *American Journal of Mental Deficiency, 79,* 417–423.

Hodapp, R. M. (1995). Parenting children with Down syndrome and other types of mental retardation. In M. Bornstein (Ed.), *Handbook of parenting. Vol. 1.* (pp. 233–253). Hillsdale, NJ: Lawrence Erlbaum Associates.

Hodapp, R. M. (1996). Down syndrome: Developmental, psychiatric, and management issues. *Child and Adolescent Psychiatric Clinics of North America, 5,* 881–894.

Hodapp, R. M. (1997). Direct and indirect behavioral effects of different genetic disorders of mental retardation. *American Journal on Mental Retardation, 102,* 67–79.

Hodapp, R. M. (1998). *Development and disabilities: Intellectual, sensory, and motor impairments.* New York: Cambridge University Press.

Hodapp, R. M. (1999). Indirect effects of genetic mental retardation disorders: Theoretical and methodological issues. *International Review of Research in Mental Retardation, 22,* 27–50.

Hodapp, R. M., & Dykens, E. M. (1994). Mental retardation's two cultures of behavioral research. *American Journal on Mental Retardation, 98,* 675–687.

Hodapp, R. M., Dykens, E. M., & Masino, L. L. (1997). Families of children with Prader-Willi Syndrome: Stress-support and relations to child characteristics. *Journal of Autism and Developmental Disorders, 27,* 11–24.

Hodapp, R. M., Evans, D. W., & Gray, F. L. (1999). Intellectual development in children with Down syndrome. In J. Rondal, J. Perera, & L. Nadel (Eds.), *Down syndrome: A review of current knowledge* (pp. 124–132). London: Whurr.

Hodapp, R. M., & Fidler, D. J. (1999). Special education and genetics: Connections for the 21st century. *Journal of Special Education, 33*, 130–137.

Hodapp, R. M., Fidler, D. J., & Smith, A. C. M. (1998). Stress and coping in families of children with Smith Magenis syndrome. *Journal of Intellectual Disability Research, 42,* 331–340.

Hodapp, R. M., Wijma, C. A., & Masino, L. L. (1997). Families of children with 5p- (cri du chat) syndrome: Familial stress and sibling reactions. *Developmental Medicine and Child Neurology, 39,* 757–761.

Holm, V. A., Cassidy, S. B., Butler, M. G., Hanchet, J. M., Greenswag, L. R., Whitman, B. Y., & Greenberg, F. (1993). Prader-Willi syndrome: Consensus diagnostic criteria. *Pediatrics, 91,* 398–402.

Holroyd, J., & MacArthur, D. (1976). Mental retardation and stress on parents: A contrast between Down's syndrome and childhood autism. *American Journal of Mental Deficiency, 80,* 431–436.

Hornby, G. (1995). Fathers' views of the effects on their families of children with Down syndrome. *Journal of Child and Family Studies, 4,* 103–117.

Kasari, C., & Bauminger, N. (1998). Social and emotional development in children with mental retardation. In J. A. Burack, R. M. Hodapp, & E. Zigler (Eds.), *Handbook of mental retardation and development* (pp. 411–433). New York: Cambridge University Press.

Kasari, C., & Freeman, S. F. N. (in press). Task-related social behavior in children with Down syndrome. *American Journal on Mental Retardation.*

Kasari, C., Freeman, S. F. N., Mundy, P., & Sigman, M. (1995). Attention regulation by children with Down syndrome: Coordinated joint attention and social referencing. *American Journal on Mental Retardation, 100,* 128–136.

Kasari, C., & Hodapp, R. M. (1996). Is Down syndrome different? Evidence from social and family studies. *Down Syndrome Quarterly, 1*(4), 1–8.

Kasari, C., & Sigman, M. (1997). Linking parental perceptions to interactions in young children with autism. *Journal of Autism and Developmental Disorders, 27,* 39–57.

Meyers, B. A., & Pueschel, S. M. (1991). Psychiatric disorders in persons with Down syndrome. *Journal of Nervous and Mental Disease, 179,* 609–613.

Miller, J. F. (1992). Lexical development in young children with Down Syndrome. In R. Chapman (Ed.), *Processes in language acquisition and disorders* (pp. 202–216). St. Louis: Mosby.

Mink, T., Nihira, K., & Meyers, C. E. (1983). Taxonomy of family life styles. I. Home with TMR children. *American Journal of Mental Deficiency, 87,* 484–497.

Opitz, J. R. (1996, March). *Historiography of the causal analysis of mental retardation.* Speech to the 29th annual Gatlinburg Conference on Research and Theory in Mental Retardation, Gatlinburg, TN.

Pitcairn, T. K., & Wishart, J. G. (1994). Reactions of young children with Down syndrome to an impossible task. *British Journal of Developmental Psychology, 12,* 485–489.

Pueschel, S. R. (1990). Clinical aspects of Down syndrome from infancy to adulthood. *American Journal of Medical Genetics, 7* (Supp.), 52–56.

Pueschel, S. R., Gallagher, P. L., Zartler, A. S., & Pezzullo, J. C. (1987). Cognitive and learning processes in children with Down syndrome. *Research in Developmental Disabilities, 8,* 21–37.

Rosen, M. (1993). In search of the behavioral phenotype: A methodological note. *Mental Retardation, 31,* 177–178.

Sanders, J. L., & Morgan, S. B. (1997). Family stress and adjustment as perceived by parents of children with autism or Down syndrome: Implications for intervention. *Child and Family Behavior Therapy, 19,* 15–32.

Seltzer, M. M., Krauss, M. W., & Tsunematsu, N. (1993). Adults with Down Syndrome and their aging mothers: Diagnostic group differences. *American Journal on Mental Retardation, 97,* 496–508.

Thomas, V., & Olsen, D. H. (1993). Problem families and the circumplex model: Observational assessment using the Clinical Rating Scale (CRS). *Journal of Marital and Family Therapy, 19,* 159–175.

Udwin, O., Yule, W., & Martin, N. (1987). Cognitive abilities and behavioral characteristics of children with idiopathic infantile hypercalcaemia. *Journal of Child Psychology and Psychiatry, 28,* 297–309.

Weisz, J. R. (1981). Learned helplessness in black and white children identified by their schools as retarded and non-retarded: Performance deterioration in response to failure. *Developmental Psychology, 17,* 499–508.

Wijma, C. A., & Hodapp, R. M. (2001). Siblings of children with 5p- versus Down syndrome. Manuscript submitted for publication.

Wishart, J. G., & Johnston, F. H. (1990). The effects of experience on attribution of a stereotyped personality to children with Down's syndrome. *Journal of Mental Deficiency Research, 34*, 409–420.

Wisniewski, K. E., Kida, E., & Brown, W. T. (1996). Consequences of genetic abnormalities in Down's syndrome on brain structure and function. In J. A. Rondal, J. Perera, L. Nadel, & A. Comblain (Eds.), *Down's syndrome: Psychological, psychobiological, and socio-educational perspectives* (pp. 21–42). London: Whurr.

Zebrowitz, L. A. (1997). *Reading faces: Window to the soul?* Boulder, CO: Westview Press.

Zebrowitz, L. A., Olson, K., & Hoffman, K. (1993). Stability of babyfaceness and attractiveness across the life span. *Journal of Personality and Social Psychology, 64*(3), 453–466.

Zebrowitz, L. A., & Montepare, J. M. (1992). Impressions of babyfaced individuals across the life span. *Developmental Psychology, 28*, 143–152.

Zigler, E. (1971). The retarded child as a whole person. In H.E. Adams & W.K. Boardman (Eds.), *Advances in experimental clinical psychology* (pp. 47–121). Oxford: Pergamon.

6

Personality and Psychopathology: New Insights From Genetic Syndromes

Elisabeth M. Dykens

Neuropsychiatric Institute, University of California, Los Angeles

Recent advances in molecular genetics and the Human Genome Project provide new opportunities to study the behavior of people with mental retardation syndromes. Indeed, over 750 mental retardation syndromes have now been identified (Opitz, 1996), and people with genetic diagnoses may comprise up to 40 to 50% of those with mild to severe mental retardation living in both institutionalized and community settings (e.g., Dereymaeker, Fryns, Haegerman, Deroover, and Van den Berghe, 1988; Matilanen, Airaksinen, Monen, Launiala, & Kaariainen, 1995). The time is thus ripe for researchers to study the behavior of people with both previously and newly described mental retardation syndromes.

However, surprisingly few behavioral researchers study distinctive genetic etiologies, instead favoring heterogenous subject groupings (Dykens, 1995; Hodapp & Dykens, 1994). This de-emphasis on genetic syndromes is readily seen in the field's journals and publications. Aman (1991a), for example, published a comprehensive bibliography of articles published between 1970 and 1990 on behavioral and emotional disorders in persons with mental retardation. Over this 20-year period, only 11% (41 out of 375) of articles in the bibliography were devoted to people with specific syndromes, and most of these ($n = 24$) were on Down syndrome. The vast majority of articles (89%) used heterogenous groups of subjects. These very same percentages were also seen in a more recent review of psychopathology articles from 1990 to 1996 (Dykens, 1996).

In personality studies as well, mixed-group designs have predominated. Some early personality researchers classified people into two, broadly defined groups—those with different types of organic etiologies and those with cultural-familial mental retardation (Balla, Styfco, & Zigler, 1971; Zigler, 1967). Yet, for the most part studies paid little attention to etiology. As a result, researchers know more about personality and psychopathology in the general population of people with mental retardation than they do in people with distinctive genetic etiologies.

Without psychologists or other behavioral experts to take the lead, most behavioral observations of people with syndromes have been made by clinical geneticists, genetics counselors, and pediatricians. Because these clinicians routinely evaluate patients for genetic disorders, they are well positioned to make observations across people with the same condition. But most of these biomedical workers are more expert in observing medical or physical functioning than they are in assessing complex behavior. Left to their own devices, these researchers typically describe behavior in rather superficial ways, relying on labels such as *pleasant and outgoing, friendly, shy,* or *placid.*

Although preliminary, these observations have piqued the curiosity of psychologists and other researchers, who have joined forces with geneticists and taken work on behavioral phenotypes many steps further (Dykens, 1995). This chapter reviews some of this work, focusing primarily on personality and psychopathology in people with mental retardation syndromes, or *direct effects* (Dykens, Hodapp, & Finucane, 2000). In a related chapter, Hodapp (chap. 5, this volume) focuses on how personality and other characteristics set the stage for interactions with others, or so-called *indirect effects.* Hodapp's chapter focuses on indirect effects of children Down syndrome, while this chapter touches on personality and psychopathology in a broad array of syndromes.

In this chapter, then, I first justify my rationale for discussing both personality and psychopathology and then make brief mention of these two constructs in people with several different syndromes. I then provide a more in-depth review of personality and psychopathology in four syndromes: fragile X syndrome, Prader-Willi syndrome, Down syndrome, and Williams syndrome. After the syndrome review, the chapter discusses both the disadvantages and the advantages of syndrome-specific personality research. In particular, I propose that personality research may stereotype people with syndromes and discuss how this risk is offset by within-syndrome behavioral variability.

WHY REVIEW PSYCHOPATHOLOGY ALONG WITH PERSONALITY?

One set of reasons for reviewing both the psychopathology and the personality constructs in the same chapter is practical, based on measurement issues, and another set of reasons is conceptual. Practically speaking, personality motivation has yet to be widely studied in people with genetic mental retardation syndromes. Instead, most syndrome-specific studies, though rare relative to mixed group studies, focus on psychopathology or maladaptive behavior. This emphasis on psychopathology is understandable in light of the clinical urgency associated with some syndromic behaviors, such as hyperphagia in Prader-Willi syndrome or extreme self-injury in Lesch-Nyan syndrome.

Prompted in part by these and other clinical urgencies, researchers have developed a wealth of measures designed specifically to assess behavioral and emotional dysfunction in people with mental retardation (see Aman, 1991b, for a review). Many of these have well-established reliability and validity and include normative data from subjects with mixed etiologies of mental retardation. These tools have facilitated a wealth of research in psychopathology, including large-scale screenings of at-risk individuals, prevalence studies, and treatment outcome studies.

In contrast, none of the available, widely used objective or projective personality measures are normed on people with mental retardation. Furthermore, people with mental retardation may have difficulty understanding items on standard, objective personality measures and fall prey to acquiescence or response biases (e.g., Zetlin, 1985). Not surprisingly, then, little support is found for administering certain objective personality tests to people with mental retardation, such as the Sixteen Personality Factor Questionnaire (Spirrison, 1992) or a short form of the Minnesota Multiphasic Personality Inventory (MMPI; McDaniel, 1997).

Although projective personality techniques circumvent problems in objective testing, they are also problematic. The Rorschach inkblots, for example, have yet to be normed on people with mental retardation. Furthermore, many people with developmental delay have difficulty with the abstract, verbal, and integrative demands of the Rorschach, and their associations tend to be concrete and impoverished. The Thematic Apperception Test (TAT) remains popular among clinicians, yet lacks a valid scoring system for people with or without mental retardation (see Worchel & Dupree, 1990, for a review). The draw-a-person task, while conceptually and verbally less demanding than the Rorschach or TAT, does not appear to be a valid test of personality or psychopathology in adults with mental retardation (Dykens, 1996).

Although the situation looks grim, three new tools have recently been introduced to the field that can potentially change the face of personality research in the years ahead. All are geared for people with mental retardation. One is a story-telling task similar to the TAT, the Apperceptive Personality Test/ Mental Retardation (S. Reiss, Benson, & Szyszko, 1993), which is scored on the basis of both open-ended responses and a structured inquiry. Remaining measures are informant-based. The EZ-Yale Personality Questionnaire (Zigler & Bennett-Gates, in press) assesses five personality styles that Zigler postulated are highly characteristic of children with mental retardation. The Reiss Profiles of Fundamental Goals and Motivation Sensitivities for Persons with Mental Retardation (S. Reiss & Havercamp, 1998) assess 15 motivational domains consistently seen in people with or without mental retardation. Table 6.1 lists the various personality domains tapped by each of these three measures. These newly developed tools

TABLE 6.1
*Domains of Functioning in Three New Personality
Measures for People With Mental Retardation*

Apperception Personality Test/MR

Global self-esteem	Anger	Immature thinking
Body image	Mood	Denial
Intellectual	Negative	Interpersonal
defensiveness	thinking	attitudes
Aggression	Basic trust	Validity
Sociability		
Optimism		

EZ Yale Personality Questionnaire
Positive reaction tendency
Negative reaction tendency
Expectancy of success
Effectance motivation
Outerdirectedness

Reiss Profile of Fundamental Goals and Motivation Sensitivities

Vengeance	Sex	Curiosity
Helping others	Physical exercise	Attention
Food	Frustration	Anxiety
Rejection	Order	Morality
Pain	Independence	Social contact

hold much promise for future research on personality profiles in people with genetic mental retardation syndromes.

Beyond the practical concerns with measurement, there are also conceptual reasons for linking personality to psychopathology. The boundaries between personality and psychopathology are often blurry and have yet to be clearly established in people with or without mental retardation. Personality problems have long been considered a risk factor for psychopathology in people in the general population. Though many people with psychiatric disorders indeed show associated personality traits, the causal direction of these relationships is unclear. It is uncertain, for example, if the rigid and orderly personality style of people with obsessive-compulsive disorder is a by-product of the disorder itself or is a contributor to the onset of the disease. Other people have full-blown personality disorders, described in the *American Psychology Association Diagnostic and Statistical Manual* (4th ed.; *DSM-IV*) as "an enduring pattern of inner experience and behavior that deviates markedly from the expectations of the individual's culture, is pervasive and inflexible, has an onset in adolescence or early adulthood, is stable over time, and leads to distress or impairment" (p. 629).

As with the general population, people with mental retardation may show the full range of personality disorders, including antisocial personality disorder (Hurley & Sovner, 1995) and paranoid personality disorder (e.g., S. Reiss, 1992). Other individuals may not meet *DSM-IV* criteria for full-blown personality disorders, but instead show maladaptive personality styles or traits. Some of these traits may set the stage for full-blown psychiatric disorders (Dykens, 1999). Zigler and colleagues, for example, postulated that people with mental retardation often show low self-esteem, low expectancy of success, and outerdirected personality styles that are secondary to their many encounters with interpersonal and academic failure (see Zigler, chap. 1, this volume, for a review). These styles, in turn, may render some people more vulnerable to sadness, depression, impulsivity, attention deficits, and dependent personality disorders (Dykens, 1999).

In a more comprehensive theory, S. Reiss and Havercamp (1996) postulated that aberrant behaviors result when people with or without mental retardation show unusually high or low sensitivities to 15 different fundamental human motivations. Developing a theory based on individual differences and reinforcing effectiveness, they proposed that people are at risk for psychopathology or socially inappropriate behaviors in their quest to satisfy one or more aberrant moivations (see Reiss, chap. 8, this volume).

Here, then, both personality and psychopathology in people with different syndromes are reviewed for practical reasons, primarily the preponderance of psychopathology relative to personality measures and studies. They are also reviewed for conceptual reasons, appreciating that links between personality and psychopathology have yet to be fully understood in people with or without mental retardation.

SYNDROME REVIEW

For some syndromes, preliminary personality or maladaptive behavior observations have been informally made by geneticists or clinicians. Other syndromes, however, have been extensively and formally studied by psychologists and other behavioral researchers. Table 6.2 summarizes personality and psychopathology findings from both informal and formal observations in 19 different syndromes.

Table 6.2 illustrates many of the previously made points on personality and psychopathology. First, personality is often described superficially, with adjectives or phrases that border on being stereotypical. Examples include placid or good-natured in Cornelia de Lange syndrome, friendly and happy in cri-du-chat syndrome, and loving and sociable in Rubinstein-Taybi syndrome. Although the issue of stereotyping is discussed at the end of the chapter, note that studies have yet to verify these global personality impressions in most syndromes.

Second, Table 6.2 shows that more consistent mention is made of maladaptive or psychiatric problems than of personality features. Reasons for this disparity were discussed earlier and are likely related to clinical urgency and measurement issues. Third, behavioral studies are unevenly distributed across syndromes. Although not readily apparent in Table 6.2, some syndromes have few behavioral studies, such as 5p- syndrome or Lowe syndrome, while other syndromes have been thoughtfully examined. Considerable work has focused, for example, on problems with social relating in males and females with fragile X syndrome (see Dykens & Volkmar, 1997, for a review) and on depression and Alzheimer-type dementia in adults with Down syndrome (see Hodapp, 1996, for a review).

It is often unclear why some syndromes have received more behavioral research than others. In some cases, dramatic breakthroughs in the genetic understandings of syndromes have

TABLE 6.2

Characteristic Personality Features and Maladaptive Behavior in 19 Mental Retardation Syndromes

Syndrome	Prevalence/Genetics	Personality, Maladaptive, and Psychiatric Features
Angelman[a]	1/20,000 maternal del 15q11–q13	Affectionate, sociable, cheerful, overactive, overexcited, poor concentration, bouts of laughter, seizures, ataxic movements
Cornelia de Lange[b]	1/10,000–40,000 autosomal dominant ?3q26.3	Placid, good-natured, not talkative, mild to severe self-injury, autistic features, aggression, restless, irritable, overactive
5p-[c]	1/50,000 del 5p15	Friendly, happy, placid, overactivity, poor concentration, self-stimulatory behaviors, self-injury, infantile cat-like cry
Down[d]	1/800 trisomy 21 in 95% cases	Sociable, outgoing, friendly, stubborn, attention deficits, overactivity, noncompliance, depression and Alzheimer-type dementia in adults
Duchenne Muscular Dystrophy[e]	1/3,500 males X-linked, xp1	Isolative, withdrawn, anxiety, depressed mood, poor peer relationships, features more pronounced in older boys, and boys with lower IQs

Fragile X[f]	1/1,250–4,000 males 1/2,500 females	Shy, withdrawn, social anxiety, extreme shyness, gaze avoidance, stereotypies, self-injury, overactivity, attention deficits
Hunter[g]	1/100,000 X-X-linked Xq28	With accumulation of mucopoly saccharides, speech loss, inattention, restless, stubborn, aggressive, apathetic & sedentary over time
Klinefelter[h]	1/1,000 males 47,XXXY	Introverted, passive, withdrawn, insecure, apprehensive, adults can be aloof, uncooperative, with impulse control & social adjustment problems
Lesch-Nyhan[i]	1/380,000 males X-linked recessive Xq26–27	Compulsive self-injury, especially lip, finger, and mouth biting, physical and verbal aggression
Lowe[j]	1/200,000 males X-linked recessive Xq24–26	Self-injury, stereotypies some secondary to visual impairments, temper tantrums, screaming
Neuro-fibromatosis-1[k]	1/2,500–4,000 Autosomal dominant 17q11.2	Anxiety, poor self-esteem, withdrawal, inattention, disruptive behavior, some secondary to degree of cosmetic disfigurement and cognitive delay
Noonan[l]	1/1,000–2,500 Autosomal dominant 12q22–qter	Affable nature, lovable, overemotional, overly concerned with others, perseveration, immature, stubborn, poor peer relationships

(continued)

TABLE 6.2 (continued)

Characteristic Personality Features and Maladaptive Behavior in 19 Mental Retardation Syndromes

Syndrome	Prevalence/Genetics	Personality, Maladaptive, and Psychiatric Features
Phenylketonuria[m]	1/10,000 Autosomal recessive 12q22–q24.1	Untreated: hyperactivity, stereotypies, lability, aggression, self-injury Treated: restless, some problems concentrating, isolative, anxious
Prader-Willi[n]	1/15,000–20,000 Paternal del 15 q11–q13	Friendly, self-centered, stubborn, tantrums, food preoccupations & seeking, skin-picking, non-food compulsions, impulsivity, sadness
Rett[o]	1/15,000 females X-linked dominant	Hand-wringing, stereotypies, screaming, panic, anxiety, hyperventilation seizures, autistic-like withdrawal, predictable regressive course
Rubinstein-Taybi[p]	1/125,000 Autosomal dominant ?16p13.3	Happy, loving, sociable, self-stimulatory behaviors, self-injury, intolerance for loud noise, lability
Smith-Magenis[q]	1/50,000 Del 17p11.2	Attention seeking, overactivity, profound sleep disturbance, inattention, stereotypies, self-injury (head-banging, nail-yanking, bodily insertions)

Turner[r]	1/2,000 females 45, XO	Withdrawn, anxiety, poor self-esteem, social adjustment problems, immaturity, lack of assertiveness, average IQ range
Williams[s]	1/20,000–25,000 Del 7q11.23	Sociable, charming, friendly, talkative, interested in feelings of others, attention deficits, hyperactivity, anxiety, fears, sadness, depression

[a]Williams et al., 1995; [b]Hawley, Jackson, & Kurnit, 1985; [c]Dykens & Clarke, 1997; [d]Hodapp, 1996; [e]Fitzpatrick, Barry, & Garvey, 1986; [f]Dykens, Hodapp, & Leckman, 1994; [g]Bax & Colville, 1995; [h]Mandoki, Sumner, Hoffman, & Riconda, 1991; [i]Anderson & Earnst, 1994; [j]Kenworthy, Parke, & Charnas, 1993; [k]Riccardi, 1992; [l]Sharland, Burch, McKenna, & Paton, 1992; [m]Smith, Beasley, Wolff, & Ades, 1988; [n]Dykens & Cassidy, 1999; [o]Van Acker, 1991; [p]Hennekman et al., 1992; [q]Smith, Dykens, & Greenberg, in press; [r]McCauley, Ross, Kushner, & Cutler, 1995; [s]Pober & Dykens, 1996.

293

sparked the curiosity of behavioral researchers. This is true in fragile X syndrome, the first human disease associated with a trinucleotide repeat, and in Prader-Willi syndrome, the first known human disease associated with genomic imprinting. As we discuss later, behavioral work in these syndromes takes advantage of genetic advances, thus allowing researchers to identify distinctive behavioral phenotypes in these disorders, as well as to link these findings to genetic status.

Behavioral research in other syndromes may be driven by clinical necessity, as in Lesch-Nyan syndrome or Smith-Magenis syndrome, or simply by the availability of subjects, as in the highly prevalent Down syndrome. Yet very little is known about the behavior of people with the hundreds of syndromes that are less genetically well understood, less clinically involved, or less prevalent. While it is a methodologic challenge to study people with rare conditions, other obstacles to the work include a leeriness about genetics from behavioral workers and concerns that genetic diagnoses are nonsignificant or invite stigma (Dykens & Hodapp, 1999). Hence, approximately 90% of behavioral mental retardation studies use subjects with heterogenous or mixed etiologies (Dykens, 1996; Hodapp & Dykens, 1994, 2000), with few researchers taking up the challenge to study rare genetic disorders. Indeed, one may wonder if some of these unexplored syndromes might have behavioral or developmental phenotypes just as intriguing as fragile X syndrome, Down syndrome, or other well-described conditions.

Appreciating that researchers know precious little about behavior in most mental retardation syndromes, four of the syndromes listed in Table 6.2 are now reviewed in more detail. These syndromes have rich or growing behavioral databases and include fragile X syndrome, Prader-Willi syndrome, Down syndrome, and Williams syndrome. Although not representative of all 750 known mental retardation syndromes, these disorders show the advantages of syndrome-based behavioral research and may ultimately spark more research interest in other syndromes as well.

Fragile X Syndrome

Fragile X syndrome, the most common inherited cause of mental retardation, results in a wide range of learning and behavioral problems, with males being more often and severely affected than females (see Dykens, Hodapp, & Leckman, 1994, for a review). The recently discovered fragile X gene (FMR-1) represents a newly identified type of human disease caused by an amplification (or excessive repetition) of three nucleotide sequences (CGG) that make up DNA. Above a certain threshold of these triplet repeats, people are fully affected with the syndrome. Below that number (and above the normal threshold), they show premutations. Persons with premutations may be affected or unaffected carriers of the syndrome, depending on the mode of inheritance and other genetic factors (see Caskey, Pizzuti, Fu, Fenwick, & Nelson, 1992, for a review).

Males. Case reports in the early 1980s described a handful of fully affected boys who met diagnostic criteria for autistic disorder. These subjects showed language and developmental delay, stereotypies, perseveration, poor eye contact, and tactile defensiveness. Excited by the possibility of a common genetic cause of autism, many researchers became caught up with linking the two disorders. This work either diagnosed autism among males with fragile X or screened autistic samples for the fragile X marker. Highly variable prevalence rates resulted from this work, due primarily to discrepancies in diagnostic criteria for autism (see Dykens & Volkmar, 1997, for a review).

This flurry of research faded as new studies emerged suggesting that, different from autism, many males showed a willingness to interact with others coupled with social and performance anxiety and mutual gaze aversion (Bregman, Leckman, & Ort, 1988; Cohen, Vietze, Sudhalter, Jenkins, & Brown, 1989). Controlled studies and meta-analyses (Einfeld, Molony, & Hall, 1989; Fisch, 1992) now suggest that only about 5–15% of males with fragile X have full-blown autistic disorder. Instead, the majority of affected males can be placed on a spectrum of social anxiety, shyness, avoidance, and gaze aversion. While some of these boys have anxiety disorders (Bregman et al., 1988) or Pervasive Developmental Disorder-Not Otherwise Specified (PDD-NOS) (A. L.

Reiss & Freund, 1990), others may simply show slow-to-warm temperament styles, including shyness or social withdrawal (Kerby & Dawson, 1994).

In addition to these difficulties, hyperactivity and attention deficits are seen in the vast majority of clinic-referred boys with fragile X syndrome (Bregman et al., 1988; Hagerman, 1996) and ADHD symptoms are higher among boys with fragile X relative to control subjects (Baumgardner, A. L. Reiss, Freund, and Abrams, 1995). While hyperactivity may diminish with age, inattention seems to persist even with advancing age (Dykens, Leckman, Paul, & Watson, 1988).

Females. As with males, many females with fragile X syndrome show variable levels of social dysfunction, primarily shyness, gaze aversion, and social anxiety. Often these problems are more pronounced in females than males. Many women with fragile X syndrome meet clinical criteria for schizotypal disorder, showing interpersonal discomfort and difficulties in communication and social relationships. Fully affected women (with CGG repeats in excess of 200) are more likely to have schizotypal disorder or schizotypal features than women with a premutation (with 50 to 200 repeats) or appropriately matched nonfragile X control women (Freund, A. L. Reiss, Hagerman, & Vinogradov, 1992; A. L. Reiss, Hagerman, Vinogradov, Abrams, & King, 1988; Sobesky, Porter, Pennington, & Hagerman, 1995). Although shyness is thus a central feature of the fragile X behavioral phenotype, affected females may also show increased risks of depression, even as compared to nonfragile X mothers of developmentally delayed children (Freund et al., 1992; A. L. Reiss et al., 1988).

Girls with fragile X have lower prevalence rates of ADHD relative to boys with fragile X, but higher rates relative to the general population. Many suffer more from inattention than hyperactivity, though one study found that at least 50% of the sample of girls with fragile X had ADHD (Lachiewicz, 1992). Among adults, problems in attending and in sustaining effort have been found in the neuropsychological profiles of women who carry the FMR-1 gene, which may contribute to problems in math, abstract reasoning, and planning (e.g., Mazzocco, Hagerman, Cronister-Silverman, & Pennington, 1992).

Fragile X syndrome thus involves vulnerabilities toward shyness, gaze aversion, social anxiety, avoidant disorders, schizotypal disorder, ADHD, PDD-NOS, and, more rarely, autistic disorder. These difficulties vary in severity, but are typically found in persons across the IQ spectrum, from those with moderate mental retardation to those with mild learning disabilities. Many specific interventions are suggested from these findings, including an emphasis on individualized learning or tasks; minimizing auditory or visual distractors at home, school, or work; and reducing the flow of people through work and living settings. Many females with fragile X also benefit from psychotherapy and from at-home supports, especially when mothers are mildly affected with the syndrome or have multiple children affected with the disorder (see Dykens & Hodapp, 1997).

Prader-Willi Syndrome

First identified over 40 years ago, Prader-Willi syndrome is best known for its food-related characteristics. Whereas babies invariably show hypotonia and pronounced feeding-sucking difficulties, young children between 2 and 6 years of age develop hyperphagia and food seeking behavior such as food foraging and hoarding (see Dykens & Cassidy, 1999, for a review). Hyperphagia is likely associated with a hypothalamic abnormality resulting in a lack of satiety (Holland, Treasure, Coskeran, & Dallow, 1995; Swaab, Purba, & Hofman, 1995). Food preoccupations are life long, and without prolonged dietary management, affected individuals invariably become obese. Indeed, complications of obesity remain the leading cause of death in this syndrome.

Although obsessive thoughts about food are invariably seen, a remarkably high proportion of persons also show nonfood obsessions and compulsive behaviors (Dykens, Leckman, & Cassidy, 1996). These nonfood symptoms include skin-picking, hoarding, needing to tell, ask, or say things, and having concerns with symmetry, exactness, ordering, arranging, cleanliness, and sameness in daily routine. Often these symptoms are associated with distress or adaptive impairment, suggesting marked risks of obsessive-compulsive disorder in this population (Dykens et al., 1996).

In addition, many children and adults with Prader-Willi syndrome show high rates of temper tantrums, aggression, stubbornness, underactivity, excessive daytime sleepiness, and emotional lability, even compared to others with mental retardation (Dykens & Kasari, 1997). These impulsive behaviors, coupled with food seeking, often lead people to need more restrictive levels of care than would be predicted by their mild levels of mental retardation (Dykens, 1999).

Studies to date have generally used psychiatric nosology or standard psychopathology measures to describe the food and nonfood features of Prader-Willi syndrome. Research is now underway that examines these same obsessive-compulsive and impulsive tendencies from a personality-motivation framework. In ongoing work, my colleagues and I are comparing motivational profiles of adults with Prader-Willi syndrome to other adults with developmental delay (Dykens & Rosner, 1999). Using the newly developed Reiss Profiles of Fundamental Goals and Motivation Sensitivities (S. Reiss & Havercamp, 1998), we find significant between-group differences in certain motivational needs. Not surprisingly, relative to controls, subjects with Prader-Willi syndrome are much more motivated by food, as well as by needs for orderliness and curiosity, especially in solving puzzles. In addition, they are easily slighted and more responsive to rejection and frustration. Problem behaviors such as temper outbursts, compulsivity, and food seeking can thus be predicted from these unusually high or low motivational styles.

Personality and psychopathology may be associated with the individual's genetic variant of Prader-Willi syndrome. Most cases of Prader-Willi syndrome (about 70%) are caused by a paternally derived deletion on the long arm of chromosome 15 [del 15(q11–q13)]. Remaining cases are attributed to maternal uniparental disomy (UPD) of chromosome 15, in which both members of the chromosome 15 pair come from the mother (Nicholls, Knoll, Butler, Karam, & LaLande, 1989). In either case, there is an absence of the paternally derived contribution to this specific region of the genome. When missing information in this same region of chromosome 15 is maternally derived, it results in a completely different and more severe developmental disorder, Angelman's syndrome (see Cassidy, 1992, for a review). Prader-

Willi syndrome is thus the first known human disease to show the effects of genomic imprinting, or the idea that genes are modified and expressed differently depending on whether they are inherited from the mother or the father.

Preliminary findings suggest some behavioral differences between Prader-Willi syndrome cases due to paternal deletion versus maternal UPD. Cases with deletions may show lower IQs and more frequent or severe problem behaviors, such as skin-picking, hoarding, temper tantrums, overeating, and social withdrawal (Dykens, Cassidy, & King, 1999). Although a dampening of symptom severity is suggested in many UPD cases, occasional cases of more severe problems in UPD, primarily autistic-like features and relatively low IQ's, are also observed.

Many people with Prader-Willi syndrome, then, are at increased risk for obsessive-compulsive, impulse control, and affective disorders. Yet even those who do not meet diagnostic criteria for these full-blown psychiatric disorders have salient vulnerabilities for specific motivational profiles that are likely to lead to aberrant behavior. Future research is needed to clarify if either psychiatric disorders or motivational profiles differ across those with paternal deletions versus maternal UPD. In the meantime, data inform interventions, suggesting pharmacologic and behavioral treatments for obsessions, compulsions, and impulsivity that complement life-long needs for dietary interventions and food restrictions (see Dykens & Hodapp, 1997, for a review).

Down Syndrome

Persistent personality stereotypes depict persons with Down syndrome as cheerful, friendly, eager to please, and affectionate—the so-called Prince Charming syndrome (Gibbs & Thorpe 1983; Hodapp, chap. 5, this volume; Menolascino, 1965). Some findings, however, call this stereotype into question. Many mothers, for example, describe their children with Down syndrome as having a wide range of personality features (Rogers, 1987), and the temperaments of some children with Down syndrome are active, distractible, and difficult (Ganiban, Wagner, & Cicchetti, 1990). Still, fathers often spontaneously remark on their child's sociability (Hornby, 1995), and the temperaments of many children with

Down syndrome have been described as easygoing (Ganiban et al., 1990). Even with these equivocal findings, the personality stereotype persists, with parents and researchers alike often remarking that children and adults with Down syndrome are extraordinarily charming and eager to please.

Yet these endearing features do not necessarily protect these same individuals from showing behavioral problems such as stubbornness, defiance, aggressive behavior, and psychopathology. Children with Down syndrome have elevated behavioral problems relative to their siblings without developmental delay (Gath & Gumley, 1986; Pueschel, Bernier, & Pezzullo, 1991). About 13 to 15% of children with Down syndrome appear to have significant behavioral difficulties. Prevalence estimates are higher and more variable in studies of children and adolescents, ranging from 18 to 38% (Gath & Gumley, 1986; Menolascino, 1965; Meyers & Pueschel, 1991). Primary problems include disruptive disorders such as ADHD, oppositional and conduct disorders, and, occasionally, anxiety disorders (Gath & Gumley, 1986; Myers & Pueschel, 1991). In contrast to the externalizing disorders of childhood, adults with Down syndrome are particularly vulnerable to depressive disorders (Callacott, Cooper, & McGrother, 1992; Meyers & Pueschel, 1991; Warren, Holroyd, & Folstein, 1989). Depression in Down syndrome is often characterized by passivity, apathy, withdrawal, and mutism, and several cases of major depressive disorder have now been well described (Dosen & Petry, 1993; Sovner, Hurley, & LaBrie, 1985; Warren et al., 1989). Prevalence estimates of affective disorders among adults with Down syndrome range from 6 to 11% (Collacott et al., 1992; Myers & Pueschel, 1991), many times higher than the 1 to 3% rates seen in the general population of persons with mental retardation (Lund, 1985; Menolascino, Levitas, & Greiner, 1986).

It is not yet known why adults with Down syndrome appear vulnerable to depression. One hypothesis implicates dementia. Almost all persons with Down syndrome over age 35 to 40 show neuropathological signs of Alzheimer's disease (Zigman, Schupf, Zigman, & Silverman, 1993), yet not all adults with Down syndrome develop the behavioral correlates of Alzheimer-type dementia, and the risk for doing so dramatically increases with advancing age. Some researchers find rates of dementia as high as 55% in persons aged 40 to 50 years and 75% in persons aged 60 years and older (Lai & Williams, 1989). Collectively, however, most studies suggest that less than 50% of adults aged 50 years or more show symptoms of dementia (Zigman et al., 1993).

Given the overlap in many clinical symptoms of depression and dementia, difficulties often arise in distinguishing these two disorders (e.g., Pary, 1992). In some cases, dementia and depression co-exist (e.g., Szymanski & Biederman, 1984). In other cases, persons diagnosed with depression may actually be showing early signs of dementia (Pary, 1992). In still others, it may be that diagnoses of dementia are overshadowing depressive conditions. In this vein, Warren et al. (1989) reported five cases of adults with Down syndrome referred for apparent dementia who were instead successfully treated for major depression.

Thus, while only a relatively small number of children with Down syndrome show disruptive behavior or other disorders, adults with Down syndrome are at considerable risk for depression and dementia. Aside from these two disorders, the overall rate of psychiatric illness in the population of persons with Down syndrome is low relative to other groups (Callacott et al., 1992; Grizenko, Cvejic, Vida, & Sayegh, 1991; Meyers & Pueschel, 1991). As such, persons with Down syndrome rarely show disorders such as Tourette's syndrome, anorexia nervosa, autism, mania, schizophrenia, or personality disorders (Barbas, Wardell, Sapiro, & Matthews, 1986; Bregman & Volkmar, 1988; Cook & Leventhal, 1987). While sociable, charming personalities may be associated with lower rates of psychopathology, the interplay between personality and psychopathology has not yet been studied in children or adults with Down syndrome.

Williams Syndrome

Williams syndrome, first identified in 1961 (Williams, Barratt-Boyes, & Lowe, 1961), is caused by a microdeletion on one of the chromosome 7s that includes the gene for elastin (Ewart et al., 1994). Persons with Williams syndrome often show hyperacusis, cardiovascular disease, hypercalcemia, neuromuskeletal and renal abnormalities, and characteristic facial features described as elfin-like, cute, and appealing (see Morris & Mervis, 1999, and Pober & Dykens, 1996, for reviews). Some of the syndrome's medical complications and facial features are likely associated with elastin insufficiency.

Williams syndrome is perhaps best known for its cognitive-linguistic profile. Many people with Williams syndrome show pronounced weaknesses in perceptual and visual-spatial functioning and relative strengths in expressive language. This relative sparing of linguistic functioning is seen in many aspects of language, including syntax and semantics (e.g., Bellugi, Marks, Bihrle, & Sabo, 1988); narrative enrichment strategies involving affective prosody and a sense of drama (e.g., Reilly, Klima, & Bellugi, 1990); and a reliance on stereotypic adult, social phrases (Udwin & Yule, 1990). But not all persons with the syndrome show strengths in grammar or *hyperverbal speech*, and this profile is now open to considerable debate (for reviews see Dykens et al., 2000, and Mervis, Morris, Bertrand, & Robinson, 1999).

Although researchers disagree on the pervasiveness of expressive language strengths, they are more apt to concede that most individuals with Williams syndrome show marked visual-perceptual difficulties, especially in written tasks requiring integrating parts into a whole (Dykens, Rosner, & Ly, in press; Mervis et al., 1999). Yet despite these weaknesses, many youngsters with Williams syndrome do well on facial recognition tasks (Bellugi, Wang, & Jernigan, 1994). This strength is consistent with informal clinical observations of subjects with Williams syndrome subjects as being "acutely attentive to the emotional states of others" (Bellugi et al., 1994, p. 35) and as "responsive to any and all facial cues" (p. 46). These strengths suggest a low probability of psychiatric disorders involving an inability to read social cues, such as autism or PDD-NOS (see Dykens & Volkmar, 1997, for a review).

In contrast to work on cognitive-linguistic profiles, studies have yet to fully examine the personality or psychiatric features of people with Williams syndrome. Early, informal descriptions of people with Williams syndrome hinted at a "classic" Williams syndrome personality, and research is beginning to support many of these impressions. Many people with Williams syndrome are pleasant, unusually friendly, affectionate, loquacious, engaging, and interpersonally sensitive and charming (e.g., Dilts, Morris, & Leonard, 1990). Such qualities may change over the course of development, with adults being more withdrawn and less overly friendly than children (Gosch & Pankau, 1997). Yet relative to others, even adults with Williams syndrome have shown a strong, social orientation including heightened motivation to help others and sensitivities to other peoples' feelings (Dykens & Rosner, 1999). Despite their empathic streak, however, persons with Williams syndrome were less likely to have friends.

Although sociability has generally been viewed as a strength, these features may also reflect social disinhibition characteristic of people who are anxious, impulsive, and overly aroused. Indeed, salient problems in Williams syndrome include anxiety, as well as hyperactivity and inattentiveness (e.g., Einfeld, Tonge, & Florio, 1997; Preus, 1984; Tomc, Williamson, & Pauli, 1990). Such problems are elevated relative to others with mental retardation, with generalized anxiety and worry often focusing on anticipated or future events, imagined or real disasters, somatic concerns, and other preoccupations. Indeed, compared to others with delay, I have found high rates of anxiety and specific fears in persons with Williams syndrome, as well as marked increased risks of specific phobias (Dykens, 1999). While fears seem to persist over time, overactivity and restlessness may decrease with age; other difficulties such as depression or sadness may be more common among adults than among children (Dykens, 1999; Gosch & Pankau, 1997; Pober & Dykens, 1996).

It is unknown how the cognitive-linguistic profile in Williams syndrome might mediate the expression of anxiety, fears, inattention, or hyperactivity and how all these relate to the musical talents sometimes shown by persons with this syndrome. To the extent that verbal comprehension and expressivity are indeed strengths, they may help the person with Williams syndrome to accurately express their thoughts and feelings. Strengths in verbal expressivity may thus bode well for increased treatment accessibility in the Williams syndrome population. Findings also suggest the need to appropriately channel sociability via social skills training, the use of team or buddy systems at school or work, and group therapies (see Dykens et al., 2000; Dykens & Hodapp, 1997, for a review).

SYNDROME SUMMARY

Across all four syndromes, then, heightened vulnerabilities toward specific personalities and psychopathologies are found. Shyness, social anxiety, and schizotypal features are prominent in males and females with fragile X syndrome, while sociability, overly friendliness, and increased empathy toward the feelings and facial expressions of others seem characteristic of people with Williams syndrome. Children and adults with Down syndrome also have a charming, affable, and sociable personality. Although many take issue with the accuracy of these descriptors, the stereotypical Down syndrome personality has persisted for over 100 years. However, these endearing features do not prevent some children from showing disruptive behavior or attention deficit disorders or some adults from showing depressive features and clinical signs of Alzheimer-type dementia. Finally, people with Prader-Willi syndrome often obsess about food and nonfood topics and engage in a variety of repetitive, compulsive-like behaviors. Relative to others with mental retardation, they are more likely to be easily slighted and frustrated, show stubbornness and temper outbursts, and have needs for orderliness.

Future research needs to focus on which behavioral features are unique vs. shared across various syndromes. While some features seem unique, as in hyperphagia in Prader-Willi syndrome, others features are shared with people with and without syndromes, such as anxiety, attention deficits, and hyperactivity. Importantly, even though syndromes may share a certain trait, there are likely to be qualitative differences in how they are expressed. For example, many people with Williams syndrome or Prader-Willi syndrome show obsessive thinking. Yet, on closer examination, researchers are now finding that obsessiveness in Williams syndrome is characterized by excessive worries and fears (Dykens, 2001), whereas obsessive thinking in Prader-Willi syndrome focuses on food, needs to tell or ask things, and a host of nonfood compulsive-like behaviors (Dykens et al., 1996). Better understandings of behavioral similarities and differences across syndromes are needed before researchers classify people together into heterogenous subject groupings.

WITHIN-SYNDROME VARIABILITY

Not all persons with fragile X, Prader-Willi, Down, or Williams syndromes show the characteristic features reviewed in this chapter. Furthermore, if they do show them, it may not be to the same extent or at the same point in development. In these ways, then, a behavioral phenotype is viewed as the "heightened probability or likelihood that people with a given syndrome will exhibit certain behavioral and developmental sequelae relative to those without the syndrome" (Dykens, 1995, p. 523).

While much phenotypic research emphasizes how people with the same genetic syndrome behave or look alike, one of the most exciting aspects of phenotypic work involves uncovering the reasons people with the same syndrome differ one from the other and discovering the combination of molecular genetic, environmental, and psychosocial factors that contribute to within-syndrome individual differences. For most syndromes, researchers do not yet know the answers, yet considerable progress is being made in studies that link within-syndrome behavioral variability to genetic status. Unlike early thinking, for example, it is now appreciated that people can have 5p- syndrome without showing the syndrome's characteristic infantile cat-like cry (Gersh et al., 1995). In females with fragile X syndrome, variability in cognitive and behavioral expressions is related to the ratio of the number of normally active X chromosomes relative to the total active plus inactive X chromosomes and the amount of FMR-1 protein being produced (see Hagerman, 1996, for a review). In Prader-Willi syndrome, preliminary findings suggest some behavioral differences in cases with paternal deletion versus maternal uniparental disomy (Dykens, Cassidy, & King, 1998).

Other sources of within-syndrome variance may be both similar and different across syndromes. For example, while age is associated with increased sadness or depressive features in Down and Prader-Willi syndromes, other correlates of personality or psychopathology may be relatively unique. Degree of obesity may prove a unique correlate of some emotional problems in Prader-Willi syndrome (Dykens & Cassidy, 1995), and gender may prove a significant factor in explaining differences in empathy and morality in adults with Williams syndrome (Dykens, in preparation). Understanding both the genetic and the psychosocial correlates of within-syndrome variability is one of the biggest challenges facing phenotypic researchers in the years ahead.

STEREOTYPING

Without an appreciation of within-syndrome variability, phenotypic work runs the risk of making gross overgeneralizations about people. These overgeneralizations or stereotypes may have accurate or faulty bases, but regardless of their roots, they have potentially damaging consequences. One destructive personality stereotype, for example, concerns males with XYY syndrome. Early researchers found increased rates of XYY males in prisons or psychiatric hospitals and concluded that males with an extra Y chromosome were predisposed to violent, aggressive, criminal behavior (Jacobs et al., 1965). Subsequent studies, correcting for sample bias, found little support linking antisocial behavior or criminality to XYY males (e.g., Borgaonkar & Shah, 1974). Some of these males, however, may show attention deficits, distractibility, oppositionality, and other problem behaviors (Waltzer, Bashir, & Silbert, 1991).

Stereotypes may also do more harm than good in the clinical setting. The Down syndrome personality stereotype, for example, may actually contribute to professionals overlooking certain psychiatric diagnoses in persons with Down syndrome, such as depression or autism. Although comorbid Down syndrome and autism is rare, with just a few cases reported in the literature, all cases were diagnosed later than usual, in late childhood, adolescence, or adulthood (see Dykens & Volkmar, 1997, for a review). This diagnostic overshadowing created undue stress for families and prevented them from using interventions and supports available to those with an autistic child. Similarly, clinicians need to ensure that the overly friendly, charming personality style of persons with Williams syndrome does not mask their possible underlying feelings of anxiety, worry, or sadness. Mental health and other professionals thus need to consider the full range of problems or psychiatric diagnoses in their patients or clients, even diagnoses that are inconsistent with a syndrome's personality characteristics.

Other potentially damaging effects of stereotypes are captured in the nicknames of some syndromes. Typically these nicknames pick up on a salient physical or behavioral aspect of a syndrome, and they can be quite pejorative. For the most part, these terms have evolved over the years into less disparaging labels. For example, people now favor neurofibromatosis over "elephant man's disease," Angelman syndrome over "the happy puppet syndrome," Down syndrome over "mongolism," and 5p-syndrome over cri-du-chat or the "cat cry" syndrome. Yet even with this shift in labels, overgeneralizations persist about people with syndromes. We often see this, for example, when well-meaning colleagues learn of my and my colleagues' work in Prader-Willi syndrome and remark, "Oh, they're the ones that are fat and can't stop eating." In fact, some people with Prader-Willi syndrome never become obese, and others maintain their ideal weights for years at a time. Furthermore, the drive for food varies across people and in the same person over the course of development.

We thus end with a cautionary note. Research is just underway on the behavioral phenotypes of people with genetic mental retardation syndromes, and within this context, there are many more studies on psychopathology than on personality. The conceptual ties between psychopathology and personality are not well understood, but this may very well change with the arrival of several new personality measures developed specifically for people with mental retardation.

In using these or other measures, syndromic research needs to adopt a two-pronged approach. First, many more between-group studies are needed that differentiate unique versus shared qualities across syndromes. In doing so, researchers must avoid potentially damaging overgeneralizations such as assuming that all people with Williams syndrome are sociable or that all people with fragile X syndrome are painfully shy. To accomplish this, the second approach is needed, which examines sources of within-syndrome variability, including genetic, developmental, and psychosocial reasons for individual differences. This two-pronged approach holds much promise for better understanding gene-behavior relationships (Dykens & Hodapp, 1999) and for generating syndrome-specific treatment recommendations (Dykens & Hodapp, 1997; Hodapp & Dykens, 1992). A blending of between- and within-syndrome research approaches also ensures that researchers do not oversimplify the behavioral richness and complexity of people with different genetic diagnoses.

ACKNOWLEDGMENT

The author thanks Robert M. Hodapp for his helpful comments on an earlier draft of this manuscript.

REFERENCES

Aman, M. G. (1991a). *Working bibliography on behavioral and emotional disorders and assessment instruments in mental retardation.* Rockville, MD: U.S. Department of Health and Human Services.

Aman, M. G. (1991b). *Assessing psychopathology and problem behaviors in persons with mental retardation: A review of available instruments.* Rockville, MD: U.S. Department of Health and Human Services.

American Psychiatric Association. (1994). *Diagnostic and statistical manual of mental disorders* (4th ed.). Washington, DC: Author.

Anderson, L. T., & Earnst, M. (1994). Self-injury in Lesch-Nyhan disease. *Journal of Autism and Developmental Disorders, 24,* 67–81.

Balla, D., Styfco, S., & Zigler, E. (1971). Use of the opposition concept and outerdirectedness in intellectually average, familial retarded, and organically retarded children. *American Journal of Mental Deficiency, 75,* 863–880.

Barbas, G., Wardell, B., Sapiro, M., & Matthews, W. S. (1986). Coincident Down's and Tourette syndromes: Three case reports. *Journal of Child Neurology, 1,* 358–360.

Baumgardner, T. L., Reiss, A. L., Freund, L. S., & Abrams, M. T. (1995). Specification of the neurobehavioral phenotypes in males with fragile X syndrome. *Pediatrics, 95,* 744–752.

Bax, M. C. O., & Colville, G. (1995). Behavior in mucopolysaccharide disorders. *Archives of Diseases in Childhood, 73,* 77–81.

Bellugi, U., Marks, S., Bihrle, & Sabo, H. (1988). Dissociation between language and cognitive functions in Williams syndrome. In D.

Bishop & K. Mogfont (Eds.), *Language Development in Exceptional Circumstances* (pp 177–189). London: Churchill Livingstone.

Bellugi, U., Wang, P., & Jernigan, T. L. (1994). Williams syndrome: An unusual neuropsychological profile. In S. H. Browman & J. Grafram (Eds.), *Atypical cognitive deficits in developmental disorders* (pp 23–56). Hillsdale, NJ: Lawrence Erlbaum Associates.

Borgaonkar, D. S., & Shah, S. A. (1974). The XYY chromosome: Male or syndrome? *Progress in Medical genetics, 10,* 135–222.

Bregman, J. D., Leckman, J. F. & Ort, S. I. (1988). Fragile X syndrome: Genetic predisposition to psychopathology. *Journal of Autism and Developmental Disorders, 18,* 343–354.

Bregman, J. D., & Volkmar, F. F. (1988). Autistic social dysfunction and Down syndrome. *Journal of the American Academy of Child and Adolescent Psychiatry, 27,* 440–441.

Caskey, C. T., Pizzuti, A., Fu, Y. H., Fenwick, R. G., & Nelson, D. L. (1992). Triplet repeat mutations in human disease. *Science, 256,* 784–789.

Cassidy, S. B. (Ed). (1992). *Prader-Willi syndrome and other chromosome 15q deletion disorders.* Berlin: Springer-Verlag.

Cohen, I. L., Vietze, P. M., Sudhalter, V., Jenkins, E. C., & Brown, W. T. (1989). Parent-child dyadic gaze patterns in fragile X males and in non-fragile X males with autistic disorder. *Journal of Child Psychology and Psychiatry, 30,* 845–856.

Collacott, R. A., Cooper, S. A., & McGrother, C. (1992). Differential rates of psychiatric disorders in adults with Down's syndrome compared with other mentally handicapped adults. *British Journal of Psychiatry, 161,* 671–674.

Cook, E. H., & Leventhal, B. L. (1987). Down's syndrome with mania. *British Journal of Psychiatry, 145,* 195–196.

Dereymaeker, A. M., Fryns, J. P., Haegeman, J., Deroover, J., & Van den Berghe, H. (1988). A genetic diagnostic survey in an institutionalized population of 158 patients. *Clinical Genetics, 34,* 126–134.

Dilts, C. V., Morris, C. A., & Leonard, C. O. (1990). Hypothesis for development of a behavioral phenotype in Williams syndrome. *American Journal of Medical Genetics, 6,* 126–131.

Dosen, A. & Petry, D. (1993). Treatment of depression in persons with mental retardation. In R. J. Fletcher & A. Dosen (Eds.), *Mental health aspects of mental retardation: Progress in assessment and treatment* (pp. 242–260). New York: Lexington.

Dykens, E. M. (1995). Measuring behavioral phenotypes: Provocations from the "new genetics". *American Journal on Mental Retardation, 99,* 522–532.

Dykens, E. M. (1996a). DNA meets DSM: The growing importance of genetic syndromes in dual diagnosis. *Mental Retardation, 34,* 125–127.

Dykens, E. M. (1996b). The Draw-a-Person task in persons with mental retardation: What does it measure? *Research in Developmental Disabilities, 17,* 1–3.

Dykens, E. M. (1999a). Personality-motivation: New ties to psychopathology, etiology, and intervention. In E. Zigler & D. Bennett-Gates (Eds.), *Personality development in individuals with mental retardation* (pp. 249–270). New York: Cambridge University Press.

Dykens, E. M. (1999b). Prader-Willi syndrome: Toward a behavioral phenotype. In H. Tager-Flusberg (Ed.), *Neurodevelopmental disorders* (pp. 137–154). Cambridge, MA: MIT Press.

Dykens, E. M. (2001). *Anxiety, fears and phobias in persons with Williams syndrome.* Under review, submitted for publication.

Dykens, E. M., & Cassidy, S. B. (1995). Correlates of maladaptive behavior in children and adults with Prader-Willi syndrome. *American Journal of Medical Genetics, 69,* 546–549.

Dykens E. M., & Cassidy, S. B. (1999). Prader-Willi syndrome. In S. Goldstein & C. R. Reynolds (Eds.), *Handbook of neurodevelopmental and genetic disorders in children* (pp. 525–554). New York: Guilford Press.

Dykens, E. M., Cassidy, S. B., & King, B. H. (1999). Maladaptive behavior differences in Prader-Willi syndrome associated with paternal deletion versus maternal uniparental disomy. *American Journal on Mental Retardation, 104,* 67–77.

Dykens, E. M., & Clarke, D. J. (1997). Correlates of maladaptive behavior in individuals with 5p- (cri du chat) syndrome. *Developmental Medicine and Child Neurology, 75,* 752–756.

Dykens, E. M., & Hodapp, R. M. (1997). Treatment issues in genetic mental retardation syndromes. *Professional Psychology: Research and Practice, 28,* 263–270.

Dykens, E. M., & Hodapp, R. M. (1999). Behavioural phenotypes: Toward new understandings of people with developmental disabilities. In N. Bouras (Ed.) *Psychiatric and behavioural disorders in developmental disabilities*(2nd ed., pp. 96–108). Cambridge, UK: Cambridge University Press.

Dykens, E. M., Hodapp, R. M., & Finucane, B. M. (2000). *Genetics and mental retardation syndromes: A new look at behavior and treatments*. Baltimore: Paul H. Brookes.

Dykens, E. M., Hodapp, R. M., & Leckman, J. F. (1994). *Behavior and development in fragile X syndrome*. Thousand Oaks, CA: Sage.

Dykens, E. M., & Kasari, C. (1997). Maladaptive behavior in children with Prader-Willi syndrome, Down syndrome, and non-specific mental retardation. *American Journal on Mental Retardation, 102,* 228–237.

Dykens, E. M., Leckman, J. F., & Cassidy, S. B. (1996). Obsessions and compulsions in Prader-Willi syndrome. *Journal of Child Psychology and Psychiatry, 37,* 995–1002.

Dykens, E. M., Leckman, J. F., Paul, R., & Watson, M. (1988). The cognitive, adaptive and behavioral functioning of fragile X and non-fragile X retarded men. *Journal of Autism and Developmental Disorders, 18,* 41–52.

Dykens, E. M., & Rosner, B. A. (1999). Refining behavioral phenotypes: Personality-motivation in Prader-Willi and Williams syndromes. *American Journal on Mental Retardation, 104,* 158–169.

Dykens, E. M., Rosner, B. A., & Ly, T. M. (2000). *Drawings by individuals with Williams syndrome: Are people different from shapes?* Manuscript submitted for publication.

Dykens E. M., & Volkmar, F. R. (1997). Medical conditions associated with autism. In D. J. Cohen & F. R. Volkmar (Eds.), *Handbook of Autism and Pervasive Developmental Disorders (2nd ed.,* pp. 388–407). New York: John Wiley.

Einfield, S. L., Molony, H. & Hall, W. (1989). Autism is not associated with the fragile X syndrome. *American Journal of Medical Genetics, 34,* 187–193.

Einfeld, S. L., Tonge, B. J., & Florio, T. (1997). Behavioral and emotional disturbance in individuals with Williams syndrome. *American Journal on Mental Retardation, 102,* 45–53.

Ewart, A. K., Morris, C. A., Atkinson, D., Jin, W., Sternes, K., Spallone, P., Stock, A. D., Leppart, M., & Keating, M. (1994). Hemizygosity at the elastin locus in a developmental disorders, Williams syndrome. *Nature Genetics, 5,* 11–16.

Fisch, G. S. (1992). Is autism associated with the fragile X syndrome? *American Journal of Medical Genetics, 43,* 47–55.

Fitzpatrick, C., Barry, C., & Garvey, C. (1986). Psychiatric disorder among boys with Duchenne muscular dystrophy. *Developmental medicine and Child Neurology, 28,* 589–595.

Freund, L., Reiss, A. L., Hagerman, R. J., & Vinogradov, S. (1992). Chromosome fragility and psychopathology in obligate female carriers of the fragile X chromosome. *Archives of General Psychiatry, 49,* 54–60.

Ganiban, J., Wagner, S., & Cicchetti, D. (1990). Temperament and Down syndrome. In D. Cicchetti & M. Beeghly (Eds.), *Children with Down syndrome: A developmental perspective* (pp. 63–100). New York: Cambridge University Press.

Gath, A. & Gumley, D. (1986). Behaviour problems in retarded children with special reference to Down's syndrome. *British Journal of Psychiatry, 149,* 151–156.

Gersh, M., Goodart, S. A., Pasztor, L. M., Harris, D. J., Weiss, L., & Overhauser, J. (1995). Evidence for a distinct region causing a cat-like cry in patients with 5p deletions. *American Journal of Human Genetics, 56,* 1404–1410.

Gibbs, M. V., & Thorpe, J. G. (1983). Personality stereotype of noninstitutionalized Down syndrome children. *American Journal of Mental Deficiency, 87,* 601–605.

Gosch. A., & Pankau, R. (1997). Personality characteristics and behaviour problems in individuals of different ages with Williams syndrome. *Developmental Medicine and Child Neurology, 39,* 527–533.

Grizenko, N., Cvejic, H., Vida, S., & Sayegh, L. (1991). Behavior problems in the mentally retarded. *Canadian Journal of Psychiatry, 36,* 712–717

Hagerman, R. J. (1996). Fragile X syndrome. *Child and Adolescent Psychiatric Clinics of North America, 5,* 895–912.

Hawley, P. P, Jackson, L. G., Kurnit, D. M. (1985). Sixty-four patients with Brachmann-de lange syndrome: A survey. *American Journal of Medical genetics, 20,* 453–459.

Hennekman, R. C., Baselier, A. C., Beyaet, E., Bos, A., Blok, J. B., Jansma, H. B., Thorbecke-Nilsen, V. V., & Verrman, H. (1992). Psychological and speech studies in Rubinstein-Taybi syndrome *American Journal on Mental Retardation, 96,* 645–660.

Hodapp, R. M. (This volume). Etiology and personality-motivation: Direct and indirect effects.

Hodapp, R. M. (1996). Down syndrome: Developmental, psychiatric, and management issues. *Child and Adolescent Psychiatric Clinics of North America, 5,* 881–894.

Hodapp, R. M., & Dykens, E. M. (1992). The role of etiology in the education of children with mental retardation. *McGill Journal of Education, 27,* 165–173.

Hodapp, R. M., & Dykens, E. M. (1994). Mental retardation's two cultures of behavioral research. *American Journal on Mental Retardation, 98,* 675–687.

Hodapp, R. M., & Dykens, E. M. (2000). *The two cultures revisited: Behavioral research in genetic mental retardation syndromes.* Manuscript submittedfor publication.

Holland, A. J., Treasure, J., Coskeran, P., & Dallow, J. (1995). Characteristics of the eating disorder in Prader-Willi syndrome: Implications for treatment. *Journal of Intellectual Disability Research, 39,* 373–381.

Hornby, G. (1995). Fathers' views of the effects on their families of children with Down syndrome. *Journal of Child and Family Studies, 4,* 103–117.

Hurley, D. A., & Sovner, R. (1995). Six cases of patients with mental retardation who have antisocial personality disorder. *Psychiatric services, 46,* 828–831.

Jacobs, P. A., Brunton, M., Melville, M. M., Brittan, R. P., & McClemont, W. F. (1965). Aggressive behaviour, mental sub-normality, and the XYY male. *Nature, 208,* 1351–1352.

Karmiloff-Smith, A., Grant, J.,Berthoud, J., Davies, M., Howline, P., & Udwin, O. (1977). Language and Williams syndrome: How intact is "intact'? *Child Development, 68,* 246–262.

Kenworthy, L., Parke, T., & Charnas, L.R. (1993). Cognitive and behavioral profiles of the occulocerebrorenal syndrome of Lowe. *American Journal of Medical genetics, 46,* 297–303.

Kerby, D. S., & Dawson, B. (1994). Autistic features, personality, and adaptive behavior in males with the fragile X syndrome and no autism. *America Journal on Mental Retardation, 98,* 455–462.

Lachiewicz, A. M. (1992). Abnormal behavior of young girls with fragile X syndrome. *American Journal of Medical Genetics, 43,* 72–77.

Lai, F., & Williams, R. S. (1989). A prospective study of Alzheimer disease in Down syndrome. *Archives of Neurology, 46,* 849–853.

Lund, J. (1985). The prevalence of psychiatric morbidity in mentally retarded adults. *Acta Psychiatria Scandanavia, 72,* 563–570.

Mandoki, M. W., Sumner, G. S., Hoffman, R. P., & Riconda, D. L. (1991). A review of Klinefelter's syndrome in children and adolescents. *Journal of the American Academy of Child and Adolescent Psychiatry, 30,* 167–172.

Matilanen, R., Airaksinen, E., Monen, T., Launiala, K., & Kaariainen, R. (1995). A population based study on the causes of mild and severe mental retardation. *Acta Paediatrica, 84,* 261–266.

Mazzocco, M. M., Hagerman, R. J., Cronister-Silverman, A. & Pennington, B. F. (1992). Specific frontal lobe deficits among women with the fragile X gene. *Journal of the American Academy of Child and Adolescent Psychiatry, 31,* 1141–1148.

McCauley, E., Ross, J. L., Kushner, H., & Cutler, G. (1995). Self-esteem and behavior in girls with Turner syndrome. *Developmental Medicine and Behavioral Pediatrics, 16,* 82–88.

McDaniel, W. F. (1997). Criterion-related diagnostic validity and test-retest reliability of the MMPI-168 (L) in mentally retarded adolescents and adults. *Journal of Clinical Psychology, 53,* 485–489.

Menolascino, F. J. (1965). Psychiatric aspects of mongolism. *American Journal of Mental Deficiency, 69,* 653–660.

Menolascino, F. J., Levitas, A., & Greiner, C. (1986). The nature and types of mental illness in the mentally retarded. *Psychopharmacology Bulletin, 22,* 1060–1071.

Mervis, C. B., Morris, C. A., Bertrand, J., & Robinson, B. F. (1999). Williams syndrome: Findings from an integrated program of research. In H. Tager-Flusberg (Ed.), *Neurodevelopmental* disorders (pp. 65–110). Cambridge, MA: MIT Press.

Meyers, B. A. & Pueschel, S. M. (1991). Psychiatric disorders in persons with Down syndrome. *Journal of Nervous and Mental Disease, 179,* 609–613.

Morris, C. A., & Mervis, C. B. (1999). Williams syndrome. In S. Goldstein & C. R. Reynolds (Eds.), *Handbook of neurodevelopmental and genetic disorders in children.* New York: Guilford Press.

Nicholls, R. D., Knoll, J. H., Butler, M. G., Karam, S., & LaLande, M. (1989). Genetic imprinting suggested by maternal heterodisomy in non-deletion Prader-Willi syndrome. *Nature, 16,* 281–285.

Opitz, J. (1996, March). *Historiography of the causal analysis of mental retardation.* Speech to the 29th Annual Gatlinburg Conference on Research and Theory in Mental retardation, Gatlinburg, TN.

Pary, R. (1992). Differential diagnosis of functional decline in Down syndrome. *The Habilitative Mental Healthcare Newsletter, 11,* 37–41.

Pober, B. R., & Dykens, E. M. (1996). Williams syndrome: An overview of medical, cognitive and behavioral features. *Child and Adolescent Psychiatric Clinics of North America, 5,* 929–944.

Preus, M. (1984). The Williams syndrome: Objective definition and diagnosis. *Clinical Genetics, 25,* 422–428.

Pueschel, S. M., Bernier, J. C., & Pezzullo, J. C. (1991). Behavioral observations in children with Down's syndrome. *Journal of Mental Deficiency Research, 35,* 502–511.

Reilly, J., Klima, E. S., & Bellugi, U. (1990). Once more with feeling: Affect and language in atypical populations. *Development and Psychopathology, 2,* 367–391.

Reiss, A. L. & Freund, L. (1990). Fragile X syndrome, DSM-III-R and autism. *Journal of the American Academy of Child and Adolescent Psychiatry, 29,* 885–891.

Reiss, A. L., Hagerman, R. J., Vinogradov, S., Abrams, M., & King, R. J. (1988). Psychiatric disability in female carriers of the fragile X chromosome. *Archives of General Psychiatry, 45,* 697–705.

Reiss, S. (1992). Assessment of a man with dual diagnosis. *Mental retardation, 30,* 1–6.

Reiss, S., Benson, B., & Szyszko, J. (1993). *Apperceptive Personality Test/Mental Retardation.* Worthington, OH: IDS.

Reiss, S., & Havercamp, S. (1996). The sensitivity theory of motivation: Implications for psychopathology. *Behavior Research Therapy, 34,* 621–632.

Reiss, S., & Havercamp, S. (1998). Toward a comprehensive assessment of fundamental motivation: Factor structure of the Reiss profile. *Psychological Assessment, 10,* 97–106.

Riccardi, V. (1992). *Neurofibromatosis: Phenotype, natural history and pathogenesis, 2nd edition.* Baltimore: Johns Hopkins University Press.

Rogers, C. (1987). Maternal support for the Down's syndrome personality stereotype: The effect of direct experience on the condition. *Journal of Mental deficiency Research, 31,* 271–278.

Sharland, M., Burch, M., & McKenna, W. M., & Paton, M. A. (1992). A clinical study of Noonan syndrome. *Archives of diseases in Children, 67,* 178–183.

Smith, I., Beasley, M. G., Wolff, O. H., & Ades, A. E. (1988). Behavior disturbance in 8–year old children with early treated phenylketonuria. *Journal of Pediatrics, 112,* 403–408.

Smith, A. C. M., Dykens, E. M., & Greenberg, F. (1998). The behavioral phenotype of Smith-Magenis syndrome. *American Journal of Medical Genetics, 81,* 186–191.

Sobesky, W. E., Porter, D., Pennington, B. F., & Hagerman, R. J. (1995). Dimensions of shyness in fragile X females. *Developmental Brain Dysfunction, 8,* 280–292.

Sovner, R., Hurley, A. D. & Labrie, R. (1985). Is mania incompatible with Down's syndrome? *British Journal of Psychiatry, 146,* 319–320.

Spirrison, C. L. (1992). Validity of the 16 PF-E experimental norms for adults with mental retardation. *Psychological Reports, 70,* 1200–1202.

Swaab, D. F., Purba, J. S., & Hofman, M. A. (1995). Alterations in the hypothalamic paraventricular nucleus and its oxytocin neurons (putatuve satiety cells) in Prader-Willi syndrome: A study of 5 cases. *Journal of Clinical Endocrinology and Metabolism, 80,* 573–579.

Szymanski, L. S., & Biederman, J. (1984). Depression and anorexia nervosa of persons with Down syndrome. *American Journal of Mental Deficiency, 89,* 246–251

Tomc, S. A., Williamson, N. K., & Pauli, R. M. (1990). Temperament in Williams syndrome. *American Journal of Medical Genetics, 36,* 345–352

Udwin, O., & Yule, W. (1990). Expressive language of children with Williams syndrome. *American Journal of Medical Genetics, 6,* 108–114.

Van Acker, R. (1991). Rett syndrome: A review of current knowledge. *Journal of Autism and Developmental Disorders, 21,* 381–406.

Walzer, S., Bashir, A. S., & Silbert, A. R. (1991). Cognitive and behavioral factors in the learning disabilities of 47,XXY and 47, XYY boys. In J. A. Evans, J. L. Hamerton, & A. Robinson (Eds.), Children and young adults with sex chromosome aneuploidy: Follow-up, clincial and molecular studies. *March of Dimes Birth Defects Foundation: Original Article Series, 26,* 45–58.

Warren, A. C., Holroyd, S., & Folstein, M. F. (1989). Major depression in Down's syndrome. *British Journal of Psychiatry, 155,* 202–205.

Williams, C. A., Zori, R. T., Henderickson, J., Stalker, H., Marum, T., Whidden, E., & Driscoll, D. J. (1995). Angelman syndrome. *Current problems in Pediatrics, 25,* 216–231.

Williams, J., Barratt-Boyes, B., Lowe, J. (1961). Supravalvular aortic stenosis. *Circulation, 24,* 1311–1318.

Worchel., F. F., & Dupree, J. L. (1990). Projective storytelling techniques. In C.R. Reynolds & R.W. Kamphus (Eds.), *Handbook of psychological and educational assessment of children: Personality, behavior, and context* (pp. 70–88). New York: Guilford Press.

Zetlin, A. G., Heriot, M. J., & Turner, J. L. (1985). Self-concept measurement in mentally retarded adults: A micro-analysis of response styles. *Applied Research in Mental Retardation, 6,* 113–125.

Zigler, E. (1967). Familial mental retardation: A continuing dilemma. *Science, 155,* 292–298.

Zigler, E., & Bennett-Gates, D. (1999). The EZYale Personality Questionnaire. In E. Zigler & D. Bennett-Gates (Eds.), *Personality development in individuals with mental retardation.* New York: Cambridge University Press.

Zigman, W. B., Schupf, N., Zigman, A., & Silverman, W. (1993). Aging and Alzheimer disease in people with mental retardation. *International Review of Research in Mental Retardation, 19,* 41–70.

7

Information Processing and Motivation in People With Mental Retardation

James P. Van Haneghan

Lisa A. Turner

University of South Alabama

Mental retardation is a developmental disability that features both motivational and cognitive components. For example, many theories of mental retardation suggest the presence of information processing deficits related to cognitive control (e.g., Merrill & Peacock, 1994), whereas others suggest thatdifferences in motivational orientation (e.g., Haywood & Switzky, 1992) are responsible for some cognitive deficits. Mental retardation is often characterized in terms of the slowing of development, suggesting that whatever motivates or energizes development proceeds more slowly (e.g., Mundy & Kasari, 1990). Many theories suggest that there are individual differences in motivational and personality factors in people with mental retardation that influence their everyday functioning regardless of the level of intellectual functioning (e.g., Merighi, Edison, & Zigler, 1990; Switzky, 1997). Hence, there appear to be motivational differences between people with mental retardation and normally developing individuals, as well motivational differences within the populations of individuals with different syndromes that cause mental retardation.

In spite of the importance of motivation to the study of mental retardation, the study of the relation between motivation and information processing in mental retardation is still in its infancy. Early theories such as theories about rigidity, the tendency to have difficulty shifting from one response to another (Kounin, 1941), or outerdirectedness, the tendency to copy others rather than rely on internally generated actions (Balla, Styfco, & Zigler, 1971), were overly inclusive in their scope and were not adequately tested (Dulaney & Ellis, 1997). Additionally, there are very few theoretical perspectives on motivation and mental retardation that link various developmental periods. For example, there is a great deal of research on the development of self-regulation in children with Down syndrome during infancy (e.g., Cicchetti & Beeghly, 1990), but there is very little work that connects that work (except by implication) with later childhood periods.

Additional difficulties in discussing motivation and information processing come from the many different constructs that are subsumed or distinguished under the categories of information processing and motivation. For example, while some theorists argue that rigidity is a function of motivational factors (e.g., Zigler & Balla, 1982), others argue that rigidity is a function of cognitive inertia (e.g., Dulaney & Ellis, 1997) that has its basis in cognitive deficits.

Only recently have researchers begun to try to differentiate and explore ways to integrate research on motivation and information processing. For example, work exploring the attributions that children with mental retardation make about their performance on memory tasks has been shown to influence their subsequent use of strategies (Turner, 1998). Researchers taking an organizational view of development (e.g., Cicchetti & Ganiban, 1990), who have examined the development of affect and self-regulation taking into account the integration of cognitive, affective, social, and biological factors, have also been instrumental in exploring the relation between information processing, affect, and motivation in young children with mental retardation.

In spite of an increasing amount of work linking motivation and information processing, there is a great deal more research and theory needed to explain more clearly information processing and motivation. For example, work with typically developing children and adults suggests that motivational and affective processes are information processes in their own right and need to be studied as such (Kuhl & Kraska, 1989). They affect working memory and thus play a role in the successful processing of information. Models of information processing in people with mental retardation have yet to take this perspective into account, although there is a movement in that direction.

Certain cognitive processes lend themselves to motivational analyses more readily than others. For example, attentional processes are influenced by motivational processes. Selective attention, or shifts from one task to another, include motivational components. Situations that involve effortful processing of information are also subject to motivational processes. The cognitive process of planning is also an example of a process that is influenced by motivational variables.

Motivational research in mental retardation has focused on trait-like characteristics of motivation orientation (e.g., intrinsic versus extrinsic motivation; e.g., Switzky, 1997) or on task or stimulus variables. It has focused on the product rather than the processes of motivational information processing. The goal of this chapter is to move beyond these constructs to develop a more integrative view of self-regulation in people with mental retardation. We have two goals for this chapter. One goal will be to review existing literature linking motivation and information processing in people with mental retardation. The second overarching goal will be to subsume ideas about motivation into a larger scheme that focuses on learning to control one's behavior. To do this, we will focus on models of self-regulation that have been discussed in the context of studying normally developing individuals. First, we will outline the more integrated perspective and the research that underlies it, and then we will discuss the existing literature, linking it to this more integrative perspective.

A MODEL OF SELF-REGULATION

Perhaps the most well-developed model of motivational information processing comes from the work of Kuhl (1994a). His model was developed during the 1980s and has its basis in contemporary work in cognitive psychology, neuroscience, and the turn of the century German psychologist Ach among others. Our goal in this chapter will be to adapt his model to the study of mental retardation. The model is complex and evolving, so our version of his ideas are an oversimplification of some very complex ideas about motivation and information processing. Also, although Kuhl's ideas are central, others' (e.g., Bargh, 1990; Barkley, 1997; Ryan, Kuhl, & Deci, 1997) ideas about self-regulation have also influenced our thinking. As we describe various components of this model, we will consider the extant mental retardation research that addresses concepts related to the model. We will also discuss potential new lines of research for people studying mental retardation, motivation, and information processing suggested by the model.

Overview of the Model

As previously noted, the model involves a discussion of self-regulation: the ability to carry out tasks or behaviors that are in the interest of the organism. Key to the model is the understanding that the interconnectivity of cognitive, self, affective, and behavioral systems is what energizes behavior (Kuhl, in press).

The success of someone in carrying out the necessary cognitive processes and behaviors to meet a goal (self-regulation) is a function of the alignment of the different systems with that goal. Figure 7.1 presents a simplified schematic of the model. The basic notion is that the ability of individuals to carry out intentions is a function of the activation of the appropriate cognitive schema and behaviors and the suppression of the inappropriate cognitive schema and behaviors. For example, when solving a mathematics word problem, students need to activate schema for planning a solution, while suppressing the impulse to just take all the numbers (relevant or irrelevant) in the problem and mindlessly apply an algorithm to them. Whether the appropriate pattern of activation and inhibition occurs is a function of the various aspects of the cognitive, self, and affective systems noted in Fig. 7.1.

In Fig. 7.1, it can be seen that there are four interrelated factors that influence whether the pattern of cognitive and behavioral activation is sufficient to successfully carry out an intention. We introduce each of these elements here and discuss them in more detail later.

FIG. 7.1.   *Diagram of the model of self-regulation and action control.*
Ideas expressed here are largely derived from the work of Kuhl (1994) and
Kuhl and Kraska (1989).

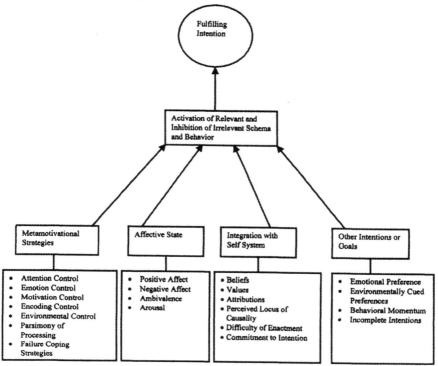

The first aspect is the presence of other competing goals or
intentions. These could be goals that are environmentally cued,
more affectively pleasurable intentions than the current goal, or
they could simply be other unfinished business that makes it difficult to concentrate on the present.

The second element has to do with the affective state of the
individual. For example, a depressed individual may have a difficult time acting because of his or her affective state. An angry
individual may act out impulsively based on environmental cues,
losing touch with the goal he or she is purported to be pursuing.

The third element of the model has to do with the self-system that an individual has developed. If a particular goal or task is consistent with the self-system, it tends to be one that is likely to be reached. According to Kuhl (2000), positive affect generated from acting in line with self-valued goals facilitates acting and tends to limit the detrimental effects of negative affect.

Finally, the fourth element concerns *metamotivational strategies* that are used to regulate behavior and cognition to facilitate the completion of an intention. For example, structuring the environment so that it is conducive to doing work is an example of a metamotivational strategy.

Kuhl (1994a) and Ryan et al. (1997) provided empirical evidence, neurobiological evidence, and evolutionary justifications for the importance of self-regulatory functioning. For example, there is evidence that people who are more planful (Gollwitzer, 1996) and intrinsically motivated achieve more and are more mentally healthy (Ryan, Sheldon, Kasser, and Deci, 1996). Ryan et al. (1997) and Kuhl (1994a) argued that there is evidence that the brain activity associated with self-regulation seems to be centered in the prefrontal cortex. Systems in the prefrontal cortex have been found to coordinate and integrate information in the service of goal-directed behavior (Barkley, 1997). Ryan et al. (1997) suggested the adaptive advantage of having a self-system that coordinates the acquisition of goals and needs. They also suggested the advantage of having a system that can parse out self versus externally driven behavior.

Being aware of self versus other can help prevent the organism from being duped into behaving particular ways. Additionally, Ryan et al. (1997) argued for the adaptive significance of intrinsic motivation and suggest that organisms that explore their environment and are curious are apt to learn more from the environment around them than organisms that are externally driven to respond only to environmental cues. They suggest this is especially true for organisms such as humans who experience a great deal of variety in the environments they inhabit. Hence, there is evidence to support the importance and centrality of self-regulation.

Typically, when self-regulation is examined, researchers oppose it with ideas about external regulation via material rewards or simply the automatic activation of cognitive schema in the presence of appropriate environmental cues. When researchers talk about cognitive processes, they are typically viewed as moving along a continuum from automatic to effortful. Generally, researchers have viewed more automatic processes as externally regulated by the presence of appropriate environmental cues.

Although much of what concerns externally cued behavior involves automatic processing of information (e.g., priming effects), the automatic processing of information does not mean that there is an absence of self-regulation. Almost any cognitive task involves both automatic and effortful elements. Whether an environmentally cued response is seen as externally based or self-regulated depends upon its context. If it is consistent with the goals the organism is pursuing, it could be viewed as self-regulated. If, however, the environmentally cued behavior is inconsistent with current goals, then it could be considered externally regulated.

More effortful processing of information also can be externally or internally regulated. For example, Kuhl (2000) described the difference between action control and self-regulated functioning. If the goal the individual is pursuing is one that is not valued by the self-system, and the motivation to carry out the task is largely external, then the effortful task is externally regulated. Ryan et al. (1996, 1997) labeled goals that are taken on by the individual but inconsistent with the self-system *introjected goals*. If the goal is part of those valued by the self-system, the effortful activity will be more likely to be self-regulated rather than controlled by environmental cues and reinforcers.

Below, we describe how cognitive processes at various levels of the information processing system are related to the model. We begin by discussing the less conscious and typically more automatic processes such as attention and we then look at higher level executive functioning.

Attention and Motivation.   Attention and motivation have been linked by a number of different researchers (Kuhl & Kraska, 1989; Simon, 1994). Attention has been defined a number of different ways, although we mention only two. First, we discuss attention in terms of orienting the individual toward particular stimuli in the environment, and second, we discuss attention in the sense of a continued focus on a particular task or stimulus. Motivation becomes important because it is goals that orient people to attend selectively to particular elements of stimuli, and it is motivation that helps maintain vigilance in carrying out a particular task.

One difficulty that arises when motivation and attention are considered is that attentional processes do not seem to be necessarily conscious processes. Consequently, one should consider some motivational processes as preconscious automatic processes directed by situational and environmental cues (Bargh, 1990). A second complexity in examining motivation and attention is that the cues and stimuli in any situation may activate multiple goals. This suggests that there are preconscious processes that prioritize the importance of goals and allow for goal shifting. For instance, the well-known cocktail party effect in which people shift their focus from one conversation to another when their name is mentioned is a good example of how goals change and attention shifts when something more central to the self is processed while carrying out another behavior. Finally, it is important to mention that a single goal usually has multiple subgoals and that these goals further focus attention and behavior in particular directions. In spite of the centrality of motivation and goals to attention, there has been very little research linking the two until recently.

There is virtually no work in the field of mental retardation that examines motivation and attention in any depth. The link between the two is often made, but not explored in detail (Tomporowski & Tinsley, 1997). And, paradoxically, those studying attentional processes often try to dismiss motivational explanations (e.g., Tomporowski & Tinsley, 1997; Dulaney & Ellis, 1997) for explanations favoring attentional or more purely cognitive constructs. However, as noted above, attention is directed by goals that are inherently motivational or intentional. Hence, exploration of the motivational basis of attentional behavior is important. Even if it is ultimately found that difficulties in attention are a function of deficits in the information processing system, researchers still benefit by exploring how the attentional system in people with mental retardation deals with goal information. To explore the motivational basis of attentional behavior, we examine discussions of automatic activation of goals, research on attention in people with mental retardation, and explorations of metamotivation.

A key component to many theories of information processing (e.g., Anderson, 1983) is that the procedures and actions needed to engage in a particular behavior are compiled in a program-like way that can be run automatically without using up a great deal of attentional resources. While substantial discussion of automaticity has taken place in light of arguments about knowledge representation and attentional resources, only recently has the discussion shifted to motivational implications of the automaticity of goal directed behavior.

Bargh (1990), Kuhl and Kraska (1989), and others noted that goals and the behaviors associated with particular goals can be automatically activated when the appropriate environmental and situational cues are present. This analysis suggests that priming a particular goal can activate behaviors and sensitivities to environmental cues pertinent to that goal, just like semantic knowledge structures can be primed (Kruglanski, 1996).

There are both good and bad consequences associated with the priming of goal related schema. The automatic priming of goals by stimuli in the environment helps to free up working memory capacity to engage in high level processing and increases behavioral momentum (i.e., further directs the schema that are activated or inhibited). Automatic priming also provides an adaptive mechanism for making very rapid shifts in attention when important environmental cues signal danger or information important to the individual.

On the other hand, when schema are activated for other goals that are not relevant to the present intention, automatic activation can disrupt performance and move the individual away from his or her goal. Thus, as it relates to Fig. 7.1, the automatic activation of information can facilitate the schema for relevant goals and inhibit schema for irrelevant goals. However, if other competing intentions are not inhibited, then the potential for disruption of goal-directed cognition and behavior by automatic environmental activation of other competing intentions is a threat to successfully carrying out the intention. Reasons why environmentally cued intentions rather than the appropriate schema are activated will be discussed as we continue to examine the model.

Kuhl (1986) and Bargh (1990) discussed a rather unique element of the processing of goal related information. That is, they both found that unfulfilled goals seem to remain active even when people are not consciously aware that they are available to fulfill. For example, Bargh (1990) noted that many times when working on a problem the solution to the problem seems to arrive in an unrelated context where a person is not necessarily deliberately considering the problem. The well-known Zeigarnik effect where a person's memory for the unfinished task is greater than his or her memory for completed tasks (Zeigarnik, 1938/1968) provides further support for the case that goals have a special status in people's memory systems. Kuhl (1986), Kuhl and Kraska (1989), and Kuhl (1994a) provided evidence that unfulfilled goals tend to take up processing capacity and make it difficult for people to pursue other goals effectively. The consumption of processing capacity may also make it likely that the individual may be susceptible to distraction by environmentally cued goals. Finally, a third element of goals is that activation of particular goals requires inhibition of other goals. Hence, inhibitory processes may be important to consider when examining information processing surrounding goals. For example, Barkely (1997) argued that inhibition is crucial to executive functioning. In order for processes such as planning, controlling emotions, and analyzing the potential efficacy of behavior, to occur, the organism has to stop and think before acting. If an individual is unable to inhibit a response these executive functions may not have time to occur.

Research in Mental Retardation.   We are not aware of any research on the information processing of goals among people with mental retardation. There is a growing body of research that suggests that people with mental retardation are slower to automatize performance than people without mental retardation. For example, Merrill, Goodwyn, and Gooding (1996) found in two experiments that people with mental retardation were slower to reach automaticity in tasks requiring them to identify whether pictures were of common objects or anomalous objects. Slower acquisition of automaticity may suggest that people with mental retardation may be slower in compiling plans to meet goals. Hence, their processing of goals may be more effortful than normally developing individuals. Furthermore, research involving people with mental retardation has also found that once a routine becomes relatively automatic, they have more difficulty suppressing that automatic behavior (Dulaney & Ellis, 1997). For example, Dulaney and Ellis (1997) found that people with mental retardation who developed skill in doing the Stroop color naming task had a difficult time switching back from naming colors to naming color words.

Research in mental retardation has also examined both positive and negative priming effects. Positive priming involves an acceleration of response when the prime is related to the target stimulus. Negative priming involves longer responses when the distractor on one trial becomes a target on the next trial. Negative priming is an example of inhibitory processes in that it is the result of attentional processing that directs attention away from distracting information.

Cha and Merrill (1994) Merrill, Cha, and Moore (1994), and Merrill and Taube (1996) examined priming in people with mental retardation. They found evidence of positive priming effects in people with mental retardation, but found mixed results when looking at negative priming (Merrill & Taube; Cha & Merrill). In two studies, they did not find negative priming, and in one study, where the negative prime involved a location, they did find negative priming effects (Merrill, Cha, & Moore). If people with mental retardation do not clearly show inhibition of goals other than the one they are currently pursuing, then they may not be able to as easily suppress irrelevant goals. If irrelevant goals are not suppressed, then they remain active and the environmental stimuli that trigger such goals may lead the individual to be distracted from the goal that is currently being pursued.

Distractibility is characteristic of many individuals with mental retardation (Tomporowski & Tinsley, 1997). Such an explanation for failures in self-regulation has been explored in relation to other developmental disorders as well. For example, Barkely (1997) proposed a model of attention deficit hyperactivity disorder

(ADHD) that centers around the detrimental effects of failures of inhibitory mechanisms on the ability of children with ADHD to self-regulate. The model was developed completely independent of Kuhl's but talks in surprisingly similar terms about the neurological underpinnings of self-regulatory failures (i.e., prefrontal lobe functioning). That is, self-regulation depends on the ability to stop, plan, and think about situations or tasks.

Another implication for work in mental retardation is that the processing of goals takes up working memory capacity. Unlike other types of information, unfulfilled goals do not appear to easily decay over time (Bargh, 1990; Kuhl, 1992; Kuhl & Kraska, 1989). Bargh cited a number of instances where goals seem to reappear to us, even after we have given up on them. Kuhl and Kraska (1989) suggested that goals that are unfulfilled actually take away from the processing capacity that an individual has to deal with additional goals. Kuhl and Kraska also noted that some individuals have a tendency to spend more time ruminating over unfulfilled goals than others. These individuals are called *state oriented*. Thus, working memory capacity is influenced by the processing of goals. If people with mental retardation have a tendency to dwell on unfulfilled goals (are state oriented), then their working memory capacity may be limited by more than some underlying neurological constraint. It may be limited by their continued processing of unfulfilled goals—something that they might be more likely to experience than their normally developing peers.

There are additional influences of goals on working memory capacity. The automation of goals may decrease the amount of working memory capacity needed to carry them out and hence leave more capacity available for other tasks. Limitations in working memory capacity have been cited as a major weakness of those with mental retardation (Merrill & Peacock, 1994; Spitz & Borys, 1984). One explanation of these limitations in working memory capacity in people with mental retardation is slowness or inability to automatize tasks (Merrill, Goodwyn, & Gooding, 1996). If one has to decide among several alternatives, each is of which is effortful, then more working memory capacity is exhausted deciding about the consequences of particular goals than would otherwise be used.

Finally, working memory capacity plays a role in determining how well an individual monitors pursuit of a particular goal and inhibits the automatic activation of another. If there is not enough attentional capacity to monitor the goal being pursued, then a goal automatically activated by an environmental cue may redirect behavior in an unintended direction. For example, imagine traveling to a new location using part of the same route you use to drive to work everyday in the car. As you are driving along you begin a heated discussion. When the cutoff point comes for you to diverge from your typical route to the new route, you forget to go in the appropriate direction and find yourself instead taking the well-learned route to work. It may be that the reported distractibility of people with mental retardation might be a function of such a process (e.g., Tomporowski & Tinsley, 1997).

As can be seen, several insights can be gained by examining more automatic regulatory processing. As noted by Bargh (1990) many routine behaviors are triggered and carried out automatically once the appropriate environmental cues are recognized. However, there are many goals cued by environments, and therefore, an additional process has to be considered in self-regulation, and that is how individuals decide upon which goal to pursue.

In some cases, the selection of one goal inhibits the processing of another, but often the goal that one wants to pursue may not necessarily be the one cued by the particular situation. For example, a sunny day may activate the intention to go to the beach, but that goal has to be put aside or reframed so that more professionally and financially rewarding goals can be pursued. Thus, the process of dealing with competing intentions is an important element of motivating behavior. These processes of decision making about goals and persisting in carrying out goals are part of what the self-regulatory system is about. It involves how individuals make decisions about what activities to pursue and, once a decision has been made, how long an individual will persist on a task. This self-regulatory system and research relating it to mental retardation are discussed later.

Autonomous Functioning

Kuhl and Kraska (1989) noted that there are a variety of determinants of the goal one chooses to pursue. Figure 7.1 illustrates these factors. One factor that influences successful pursuit of goals and intentions is the presence of other competing intentions. There are the more automatically environmentally cued behavioral tendencies, there are emotionally interesting goals to pursue, there are intentions one is already pursuing, and there are the cognitive intentions that one wants to pursue. Once a particular goal is decided upon, then there is a need to consider how to maintain pursuit of that goal (Kuhl & Kraska, 1989) and inhibit other potential intentions. Moreover, once a goal is pursued, there is a need to consider whether one is making progress toward meeting that goal. Finally, at some point in time one has to determine whether to continue to pursue an unfulfilled goal. These sets of processes join together under the rubric of self-regulation.

Given that one can assume that self-regulatory and externally cued regulatory processes compete in determining the actions of an individual, the interaction and coordination of those different systems is important to an organism for meeting its needs and desires. For example, there is a need to be able to maintain goals directed by the self-regulatory system in face of the activation of other goals suggested by the externally directed behavioral regulatory system. For instance, when writing this paper at home, the authors need to maintain the intention to write in the face of distractions such as household chores.

Kuhl and Kraska (1989) discussed the development of what they label a *motivational maintenance system* that helps to coordinate different goals and also discussed developmental and individual differences in how that motivational maintenance system influences the performance of goals and actions. The system consists of decision and maintenance processes that attempt to keep intentions and actions in equilibrium. The development of that motivational maintenance system requires the presence of a variety of motivational processing schema. On a basic level is the ability to cognitively represent intentions (Kuhl & Kraska, 1989). Other abilities mentioned by Kuhl and Kraska include a conception of impulsivity. That is, a child needs a conception of how emotionally pleasurable but distracting competing goals can lead one astray from an intended goal. As a consequence of recognizing the distractions created by emotionally attractive alternatives, children develop a sense of commitment and a recognition that one needs to stick to a goal in the face of emotionally attractive alternatives. They need to recognize that commitment to a goal may require sacrificing short-term pleasures (Mischel, 1996).

Related to the notions of impulsivity and commitment is the development of a sense of the difficulty of enacting particular intentions. Based on data reported by Kuhl and Kraska, and their review of the literature, they believe that by about age 8 or 9 years children have developed the abilities to commit to intentions and determine the difficulty of enactment.

Importance of the Self-System. According to Kuhl and Kraska, individual differences in commitment are based on how well a particular goal is integrated with the self. Integration of the goal with the self is a complex function of both one's self-concept in particular domains and the perceived internality or externality of the goal. For example, an individual is less likely to commit to a goal he or she believes that he or she does not have the ability to pursue. If an individual were to pursue that goal, it is likely that, since that individual does not believe he or she can pursue it successfully, the locus of causality for maintaining motivation to pursue the goal will be external to the individual. Hence, such a goal would not be well integrated with the self and it would be difficult for an individual to pursue such a goal. For instance, a child who believes he or she cannot do mathematics may not be very committed to doing mathematics homework and may be easily distracted from that work. Thus, in Kuhl's model, goal orientation and ability beliefs and attributions come into play in the decision to commit to a particular goal and to integrate it with the self.

Kuhl (2000) argued that the degree of integration of an intention with the self influences the regulation of affect surrounding that goal. For example, he argued that pursuing an intention that is well integrated with the self-system leads to the inhibition of negative affect after failure, thus making it easier for the individual to bounce back and persist after failure. More will be noted about the integration of goals with the self later. We will also return to issues of how theories that focus on attributions and goal orientations (e.g., Elliott & Dweck, 1988; Nicholls, 1984; Weiner, 1986) can be viewed within the context of the model outlined by Kuhl.

Research in Mental Retardation. Research on the decision processes necessary to pick a goal to pursue, on commitment to goals, and on persistence in carrying out a goal in the face of distracting alternatives among people with mental retardation is limited. Tomporowski and Tinsley (1997) reviewed research on vigilance in people with mental retardation and concluded that people with mental retardation are less vigilant in carrying out a task over time and that people with mental retardation are particularly disrupted when the processing demands of a task increase. However, Tomporowski and Tinsley reported no research that examines how people with mental retardation maintain goal commitment in the face of an attractive alternative task that could distract them. Furthermore, there is no work examining the strategies people with mental retardation use to sustain attention to a task, which is the issue discussed next.

Metamotivation

Kuhl (1986) described the development of what he labels metamotivational skills that help in the maintenance of an intention. These metamotivational skills interestingly enough are somewhat similar to some of Sternberg's contextual components of his triarcic theory of intelligence in that they involve strategies in which people take advantage of their contexts to meet goals. These metaskills involve knowledge of strategies that help to coordinate action and goals.

One skill Kuhl (1986) mentioned is active attentional selectivity. This involves directing attention toward stimuli that are related to achieving a goal and away from distractors. For instance, a child who shuts off the television so that he or she can concentrate on homework is engaging in a strategy that helps improve concentration. A second ability mentioned by Kuhl is what he labeled encoding control. This involves only processing features of stimuli or situations that are related to current goals. For instance, in a memory task where there are plants and animals and the instructions are to memorize the animals, an individual engaging in encoding control would focus rehearsal and elaborations on the animals only. A third ability mentioned is emotions control, which refers to the notion that a person's emotional states influence his or her ability to meet goals and that in order to accomplish intentions it is necessary to be able resist other emotionally tempting activities or overcome the deleterious effects of certain emotional states (e.g., depression). For example, a difficult task for children to accomplish is to learn to discipline themselves to do homework when they would rather be playing outside (a more emotionally pleasant activity). Strategies used to help make the homework more emotionally satisfying or to make the alternative less attractive emotionally are instances of emotion control. The fourth self-regulatory skill mentioned by Kuhl is motivational control. This ability involves engaging in strategies that increase the motivational basis for an intention. For instance, the motivation to complete an intention can be enhanced by increasing the importance of the task to the self. For instance, a student might increase his or her motivation to do schoolwork by thinking about the negative consequences of not completing work. A fifth self-regulatory ability involves environmental control. That is, individuals set up the environment to favor successful completion of a goal. For instance, someone trying to stop smoking might avoid situations that trigger smoking behavior. Finally, a sixth self-regulatory skill described by Kuhl involves *parsimony of information processing.* The basic notion is that in making decisions about which action of several to pursue, there becomes a point where further mulling over what to do becomes pointless. Kuhl argued that some individuals continue to mull over decisions even when mulling over the situation is fruitless. Continuing to process information under such circumstances might detract from the ability to complete an intention by exhausting processing capacity.

Research on Metamotivation and Mental Retardation. There is some evidence that some of the metamotivational concepts considered by Kuhl are part of the repertoire of people with mental retardation. For example, Levine and Langness (1985) found that people with mental retardation use some of the metamotivational skills described by Kuhl. They note, for instance, that people with mental retardation often succeed in grocery shopping by using what Kuhl called *environmental control.* That is, they arrange the environment in a way that helps them obtain their goal.

For instance, Levine and Langness talk about some people with mild mental retardation who go to the same cashier each week so that they can be sure that they will be taken care of at the store or individuals who bring large amounts of money to the store in order to avoid problems with not having enough cash to purchase their groceries. Sternberg (1987) also mentioned examples of this kind of environmental shaping by people with mental retardation in relating the contextual components of his theory of intelligence to a general theory of intellectual exceptionality.

There is also some research addressing encoding control and attentional control in people with mental retardation. Research using a directed forgetting paradigm has shown that individuals with mental retardation are slower to develop attentional and encoding control than their chronological age peers (Bray, Turner, & Hersh, 1985). Furthermore, Bray et al. (1985) report that even though there is some development of encoding control by adolescence, adolescents with mental retardation are not as effective in limiting their study to items to be tested as their chronological age peers.

State Versus Action Orientation

The major individual difference variable in Kuhl's model is the notion of state versus action orientation. Individuals who spend a great deal of time ruminating over decisions and incomplete intentions, who are preoccupied with prior failures, and who tend to not be able to maintain behavior aimed at an emotionally fulfilling goal are labeled by Kuhl as state oriented. His research concerning this construct offers alternative explanations for certain phenomenon such as learned helplessness. In addition, he used the theory to explain such motivational paradoxes as the presence of both distractibility and perseveration in individuals and overcommitment and procrastination. For example, he argued that people who are state oriented are more likely to be controlled by environmental cues and thus will continue perseverating on something that is continually cued by the environment and are distracted easily when another activity is triggered by the environment. Kuhl (1994b) developed an instrument to examine state orientation and presented evidence for three different manifestations of state orientation.

Hesitancy to Act. First, state oriented individuals are more likely to be hesitant to act. Hesitation to act can be caused by factors that lead to the disengagement of the self-regulatory system or, through the second manifestation of state orientation, preoccupation with task irrelevant or other thoughts. The self-regulatory system becomes disengaged, according to Kuhl (1994a), because of the long-term effects of an environment that does not provide opportunities for self-initiated exploration or an environment containing too much external control.

Hesitancy and Mental Retardation.   Kuhl suggested that how parents and caregivers organize the environment for a child is crucial to avoiding hesitancy to act. More will be said about this issue later. However, it should be noted that his ideas are consistent with some theories of intelligence that claim that mediated activity is important to helping children become active processors of information (Campione, Brown, & Ferrara, 1982; Feuerstein, 1980). Additionally, Haywood and Switzky's (1992) program of research on intrinsic motivation in people with mental retardation suggested that people with mental retardation are more extrinsically motivated (motivated by external forces) than people without mental retardation. An examination of the Picture Motivation Scale that has been used to measure intrinsic motivation in individuals with mental retardation indicates that some of the items on their scale reflect the tendency to *act* or to *not act*. Thus, there is evidence that some people with mental retardation tend to be externally controlled and hesitant to act. Hence, people with mental retardation are likely to be more state oriented than normally developing individuals.

Preoccupation.   The other cause of a hesitancy to act according to Kuhl (1994a) concerns the second manifestation of state orientation, preoccupation. Preoccupation both prevents the organism from acting and can disrupt the fulfillment of intentions. Preoccupation prevents effective fulfillment of intentions in a variety of ways. The main type of preoccupation discussed by Kuhl is ruminations of over past, present, or even future intentions that are unfulfilled. Such ruminations take up working memory capacity. The working memory taken up by such ruminations is less available for specifying and planning how an intention will be met. It will also make the individual more susceptible to externally cued alternative intentions. Thus, the individual may be susceptible to cognitive slips (Heckhausen & Beckmann, 1990) or even may shift totally to alternative unrelated task intentions. In addition, according to Kuhl (1994a) another type of preoccupation that can occur is an overly stringent perseveration on avoiding distractions and controlling behavior in such a way that regulation of the intended goal gets lost. Avoiding distractions becomes in itself a distraction from the intention one chooses to fulfill.

Preoccupation and Mental Retardation.   There is little research in mental retardation that addresses preoccupation as described in Kuhl's theory. It would not be surprising that such preoccupation is characteristic of children with mental retardation. There is evidence that children who present a *helpless orientation* as described by Dweck tend to perseverate on failure-related cognitions and attributions (Diener & Dweck, 1978). Given that children with mental retardation are more likely to present the pattern of beliefs that define helplessness according to Dweck (i.e., low ability beliefs and performance goals), then it is likely that children with mental retardation are more likely to be preoccupied than their normally developing counterparts. Several programs of research have suggested that such a pattern exists in people with mental retardation (see Switzky, 1997, for a review). Hence, there is indirect, but not direct, evidence that children with mental retardation are more likely to become preoccupied in the pursuit of goals.

Volatility.   The third element of state orientation is volatility. According to Kuhl, this element represents the degree to which individuals have difficulty continuing to work on a pleasurable goal or intention. State oriented people often have a difficult time staying in an action-oriented mode. For example, a child may start to play a computer game that he or she enjoys, but not persist on the task and get up and engage in some other behavior, and then come back again to the game and play again. Interestingly, Kuhl sees volatility and preoccupation as leading to two opposite effects. Volatility involves behavioral activity that puts one off-task, whereas preoccupation involves cognitive rumination that puts one off-task.

Volatility and Mental Retardation.   Again, there is little work that explores volatility in people with mental retardation. Work on vigilance has largely looked at fairly uninteresting experimental tasks (e.g., identifying letters or symbols) in exploring on task behavior (Tomporowski & Tinsely, 1997). Vigilance studies suggest that people with mental retardation are more likely to engage in off-task behavior. However, there is virtually no research that explores the ability of people with mental retardation to maintain performance on an activity that they are intrinsically interested in carrying out.

State Orientation, Attributions, and Learned Helplessness

Much of the work on motivation and cognition in children with mental retardation has focused on low ability and effort attributions as an issue influencing strategic performance of people with mental retardation (e.g., Hale, Turner, & Borkowski, 1989). Kuhl's notion of state orientation provides a useful addition to research on attributions. As Kuhl and Eisenbeiser (1986) point out, attributions about performance are correlated with performance, but may not necessarily be the determinants of performance. As an example, they note that even if someone attributes failure performance to low ability or high task difficulty (attributions that might discourage further task pursuit), individuals can draw different implications from those attributions. In particular they argue that the individual can engage in state oriented cognitions that discourage self-regulation or in action oriented cognitions that encourage self-regulation. For example, if one believes that failure was due to low ability, a state oriented cognition would involve perseveration on the incomplete intention. On the other hand, one could use low ability attributions in an action oriented fashion to suggest that on the next occasion or on a similar task one might need to try harder, take more time, or engage in other behaviors to help succeed.

The need to consider the implications of attributions as well as the attributions themselves led Kuhl to argue that attributional retraining (e.g., attempts to change attributions) will not be very effective if one does not also change the cognitions surrounding task failure and success. A suggestion that performance be attributed to effort, without a corresponding attempt to increase action oriented cognitions and decrease state oriented cognitions, may actually make matters worse according to Kuhl (1994a). An analysis of causes of failure may lead an individual already engaging in state related processing to increase rather than decrease their state oriented cognitions. Thus, according to Kuhl, learned helplessness involves more than a belief that one cannot control the outcome due to low ability or some external cause. Learned helplessness involves engaging in state related cognitions that make it difficult to pursue a new goal.

His belief that state orientation rather than lack of control explains learned helplessness better comes from several studies (e.g., Kuhl, 1981) where state and action oriented individuals work on a task that is unsolvable (e.g., an unsolvable anagram) and then on an unrelated task. He finds that state oriented individuals tend to have more difficulty dealing with the unrelated task and engage in more state related cognitive processing, even though they have no rational expectation for failure on that new task. It is the generation of state related cognitions and other manifestations of state orientation, according to Kuhl, that lead to helplessness. His model helps explain why in Dweck's (1986) theory concerning entity (ability) versus incremental (effort) beliefs about ability that children who are helpless tend to be those who not only make attributions to ability, but also have performance (externally driven) goals such as grades versus learning (intrinsically motivated) goals such as task mastery. Those individuals who are externally regulated (those with performance goals) are more likely to be engaged in state oriented processing of their intentions. Hence, learned helplessness is a function of both attributions and processing style according to Kuhl. Attributions concerning performance are in themselves inadequate to explain behavior.

Kuhl and Eisenbieser further argued that the failure of attributions and other cognitions about one's motivation to explain behavior need to be considered in light of action versus state orientation. They argued that expectancy value theories, where people act in light of their cognitive expectations of success and the intrinsic value of the activity, are inadequate because they fail to take into account the ongoing regulation of behavior. One may value a particular activity, but not engage in that activity because of state orientation or other factors that lead to an external regulation of behavior. Kuhl has evidence that state oriented individuals are less likely to engage in behavior that they value and expect to succeed in because of their style of self-regulation. For instance, in one study, Kuhl & Eisenbieser (1986) found that state oriented high school students were more likely to stay with a boring task (sorting cards) than a more interesting one (reading comics) when given a choice to switch to the more attractive one. In addition, expectancies do not always predict performance either. More action oriented motivational processing can overcome the effects of negative performance expectations. Hence, Kuhl's (1994a) discussion of self-regulation and state orientation states that researchers need to focus on more complex issues in dealing with the link between cognition and behavior.

State Orientation and Mental Retardation. Research in mental retardation has focused on three different areas that may be related to state orientation. First, much research has focused on goal orientations (Switzky, 1997). Research on goal orientation is related to state orientation in that it focuses on whether an individual tends to be driven by intrinsic competence or extrinsic contingencies. Ryan, Kuhl, and Deci, (1997) developed the notion of autonomous versus controlled motivational functioning corresponding to Kuhl's two motivational systems. These authors clarified the concept of autonomy by pointing out that autonomy does not reflect acting without regard to others and the environment, but reflects the organism's ability to organize, prioritize, facilitate, and persist in meeting its needs and desires. Their view of autonomy does not define autonomy as whether something is intrinsically versus extrinsically motivated, but rather in how well integrated a particular behavior is within the self-system. For example, one can be externally motivated to obey traffic laws, but later internalize the value of obeying laws in terms of greater traffic safety and fuel economy. In the latter case where someone has an internal reason for obeying the laws, the individual is operating autonomously even though there is initially an external reason for obeying the laws. Development of a perceived internal locus of causality is integral to autonomous function in this view.

The notion of perceived causality is important in this view as it is in other motivational theories (e.g., Dweck, 1996). However, Ryan et al.'s model makes an important distinction in that the locus of causality is sometimes external, even when it seems on the surface to be internal. They discuss the concept of introjected regulation, where there is an external locus of control for a seemingly intrinsic motivation. An introjected regulation involves attempts to take on as one's own, goals that are actually of more interest to someone else. Introjected goals are not integrated with the self-system, and consequently, they are more easily interrupted than goals that are integral to the self. What evidence is there concerning the internality versus externality of goals for people with mental retardation? Below research that focuses on goal orientation will be discussed. Both the models that have generated such research and specific studies of people with mental retardation will be discussed.

Outerdirectedness.   One theoretically relevant concept that has been studied in mental retardation research is the concept of outerdirectedness. Yando and Zigler (1979) suggested that many people with mental retardation, particularly the developmentally young and institutionalized, are more likely to imitate and model the behavior of others in solving a problem than to use their own skills and abilities to solve a problem. In other words, the individual tries to make the other person's actions and intentions their own. They do this according to Zigler et al. (1979) in order to maintain social contact with others and because of a lack of confidence in their own skills. Outerdirected behavior is an example of an introjected goal.

Goal Orientation and Mental Retardation.   External versus internal regulation is also the focus of research that examines goal orientation,that is work on whether people engage in activities for reasons that are related to task enjoyment or external rewards. There have been several different programs of research examining goal orientation under different guises. For example, Nicholls (1984) described task versus ego orientation, where individuals are motivated by their valuing of an activity (task orientation) or by their valuing of external rewards (good grades, social praise and so on, ego orientation). Dweck (1986) made a similar distinction between learning and performance goals. Students who are learning or task oriented in their goals choose challenging tasks, persist, and seek relevant feedback (Dweck & Leggett,

1988). They are more likely to engage in action related processing of goals. In contrast, students with performance or ego orientations are primarily concerned with external evaluation. They want to either show others that they are capable of success or hide information that might imply they are incapable of success (Nicholls, 1984). The implications of performance goals differ as a function of confidence or efficacy. Students who have confidence in their abilities will likely work hard to show their skills, but students who believe that they cannot succeed will try to hide this information by not working hard (Jagacinski & Nicholls, 1984).

Recently, Elliot and Harackiewicz (1996) and Skaalvik (1997) pointed out that ego orientation per se is not as problematic when an individual is focused more on reaching a goal (even if for extrinsic reasons), than on avoiding failure. Both groups of researchers found that individuals who were more focused on avoiding failure than on attaining goals were less successful in performing a task than those who were ego oriented, but focused on meeting goals and succeeding. These findings are consistent with Kuhl's ideas. According to Kuhl and Kraska (1989), attempting to avoid failure and not think about it is part of state oriented processing that can hurt performance. They argued that suppression of failure thoughts interferes with self-regulation in two ways. First, active suppression requires effortful activity that takes up working memory capacity. Second, Kuhl (1994a) argued that negative affect associated with such activity blocks positive affect that facilitates self-regulatory mechanisms. Thus, failure avoidance is detrimental to successful self-regulation

As noted earlier, performance goals and low abilities seem to be associated with state oriented processing of information. The goals that people set and the behaviors that they employ to reach those goals have dramatic implications for information processing and learning. In studies where goals have been manipulated, ego or performance goals were likely to result in shallower information processing (Graham & Golan, 1991). In contrast, learning goals were likely to result in deeper information processing (Graham & Golan, 1991) and the choice of more challenging tasks (Elliot & Dweck, 1988).

The goals that persons with mental retardation establish are likely influenced by their needs, the feedback they receive, and their beliefs. However, once the goal tendencies are established, they probably operate quite early in the chain of events and serve to activate the beliefs that are relevant to the present goals. Individual differences in goals have been studied by several research groups using somewhat different constructs: ego and task goals (Nicholls, 1984), learning and performance goals (Dweck & Leggett, 1988), and intrinsic versus extrinsic motivational orientation (Haywood & Switzky, 1986). Haywood and Switzky (1986) reported that children with mental retardation were more extrinsically motivated (and hence less intrinsically motivated) than children without retardation. That is, the children with retardation were more influenced by factors extrinsic to the task, such as social and material rewards provided by adults. The implication of the findings on extrinsic motivation is that children with mental retardation (who are extrinsically motivated) may encode and attend to different features of a task situation because of their extrinsic goals.

It also appears that goal orientation can be manipulated as a function of the task or learning situation (Koestner, Zuckerman, & Olsson, 1990). Attempts to extend these findings to children with retardation have not been completely successful. When using fairly brief verbal induction of orientations very similar to ego and task orientations, Koestner, Aube, Ruttner, and Breed (1995) found no effect on the puzzle-solving performance of children with mental retardation. Pickering (1995) found no effect on the memory performance of children with mental retardation. However, Koestner et al. did find that children who received the task oriented instructions reported more interest in the task than children who received the more ego oriented instructions. The mixed success of inducing ego versus task goals may be related to individual differences in state orientation. While it may be possible to induce action oriented thinking with such an induction, it may be difficult in the face of state oriented thinking for task related thinking to take hold. It may be in the unsuccessful case that the task motivation was introjected rather than internalized and accepted by the participants in the study.

Ryan et al. (1996) argued that self-determination and autonomous function are important contributors to mental health and well-being among people. Wehmeyer and Metzler (1995) found that people with mental retardation have little opportunity for self-determination. Furthermore, Wehmeyer,

Kelchner, and Richards (1996) found that people with mental retardation who were more self-determined tended to function better than those who were not. Hence, the link between mental health, well-being, and autonomous function appears to be true in people with mental retardation as well as in those without.

Taken together, there appear to be differences in performance between children with and children without retardation due to consistent differences in goal structures. There are also differences in goal structures within the population of people with mental retardation that lead them to be more internally or externally focused in their locus of causality for their behaviors (Switzky, 1997). Based on Kuhl's model, we might also add that autonomous functioning may be compromised by an extrinsic motivational orientation by inducing state dependent processing of goal related information. State dependent processing would then make it difficult for those individuals to self-regulate.

Beliefs About Control Among Persons With Mental Retardation. State related processing may also be related to the other area of research in mental retardation that has looked at cognitive processing and motivation, that is, the examination of beliefs about the controllability of performance. As noted by Skinner (1996) the concept of control has been used in a variety of ways, and the definitions of control often confound several factors. Most major conceptualizations of control refer, according to Skinner, to two elements: a sense of competence (one's ability or feeling of efficacy) and a sense of contingency (having the means to reach a goal). She noted that theories concerning control beliefs often confound these two constructs. Additionally, Skinner noted that not only are beliefs about control important, but so is the capacity that an individual has to control the believed cause. For example, a child may believe that effort can improve performance, but not see himself or herself as capable of that sustained effort. Although this has not been explored by Skinner or others, the notion that perhaps state related processing may be one reason why individuals may discount their effort as a reason for success or failure. For example, individuals who perseverate on unfulfilled goals or are hesitant to act may believe that they are incapable of the sustained effort necessary to carry out a difficult task, even though they believe that effort can lead to success. In some pilot work, the authors found a relationship between capacity beliefs and state orientation in college students. State oriented students were less likely to believe that they had the capability to control attributed causal variables such as effort. Research in mental retardation has examined a variety of control beliefs. Research has examined competence beliefs such as self-esteem and self-efficacy, student theories about intelligence, attributions about ability and effort in task performance, and the degree to which individuals believe that outcomes are related to controllable versus uncontrollable causes.

Skinner (1995) developed a questionnaire that assesses control beliefs. Her scale includes control beliefs, strategy beliefs, and capacity beliefs. Control beliefs refer to a person's belief that he or she can reach a certain goal (e.g., I can do well in school). Strategy beliefs (similar to attributions discussed above) refer to the means deemed necessary to reach a certain goal (e.g., To do well I must try hard), and capacity beliefs refer to one's perceived access to the strategies (e.g., I can try hard in school). Using the Skinner questionnaire, Turner (1996) reported that children and adolescents with mild mental retardation had lower capacity beliefs for effort, ability, and luck than children without retardation.

Turner (1998) reported that the ability and effort beliefs of 11- and 17-year-olds with mild and moderate mental retardation were related to persistence on a memory task. This relation held when age and IQ were controlled, indicating that these beliefs are distinct from intellectual ability. In an experimental manipulation, Hoffman and Weiner (1978) found that the performance of adults with mental retardation increased when their previous success was attributed (by the experimenter) to the participant's ability. Attributing success to effort did not result in significant performance increases. On the other hand, Turner, Dofny, and Dutka (1994) reported that experimenter attributions of improvements to the participant's effort were related to improved performance when combined with strategy training. Children with mild mental retardation who received strategy training combined with attributional training (which focused on the importance of effort) were more likely to generalize the trained strategy than were their peers who received only strategy training or only attribution training. The success of the combined training strategy-attribution training over either component individually makes it clear that strategy use and beliefs are intricately related and should be addressed in tandem.

In several studies of children's beliefs, the focus was on whether outcomes were attributed to internal or external factors. In most of these studies, children were asked to indicate which cause (internal or external) was important. This tells us little about children's beliefs in their ability to control outcomes because internal factors (e.g., effort and ability) often differ in their perceived controllability. However, these studies set the stage for the later, more detailed analyses.

Wehmeyer (1994) reported that adolescents with mental retardation attributed outcomes more to external factors than did a group of adolescents identified as at-risk for school problems. MacMillan (1969) focused specifically on attributions for failure and found that when children were prevented from completing a task, children with mental retardation blamed themselves for the noncompletion, whereas the children without mental retardation blamed the noncompletion on the external force that stopped them from working on the task. Similarly, Chan and Keogh (1974) found that boys with mental retardation were likely to attribute failure to internal causes and success to external causes. If these beliefs are related to behavior in the same ways for children with mental retardation as they are for children without mental retardation, the implications for behavior are quite negative. The attribution of success to external causes indicates that the child is not taking credit for the success and that the success will likely not increase future expectations for success (because it was caused by someone else). The implications of the attributions of failure to internal causes are less clear: If failure is attributed to effort, the implication would be to try harder next time, but if it is attributed to ability, there may be no apparent way to improve in the future.

In studies that have examined attributions of outcomes to effort and ability separately, it appears that children with retardation are less effort-oriented than their peers without retardation. Koestner et al. (1995) reported that young adolescents with mild mental retardation were less likely to attribute failure to effort than were elementary school children without retardation (an approximate mental-age-matched group). Similarly, Haleet al. (1989) reported that children with mild mental retardation attributed academic outcomes to effort less than their chronologically age matched peers. Also, Turner (1996) reported that children and adolescents with mild to moderate mental retardation rated effort as less important for academic outcomes than did children without retardation. It appears from the work cited that children with retardation are less effort oriented than their peers. However, the research findings are not completely consistent: Weisz (1979) reported similarities between children with and without retardation on their attributions of failure to effort.

Another program of research that focuses on effort versus ability is Dweck's work on the malleability of ability. Dweck (1986) reported that children differ in the degree to which they see intelligence as malleable. Some children (incremental theorists) see intelligence as something that grows and develops from effort and experience while others (entity theorists) see intelligence as stable and not amenable to change through effort. Children who hold an incremental theory of intelligence are likely to set learning goals and engage in achievement oriented behavior. In contrast, children with entity beliefs are likely to set performance goals and are at risk for developing learned helplessness if they have little confidence in their abilities. In an investigation with children with mild mental retardation, Hale et al. (1989) found that the children with mental retardation held stronger entity beliefs than did children without retardation of the same chronological age. Koestner et al. (1995) found that relative to approximate mental age matches, seventh and eighth graders with mental retardation were more likely to hold entity theories of ability.

This apparent tendency to undervalue effort and believe in an entity theory of intelligence has dramatic implications for the cognitive functioning and development of persons with mental retardation. We know that mastery related behavior supports cognitive development, whereas the tendency to undermine the importance of effort inhibits cognitive development. If the beliefs about effort are logically related to the expenditure of effort, children who see effort as relatively unimportant are likely to avoid challenging tasks, fail to persist, and fail to employ and modify learning strategies.

Additionally, without pursuit of challenge, children who devalue effort may not develop the metamotivational skills to maintain effortful behavior in the face of distractions. Additionally, devaluing of effort may lead the child to be more externally than internally regulated, thereby undermining the autonomous functioning of the motivational maintenance system. They will be controlled more by the externally cued, more automatic motivational system. In short they will not be able to pursue their own goals and intentions very effectively.

Effort beliefs are not the only ones that have the potential to impact learning and performance: Self-esteem (e.g., Harter, 1982) and self-efficacy (Bandura, 1993) may also impact children's achievement oriented behavior. The studies examining the self-esteem of children with mild mental retardation have resulted in contradictory findings (see Switzky, 1997, for a discussion); however, for the most part, it appears that students with mild mental retardation have a lower self-esteem (in at least some domains) than their peers without retardation (Chiu, 1990; Ford & Turner, 1994; Zigler, Balla, & Watson, 1972).

In Kuhl's model, self-esteem and self-efficacy variables seem to be precursors and outcomes of state versus action oriented processing of intentions. Ability attributions, as noted earlier, may have some impact on the perceived difficulty of enacting an intention. They also may have an impact on the commitment that one makes to pursuing an intention. Given low self-esteem, ability attributions, and the devaluing of effort, it is not surprising that people with mental retardation have deficits in autonomous functioning, and it is expected that future research is likely to find people with mental retardation to be more likely to engage in more state oriented versus action oriented processing of goals.

It is also not surprising based on Kuhl's theory that Hoffman and Weiner's attempts to simply change performance by suggesting that it was the individual's effort that led to successful performance failed. The attribution of effort was introjected rather than integrated with the self. That ability attributions of success made a difference in that study may be related to the social reinforcement associated with the suggested ability attribution. The success of Turner et al.'s (1994) combination of strategy training and with attribution training is consistent with Kuhl's theory in the sense that the training focused on action related cognitions (the strategy) and tied the strategy to the child's effort. The attribution was better integrated with the child's self-system and therefore was more generalizable. Kuhl's model also suggests that one needs to look at more than attributions. To increase autonomous functioning and the generalizability of strategy training, one needs to examine the amount of state related functioning that an individual engages in and increase their self-regulatory functioning. To do that means looking at ways to increase task related cognitions, planning, and positive affect associated with tasks.

Planning and Self-Regulation

An important consideration in Kuhl's model is how individuals deal with intentions. As noted above, individuals who are more state oriented tend to have difficulties in intentional processing. Kuhl and Kraska (1989) discussed the importance of specifying an intention to fulfilling it. Kuhl discussed problems in fulfilling what he labels *degenerated intentions* (vaguely specified plans for meeting goals). Hence, planning plays an important role in determining the successful fulfillment of an intention. There is a great deal of work (Gollwitzer, 1996; Mischel, 1996; Taylor & Pham, 1996) that suggests that specifying the means to goals (having a specific plan) can have a positive impact on the implementation of intentions and can facilitate the processing of information related to intentions. These researchers reported data from a variety of studies that find that when individuals have a plan: (a) information concerning a particular goal is more easily primed, (b) test performance can be improved, (c) the distracting effect of a competing goal object can be lessened, and (d) the individual will be more sensitive to environmental cues that can signal the potential to implement an intention. In short, having a specified plan can help in creating an *action orientation* toward completion of a goal. Gollwitzer (1996) argued that creating a plan can make the more effortful goal processing system work in a fashion much like the more automatic goal processing systems mentioned earlier.

Mental Retardation and Planning. Research on planning in people with mental retardation has largely focused on planning using more abstract problem solving tasks such as the Tower of Hanoi (e.g., Spitz, Minsky, & Bessellieu, 1985) by individuals with mild to moderate mental retardation. In general, the findings indicate that people with mental retardation do not seem to be able to plan as far ahead in solving such tasks as individuals without mental retardation (Spitz & Borys, 1984). If there are limitations in the abilities of people with mental retardation to plan ahead, then they are likely to be limited in their abilities to specify plans for more complex goals and would therefore be less likely to fulfill them.

One interesting note that Spitz et al. (1985) made from this research is that the amount of time spent planning the first move on the Tower of Hanoi was unrelated to successful performance in people with or without mental retardation. They suggest that it is the content of planning and task related cognitions that take place prior to making the first move, rather than the amount of time taken before the first move, that influences performance. Their suggestion is consistent with Kuhl's model in that state oriented people may be slow to act, may be caught up in preoccupation with past failures, and thus may take more time before acting, but are still ineffective in reaching a goal.

An important part to specifying a plan is having specific goals. There have been two lines of research that have explored goal setting in people with mental retardation. First, there is work in the behaviorist tradition that finds that training individuals with mental retardation to set goals has a positive effect on performance (e.g., Cole & Gardner, 1988; Moore , Agran, & Fodor-Davis, 1989). However, these investigations have not separated out why goal setting works. Consideration of planning processes and other volitional mechanisms suggested by Kuhl's model might provide further insight and perhaps lead to the development of other interventions.

One line of research that holds promise is work by Gollwitzer (1999). Gollwitzer showed in a variety of studies that by developing simple plans (what he calls implementations intentions) for when and how a goal will be attained that the probability of reaching a goal can be enhanced.

For example, a student might have as a goal the desire to complete a project. He or she is more likely to complete the project if he or she specifies times and places for working on the project. According to Gollwitzer, one advantage such simple implementation intentions have is that they specify when and how a goal will be attained. Thus, they take away the cognitive burden by specifying the appropriate situational cues for working on the goal. Having implementation intentions helps activate the appropriate schema for carrying out a task. Additionally, Gollwitzer also argued that implementation intentions can be used to help keep an individual on task in the face of distractions. For example, when working on a manuscript, an author may have the implementation intention that whenever the phone rings, he or she will let the answering machine pick it up and respond to messages later." Setting such an implementation intention helps eliminate one distraction that might take the writer off-task. We know of no research that has addressed this issue in relationship to people with mental retardation. One question that needs to be answered is whether people with mental retardation typically use implementation intentions. Another question of interest, given that implementation intentions enhance the probability of meeting goals, is whether training in implementation intentions can help people with mental retardation to be more self-regulated.

Goals and plans have also taken on more importance in the recent work of Borkowski and Thorpe (1994) who noted that underachieving children generally do not set long-term goals or have not well defined where they are going and what they want to do with their lives. Hence, they have little interest in pursuing academic work. The long-term plans people with mental retardation have for themselves may be important determinants of how much effort they put into schoolwork and whether they become more intrinsically interested in their schoolwork or have more introjected and external motivations for pursuing schoolwork.

Developmental and Contextual Determinants of Self Regulation

The discussion of Kuhl's model suggests that there are many complex processes associated with the development of self-regulation and that these processes are affective as well as cognitive in nature. Ryan et al. (1997) mentioned three different components that facilitate the development of autonomous functioning: opportunities for autonomy, opportunities to succeed at optimally challenging activities (showing competence), and opportunities for relatedness (supportive attachment to parents and other significant adults). The source for many of these components lies mostly in a secure relationship with caregivers and the degree of intersubjectivity experienced by the child and caregiver, that is, setting up the conditions such that a child feels comfortable to autonomously explore the world around him or her. Later, we outline some issues concerning whether people with mental retardation have such opportunities.

Opportunities for Autonomy and Relatedness. The desire to explore and engage in self-initiated activity originates in the early attachment between a child and his or her caregivers (Bretherton, 1985). Hence, early opportunities for autonomy depend upon the sense of relatedness experienced by children. The study of attachment relationships in children with mental retardation is complicated somewhat because it is difficult to identify many children with mental retardation at such early ages. Much of the work has involved an examination of children with Down syndrome (Cichetti, Ganiban, & Barnett, 1991). Work with children with Down syndrome has indicated that such children can develop secure attachments, but that the process is slowed somewhat by dampened levels of arousal and slower motor development (Cichetti et al., 1991). Borkowski et al. (1992) indicated that poor attachment may explain why children of teenage mothers are at risk for mental retardation and other developmental delays. Children who do not feel affectively positive and safe when exploring the world around them are less likely to learn about that world.

Central both to attachment and interest in exploring the environment is the affective system. It is important in Kuhl's theory as well. Kuhl (1994a) and Ryan et al. (1997) argued that that positive affect associated with a context is important to self-regulatory functioning and that negative affect, or lack of positive affect, is associated neurologically with a blocking of the activation of subsystems associated with self-regulation. Whitman, O'Callaghan, and Sommer (1997) argued that affect regulation is an important to optimal development. Whitman et al. (1997) noted that infants who have a difficult time in affect regulation are at risk for developmental delay. Likewise, some groups of developmentally delayed infants such as those with Down syndrome have difficulty in affect regulation. Some researchers have found that Down syndrome children have somewhat dampened affect and are more labile than normally developing children (Cichetti & Sroufe, 1978; Walden, Knieps, & Baxter, 1991). Hence, early difficulties in affect regulation may lead to later problems in self-regulation.

Opportunities to Succeed at Optimally Challenging Activities. Early in development, the presentation and sequencing of activities falls on parents and other caregivers so that they can provide an optimal level of challenge. This task involves sensitivities to the child's affect as he or she engages in activities and good observational skills to make sure the task can be understood by the child. The parent has to be sensitive to the child's "zone of proximal development" (Vygotsky, 1978). There is some evidence that parents of children at risk for developmental delay of the cultural-familial variety are less likely to structure the environment to optimize challenges for their children (e.g., poorer HOME scores, indicating a less stimulating home environment; Bradley and Caldwell, 1984). Likewise, there is evidence that some parents of children who have developmental delays are more likely be more directive and less contingent (Knieps, Walden, & Baxter, 1994) when engaging in a task with their young children (see Whitman et al., 1997, for a review). This overdirectedness may limit the opportunities for children to be autonomous and may present problems in providing children with experiences of optimal challenge that can lead to the development of a sense of competence. Changing such an interaction style is difficult, because it is not simply a function of the parents, but is often, as in Down syndrome, a complex result of the transactions between caregivers and children who are not as responsive to stimulation as normally developing children (e.g., Cichetti et al., 1991). However, there is evidence that when parents of children with Down syndrome allow their children to take the lead in interactions (act autonomously), their children are more likely to engage in further attempts at mastery (Harris, Kasari, & Sigman, 1994). For example, Harris et al. (1996) found that children with Down syndrome whose parents promote autonomous action are more likely to have larger vocabularies than more directive parents. Thus, there are both differences between children with mental retardation and children without mental retardation and differences among individuals with mental retardation.

Along with research on the origins of a preference for optimal challenge, there is a great deal of mental retardation research on mastery motivation that explores differences between the mastery motivation of children with mental retardation and of those without. Research and theory in the area of mastery motivation suggest that humans are motivated to master challenging situations. White (1959) suggested that humans have an intrinsic need to have an impact on their environment. He saw behaviors such as curiosity and exploration as expressions of this need. These behaviors reflect and support cognitive development.

There is a great deal of variability in the studies that focus on the mastery behaviors of children with mental retardation. The studies vary in age and developmental level of the participants, the type of toys used to elicit mastery, and the measurement of mastery. Even with these variations, a few things are clear. Children with developmental delays do engage in mastery behaviors (Hupp, 1995), these behaviors can be measured reliably (e.g., Hauser-Cram, 1996), they are distinct from perseveration (Hupp & Abbeduto, 1991), and they are related to some measures of parent behavior (Hauser-Cram, 1996).

The primary measures of mastery behaviors used in many of the studies include general exploration of objects, specific goal-related exploration of objects, and affect in response to producing an effect. It appears that children with developmental delays engage in mastery behaviors similar to their peers without developmental delays (Hauser-Cram, 1996). However, a few studies have reported interesting differences between children with and without developmental delays. Goodman (1981) reported that children with delays were less organized in their exploration than were children without delays who achieved similar levels of success on the task. Similarly, Rushkin, Mundy, Kasari, & Sigman (1996) reported that children with Down syndrome engaged in shorter strings of goal-oriented mastery behaviors than did their mental-age-matched peers. When investigating the mastery behaviors of older children with mental retardation, Harter and Zigler (1974) reported that the children with mental retardation were less mastery oriented than their mental-age-matched peers. In contrast, Mac Turk, Vietze, McCarthy, McQuiston, and Yarrow (1985) reported that young children with Down syndrome exhibited similar levels of persistence as their mental-age-matched peers, but varied in the organization of goal directed behaviors. Hupp (1995) even suggested that children with delays might perform slightly better than their mental-age-matched peers. It is likely that many of the differences in the mastery behaviors of children with and without retardation emerge as a function of age and experience. Children with a history of ample opportunities for developmentally appropriate mastery, coupled with caregiver support and reinforcement, may perform similarly or better than their mental-age-matched peers due to the greater amount of positive experiences. However, when children do not have these opportunities (because of their mental retardation), they may fall behind peers of the same mental age. This is a rather simplistic explanation and does not account for all of the data. As mentioned earlier, for some etiologies (e.g., Down syndrome), there may be physical attributes (e.g., muscle tone) and neurological complications (lower or heightened levels of arousal) that impede mastery behaviors and hence lead to lower rates of some mastery behaviors.

When comparing the affective response to success by children with and without delays, the findings seem to vary with subject population. Studies conducted with children with Down syndrome have indicated that children with Down syndrome show less goal-related positive affect than their mental-age-matched peers (e.g., Ruskin et al., 1994). In contrast, Hauser-Cram (1996) reported that children with nonspecified mild delays showed similar affect to their mental-age-matched peers. It is likely that the affect expressed in response to mastery is influenced by both the level of affective development and the previous attributional feedback received from important others (see the previous discussion).

The implications of mastery behaviors go far beyond the toys or situations that are being mastered. As children engage in mastery behaviors, they are gathering information that allows them to establish categories, develop schemas, and develop scripts. These early experiences require that the child assimilate new information into existing schemas and accommodate schemas to account for unanticipated stimuli and events. To master some tasks, the child must establish a goal, maintain that goal in working memory, and recognize when the goal is met. All of these activities provide opportunities for children to practice and develop their information processing skills and to develop confidence in their abilities.

Through experience with mastery attempts and feedback from important others, the child comes to see himself or herself as able or unable to control outcomes. As the child develops beliefs about his or her efficacy, these beliefs guide future behaviors. Research with school-age children has indicated that beliefs in one's ability to impact outcomes are related to persistence, seeking feedback, and seeking challenging tasks (Dweck, 1986). Children who see their behavior as affecting outcomes in positive ways are likely to engage in the behaviors necessary to master new situations. However, if it appears that behavior seldom leads to the desired goal, children are likely to remain passive and not pursue challenging situations.

Borkowski, Carr, Rellinger, and Pressley (1990) argued that motivational characteristics such as attributional beliefs, self-esteem, and self-efficacy are intimately related to information processing. Motivating beliefs are likely to promote activity with a task. This task-oriented activity provides numerous opportunities for the child to learn from a more accomplished peer or adult who may respond to the child's activity by providing a scaffold to support the child's activity and learning. This activity also provides opportunities for the child to learn about the task and to discover appropriate strategies for solving the task. Once the child becomes aware of the strategies for solving the task (through either exploration or instruction), it is the personal belief system that either energizes or inhibits strategic behavior. The child who believes that effort is important is more likely to employ the effort necessary to successfully execute the strategy. Effort and a sense of efficacy are also necessary for monitoring the effectiveness of strategies and adapting strategies to fit task demands. This connection between beliefs and strategic behavior is not a one-way street. Borkowski and colleagues argued that the relation of beliefs to behavior (e.g., strategy use and related performance) is a bidirectional relationship. The positive outcomes usually associated with effortful behaviors affirm the effort-related beliefs and sense of efficacy which in turn support future efforts and positive outcomes. For children with mental retardation, this relationship may be more precarious: If children expend their efforts on tasks that are not appropriate for their developmental level, their efforts may not result in success and this lack of success may undermine the beliefs in the importance of effort. Therefore, the child's cognitive level may put him or her at risk for failure and hence the development of beliefs that may undermine future task-related activities. If, on the other hand, children with mental retardation employ their efforts on tasks that are developmentally appropriate and receive supportive feedback, their efforts should be reflected in improved performance which then supports efficacy and effort beliefs.

CONCLUSIONS AND RECOMMENDATIONS

We have covered a great deal of ground in this chapter, considering everything from automatic processing to mastery motivation and attachment. Our coverage was so extensive because the problem of developing self-regulation requires consideration of a number of different types of cognitive and affective processing. Our goal was to think heuristically, so that information processing and motivation might be viewed from a different perspective than it has traditionally been examined. This is not to say that Kuhl's model is incompatible with other research. In fact, it helps to think about ways to elaborate research further. We now describe several agendas for research and intervention that are implied by our discussion.

Issues for Research

1. *Studies of How People with Mental Retardation Process Goals.* There is a growing body of research suggesting that people process goals differently than they do other types of information. We believe that some of the paradigms that have been used to study goals in normally developing people (e.g., priming of goal related information) could be easily adapted to people with mental retardation. It may be that people with mental retardation process goals differently than normally developing people. For example, they may have more difficulty deactivating goals they have failed to reach, thus compromising their abilities to self-regulate. They may also fail to develop implementation plans (Gollwitzer, 1999) to help increase the probability that they will meet goals.

2. Studies of State Versus Action Orientation in People With Mental Retardation.   Both Kuhl's scale measuring the different elements of state versus action orientation and direct measures of state versus action oriented thinking processes (e.g., self-talk when carrying out a task) would provide evidence whether Kuhl's construct can explain variability both among different people with mental retardation and between those with and without mental retardation. Kuhl's account of learned helplessness as a function of state related thinking as well as attributional beliefs would also be interesting to test. Finally, it would be important in such an endeavor to explore Kuhl's ideas in light of other theoretical ideas about motivation and information processing. For example, does state oriented processing explain variance that cannot be explained by the constructs of intrinsic motivation or by attributions? Thus, studies that compare the relative predictability of these new constructs in relation to others that have been examined is worthwhile. The motivational literature is cluttered with very similar sounding constructs; hence, the study of the predictability of multiple constructs is important to establishing the validity of this new perspective.

3. Studies of Metamotivation.   There has been very little attempt to examine strategies used by people with mental retardation to keep themselves on task. While it is difficult to study metamotivation because of the lack of verbal ability in people with mental retardation, it is not impossible. In fact, the measures that Kuhl and Kraska (1989) used were pictorial rather than necessarily verbal in nature. One could set up situations where metamotivational choices could be made. For example, to study attention control, the child is asked to choose a place to study. One place is noisy and the other is quiet. The choice the child makes could be used to code whether the child is using a metamotivational skill.

In addition, several simple paradigms exist for studying the ability of children to self-regulate when faced with temptations to veer off task. For instance, Mischel (1996) used a paradigm where a child can get a more attractive prize if he or she waits for a longer period of time. The child has to forgo a less attractive, but tempting, prize that he or she can have right away. Mischel used this paradigm with preschoolers to study strategies that children use to stay on task. We know of no attempt to use this paradigm to study children with mental retardation.

4. Studies of Planning.   In Kuhl's theory, the importance of planning is emphasized in leading to the actual carrying out of an intention. Further, poorly specified plans are less likely to be implemented, leading to state orientation and its accompanying disruption of self-regulation. Aside from Spitz et al.'s (1985) work, there has been little consideration of planning in research on mental retardation. Studies of everyday planning and studies of the quality of plans generated by people with mental retardation in order to reach goals would be an important means to learn about why people with mental retardation fail to meet goals. Also important is whether part of the planning process involves implementation intentions.

5. Studies of Groups With Specific Etiologies.   Given the neurological basis for some of the work reported by Kuhl (1994a), it would be interesting to explore how different etiological groups that have different underlying neurological deficits will vary in their processing of goals and intentions. For example, individuals with Smith-Magenis syndrome (Van Haneghan, Switzky, & Baxter, 1998), who have a genetic defect at Chromosone 17, have difficulty with sequential processing of information (Dykens, 1994). Could these sequential processing deficits be related to underlying problems in the neurological systems controlling self-regulation? Likewise, problems in arousal and affect systems may undercut brain systems responsible for self-regulation in children with Down syndrome (Cichetti et al., 1991).

6. Studies That Continue to Show Appreciation of Situational and Individual Differences Among Individuals With Mental Retardation.   The focus on different etiologies points out that people with mental retardation are not a uniform population and that generalizations about people with mental retardation have to be tempered by an appreciation for situational and individual differences. A good example of this comes from recent research by Baroody (1996) on the spontaneous development of arithmetic strategies by children with mental retardation. Children given the opportunity to practice sums were more likely to develop shortcut strategies than children who were not given such an opportunity. Baroody noted that the spontaneous development of strategies for solving simple addition problems belies the general belief that people with mental retardation are passive learners. His research suggests that given the appropriate context to facilitate self-regulation, such children can learn for themselves. Hence, researchers must be careful in making attributions about those with mental retardation without examining the context of their functioning.

7. Integration of Neuropsychological, Cognitive, and Behavioral Perspectives. Kuhl and his colleagues have attempted to explore the neuropsychological links of his construct of state versus action orientation to prefrontal lobe functioning. Surprisingly, mental retardation research has been slow to link neuropsychological functioning to different patterns of self-regulatory, behavioral, or cognitive functioning. Part of the issue has been that identifying specific neurological dysfunctions of people with mental retardation has been difficult. Additionally, some of the failure may have been related to the culture of mental retardation research that focused on group comparisons. Regardless of the cause, more research needs to seriously consider patterns of neuropsychological functioning in individuals with mental retardation.

8. More Studies of the Link Between Early Affect Regulation, Mastery, and Attachment With Later Self-Regulatory Functioning. A great deal of research and theoretical ideas point to early affective development as a crucial element in the development of styles of self-regulation in later life. Studies that link particular problems in early affective development with difficulties in later cognitive, social, and affective development will help provide a focus for intervention as well as research. As noted in the beginning of this chapter, those who take an organizational view of development have provided researchers with a number of tools for examining early developments. More work is needed to explore self-regulatory functioning later in childhood and in adult life.

Implications for Intervention

The three themes discussed by Ryan et al. (1997) provide an important standard for examining interventions with people with mental retardation. As noted above, there is evidence that opportunities for autonomy, competence, and relatedness are sometimes lacking in the environments of children with mental retardation. While the difficulties in theses areas are multiply determined and not simply a function of the caregiver's style, that does not preclude working with caregivers to help promote transactions with the child that support autonomy, competence, and relatedness.

Likewise, special education services that provide for these three factors will also support autonomous functioning. It is important to note also that the promotion of these three objectives does not preclude the use of external reinforcement in education and training. However, it does suggest that caregivers and teachers look at the nature of reinforcement in such a way that the child accepts the value of the externally reinforced activity. That is, it is important that the perceived locus of causality be internal and not introjected if one wants to increase self-regulation. Many individuals argue that because of many years of control by external reinforcement, people with mental retardation do not act autonomously. Kuhl's theory provides a starting point for thinking about what researchers can do to help facilitate situations where autonomous functioning rather than reaction to reinforcement is more likely in people with mental retardation. If researchers can succeed in this endeavor, then the independent functioning and quality of life of people with mental retardation can be improved.

REFERENCES

Anderson, J. R. (1983). *The architecture of cognition.* Cambridge, MA: Harvard University Press.

Balla, D., Styfco, S. J., & Zigler, E. (1971). Use of the opposition concept and outerdirectedness in intellectually-average, familial retarded, and organically retarded children. *American Journal of Mental Deficiency, 75,* 663–680.

Bandura, A. (1993). Perceived self-efficacy in cognitive development and functioning. *Educational Psychologist, 28,* 117–148.

Bargh, J. A. (1990). Auto-motives: Preconscious determinants of social interaction. In E. T. Higgins & R. M. Sorrentino (Eds.), *Handbook of motivation and cognition: Foundations of social behavior* (Vol. 2, pp. 93–130). New York: Guilford Press.

Barkely, R. A. (1997). Behavioral inhibition, sustained attention, and executive functions: Constructing a unifying theory of ADHD. *Psychological Bulletin, 121,* 65–94.

Baroody, A. J. (1996). Self-invented addition strategies by children with mental retardation. *American Journal on Mental Retardation, 101,* 72–89.

Borkowski, J. G., Carr, M., Rellinger, E., & Pressley, M. Self-regulated cognition: Interdependence of metacognition, attributions, and self-esteem. In B. Jones & L. Idol (Eds.), *Dimensions of thinking and cognitive instruction* (pp. 53–92). Hillsdale, NJ: Lawrence Erlbaum Associates.

Borkowski, J. G., & Thorpe, P. K. (1994). Self-regulation and motivation: A life-span perspective on underachievement. In D. H. Schunk & B. J. Zimmerman (Eds.), *Self-regulation of learning and performance: Issues and educational applications* (pp. 45–73). Hillsdale, NJ: Lawrence Erlbaum Associates.

Borkowski, J., Whitman, T., Wurtz Passino, A., Rellinger, E., Sommer, K., Keogh, D., & Weed, K. (1992). Unraveling the new morbidity: Adolescent parenting and developmental delays. In N. Bray (Ed.), *International review of mental retardation* (Vol. 18, pp. 159–196). San Diego, CA: Academic Press.

Bradley, R., & Caldwell, B. (1984). 174 children: A study of the relationship between home environment and cognitive development during the first 5 years. In A. Gottfried (Ed.), *Home environment and early cognitive development* (pp. 5–54). Orlando, FL: Academic Press.

Bray, N. W., Turner, L. A., & Hersch, R. E. (1985). Developmental progressions and regressions in the selective remembering strategies of EMR individuals. *American Journal of Mental Deficiency, 90,* 198–205.

Bretherton, I. (1985). Attachment theory: Retrospect and prospect. In I. Bretherton & E. Waters (Eds.), Growing points of attachment theory and research. *Monographs of the Society for Research in Child Development, 50* (1–2, Serial No. 209), 3–35.

Campione, J. C., Brown, A. L., & Ferrara, R. A. (1982). Mental retardation and intelligence. In R. J. Sternberg (Ed.), *Handbook of human intelligence* (pp. 392–490). New York: Cambridge University Press.

Cha, K. H., & Merrill, E. C. (1994). Facilitation and inhibition in visual selective attention processes of individuals with and without mental retardation. *American Journal on Mental Retardation, 98,* 594–600.

Chan, K.S., & Keogh, B.K. (1974). Interpretation of task interruption and feelings of responsibility for failure. *Journal of Special Education, 8*(2), 175–178.

Chapman, M. (1984). Intentional action as a paradigm for developmental psychology: A symposium. *Human Development, 27,* 113–114.

Chiu, L. (1990). Self-esteem of gifted, normal, and mild mentally handicapped children. *Psychology in the Schools, 27,* 263–268.

Cicchetti, D., & Beeghly, M., (Eds.). (1990). *Children with Down syndrome: A developmental perspective.* New York: Cambridge University Press.

Cicchetti, D., & Ganiban, J. (1990). The organization and coherence of developmental process in infants and children with Down's syndrome. In R. M. Hodapp, J. A. Burack, & E. Zigler (Eds.), *Issues in the developmental approach to mental retardation* (pp. 169–225). New York: Cambridge University Press.

Cicchetti, D., Ganiban, J., & Barnett, D. (1991). Contributions for the study of high-risk populations to understanding the development of emotion regulation. In J. Garber & K. A. Dodge (Eds.), *The development of emotion regulation and dysregulation* (pp. 15–48). New York: Cambridge University Press.

Cicchetti, D., & Sroufe, L. A. (1978). An organizational view of affect: Illustration from the study of Down's Syndrome infants. In M. Lewis & L. A. Rosenblum (Eds.), *The development of affect* (pp. 309–350). New York: Plenum Press.

Cole, P. G., & Gardner, J. (1988). Effects of goal-setting on the discrimination learning of children who are retarded and children who are nonretarded. *Education and Training in Mental Retardation, 23,* 192–201.

Diener, C. I., & Dweck, C. S. (1978). An analysis of learned helplessness: Continuous changes in performance, strategy, and achievement cognitions following failure. *Journal of Personality and Social Psychology, 36,* 451–462.

Dulaney, C. L., & Ellis, N. R. (1997). Rigidity in the behavior of mentally retarded persons. In W. E. McLean, Jr. (Ed.), *Ellis' handbook of mental deficiency, psychological theory, and research* (3rd ed., pp. 175–195). Mahwah, NJ: Lawrence Erlbaum Associates.

Dweck, C. S. (1986) Motivational processes affecting learning. *American Psychologist, 41,* 1040–1048.

Dweck, C. S. (1996). Implicit theories as organizers of goals and behavior. In P. M. Gollwitzer & J. A. Bargh (Eds.), *The psychology of action: Linking cognition and motivation to behavior* (pp. 69–90). New York: Guilford Press.

Dweck, C. S., & Leggett, E. L. (1988). A social-cognitive approach to motivation and personality. *Psychological Review, 95,* 256–273.

Dykens, E. (1994, Summer). Behavioral and cognitive profiles in SMS. *Spectrum, 1*(2), 7.

Elliot, A. J., & Harackiewicz, J. M. (1996). Approach and avoidance achievement goals and intrinsic motivation: A mediational analysis. *Journal of Personality and Social Psychology, 70,* 461–475.

Elliott, E. S., & Dweck, C. S. (1988). Goals: An approach to motivation and achievement. *Journal of Personality and Social Psychology, 54,* 5–12.

Feuerstein, R. (1980). *Instrumental enrichment: An intervention program for cognitive modifiability.* Baltimore: University Park Press.

Ford, S.K., & Turner, L.A. (1994). *Self-esteem of adolescents with mental retardation.* Unpublished manuscript, University of New Orleans, New Orleans, LA.

Gollwitzer, P. M. (1996). The volitional benefits of planning. In P. M. Gollwitzer & J. A. Bargh (Eds.), *The psychology of action: Linking cognition and motivation to behavior* (pp. 287–312). New York: Guilford Press.

Gollwitzer, P. M. (1999). Implementation intentions: Strong effects of simple plans. *American Psychologist, 54,* 493–503.

Goodman, J.F. (1981). The lock box: A measure of psychomotor competence and organized behavior in retarded and normal preschoolers. *Journal of Consulting and Clinical Psychology, 49*(3), 369–378.

Graham, S., & Golan, S. (1991). Motivational influences on cognition: Task involvement, ego involvement, and depth of information processing. *Journal of Educational Psychology, 83,* 187–194.

Hale, C.A., Turner, L.A., & Borkowski, J.G. (1989, March). *Attributional beliefs in mildly retarded adolescents.* Paper presented at the Gatlinburg Conference on Mental Retardation, Gatlinburg, TN.

Harris, S., Kasari, C., & Sigman, M. D. (1996). Joint attention and language gains in children with Down syndrome. *American Journal of Mental Retardation, 100,* 608–619.

Harter, S. (1982). The perceived competence scale for children. *Child Development, 53,* 87–97.

Harter, S., & Zigler, E. (1974). The assessment of effectance motivation in normal and retarded children. *Developmental Psychology, 10,* 169–180.

Hauser-Cram, P. (1996). Mastery motivation in toddlers with developmental disabilities. *Child Development, 67,* 236–248.

Haywood, H. C., & Switzky, H. N (1986). Intrinsic motivation and behavioral effectiveness in retarded persons. In N. Ellis & N. Bray (Eds.), *International review of research in mental retardation* (Vol. 14, pp. 1–46). New York: Academic Press.

Haywood, H. C., & Switzky, H. N. (1992). Ability and modifiability: What, how, and how much? In J. S. Carlson (Ed.), *Advances in cognition and educational practice: Theoretical issues: Intelligence, cognition, and assessment* (Vol. 1, Part A, pp. 25–85). New York: Academic Press.

Heckhausen, H., & Beckman, J. (1990). Intentional action and action slips. *Psychological Review, 97,* 36–48.

Hoffman, J., & Weiner, B. (1978). Effects of attributions for success and failure on the performance of retarded adults. *American Journal of Mental Deficiency, 5,* 449–452.

Hupp, S. C. (1995). The impact of mental retardation on motivated behavior. In R. H. McTurk & G. A. Morgan (Eds.), *Mastery motivation: origins, conceptualizations, and applications* (pp.221–236). Norwood, NJ: Ablex.

Hupp, S. C. & Abbeduto, L. (1991). Persistence as an indicator of mastery motivation in young children with cognitive delays. *Journal of Early Intervention, 15,* 219–225.

Jagacinski, C. M., & Nicholls, J. G. (1984). Conceptions of ability and related affects in task involvement and ego involvement. *Journal of Educational Psychology, 76,* 909–919.

Knieps, L. J., Walden, T. A., & Baxter, A. (1994). Affective expressions of toddlers with and without Down syndrome in a social referencing context. *American Journal of Mental Retardation, 99*, 301–312.

Koestner, R., Aube, J., Ruttner, J., & Breed, S. (1995). Theories of ability and the pursuit of challenge among adolescents with mild mental retardation. *Journal of Intellectual Disability Research, 39*, 57–65.

Koestner, R., Zuckerman, M., & Olsson, J. (1990). Attributional style, comparison focus of praise, and intrinsic motivation. *Journal of Research in Personality, 24*, 87–100.

Kounin, J. S. (1941). Experimental studies of rigidity: I. The measurement of rigidity in normal and feeble-minded persons. *Character and Personality, 9*, 251–272.

Kruglanski, A. W. (1996). Goals as knowledge structures. In P. M. Gollwitzer & J. A. Bargh (Eds.), *The psychology of action: Linking cognition and motivation to behavior* (pp.599–618). New York: Guilford Press.

Kuhl, J. (1981). Motivational and functional helplessness: The moderating effect of state vs. Action orientation. *Journal of Personality and Social Psychology, 40*, 155–170.

Kuhl, J. (1986). Motivation and information processing: A new look at decision making, dynamic conflict, and action control. In E. T. Higgins & R. M. Sorrentino (Eds.), *Handbook of motivation and cognition : Foundations of social behavior* (pp. 404–434). New York: Guilford Press.

Kuhl, J. (1992). A theory of self-regulation: Action versus state orientation, self-discrimination, and some applications. *Applied Psychology, 41*, 95–173.

Kuhl, J. (1994a). A theory of state and action orientations. In J. Kuhl, & J. Beckmann (Eds.), *Volition and personality: Action versus state orientation* (pp. 9–46). Seattle: Hogrefe & Huber.

Kuhl, J. (1994b). Action versus state orientation: Psychometric properties of the action control scale (ACS-90). In J. Kuhl, & J. Beckmann (Eds.), *Volition and personality: Action versus state orientation* (pp. 47–60). Seattle: Hogrefe & Huber.

Kuhl, J. (2000). A functional-design approach to motivation and self-regulation: The dynamics of personality systems interactions. In M. Boekaerts, P.R. Pintrich, & M. Zeidner (Eds.), *Self-regulation: Directions and challenges for future research* (pp. 111–207). San Diego, CA: Academic Press.

Kuhl, J., & Eisenbeiser, T. (1986). Mediating versus meditating cognitions in human motivation: action control, inertial motivation, and the alienation effect. In J. Kuhl & J. W. Atkinson (Eds.), *Motivation, thought, and action* (pp. 288–306). New York: Praeger.

Kuhl, J., & Kraska, K. (1989). Self-regulation and metamotivation: Computational mechanisms, development, and assessment. In R. Kanfer, P. L. Ackerman, & R. Cudek (Eds.), *Abilities, motivation, and methodology: The Minnesota Symposium on individual differences* (pp. 343–374). Hillsdale, NJ: Lawrence Erlbaum Associates.

Levine, H. G., & Langness, L. L. (1985). Everyday cognition among mildly retarded adults: An ethnographic approach. *American Journal of Mental Deficiency, 90,* 18–26.

MacMillan, D. L. (1969). Motivational differences: Cultural-familial retardates vs. normal subjects on expectancy for failure. *American Journal of Mental Deficiency, 74*(2), 254–258.

MacTurk, R. H., Vietze, P. M., McCarthy, M. E., McQuiston, S., & Yarrow, L. J. (1985). The organization of exploratory behavior in Down Syndrome and nondelayed infants. *Child Development, 56,* 573–581.

Merighi, J., Edison, M., & Zigler, E. (1990). The role of motivational factors in the functioning o f mentally retarded individuals. In R. M. Hodapp, J. A. Burack, E. Zigler, Eds., *Issues in the developmental approach to mental retardation* (pp. 114–134). New York: Cambridge University Press.

Merrill, E. C., Cha, K-H., & Moore, A. L. (1994). The inhibition of location information by persons with and without mental retardation. *American Journal on Mental Retardation. 99,* 207–214.

Merrill, E. C., Goodwyn, E. H., & Gooding, H. L. (1996). Mental retardation and the acquisition of automatic processing. *American Journal on Mental Retardation, 101,* 49–62.

Merrrill, E. C., & Peacock, M. P. (1994). Allocation of attention and task difficulty. *American Journal on Mental Retardation. 98,* 588–593.

Merrill, E. C., & Taube, M. (1996). Negative priming and mental retardation: The processing of distractor information. *American Journal on Mental Retardation. 101,* 63–71.

Mischel, W. (1996). From good intentions to willpower. In Gollwitzer, P. M. & Bargh, J. A. (Eds). *The psychology of action: Linking cognition and motivation to behavior.* (pp. 197–218). New York: The Giolford Press.

Moore, S. C., Agran, M., & Fodor-Davis, J. (1989). Using self-management strategies to increase the production rates of workers with severe handicaps. *Education and Training in Mental Retardation, 24*, 324–332.

Mundy, P., & Kasari, C. (1990). The similar-structure hypothesis and differential rate of development in mental retardation. In R. M. Hodapp, J. A. Burack, E. Zigler (Eds.), *Issues in the developmental approach to mental retardation* (pp. 71–92). New York: Cambridge University Press.

Nicholls, J. G. (1984). Achievement motivation: Conceptions of ability, subjective experience, task choice, and performance. *Psychological Review, 91*, 328–346.

Pickering, S.L. (1995). *Relationships of ego and task instructions, attributional beliefs, and self-esteem to cognitive performance of students with mental retardation.* Unpublished masters thesis, University of South Alabama, Mobile, AL.

Ruskin, E. M., Mundy, P. Kasari, C., & Sigman, M. (1994). Object mastery motivation of children with down syndrome. *American Journal on Mental Retardation, 98*, 499–509.

Ryan, R. M., Kuhl, J., & Deci, E. L. (1997). Nature and autonomy: An organizational view of social and neurobiological aspects of self-regulation in behavior and development. *Development and Psychopathology, 9*, 701–728.

Ryan, R. M., Sheldon, K. M., Kasser, T., & Deci, E. L. (1996). All goals are not created equal: An organizational perspective on the nature of goals and their regulation. In P. M. Gollwitzer & J. A. Bargh (Eds.), *The psychology of action: Linking cognition and motivation to behavior* (pp. 7–26). New York: Guilford Press.

Skaalvik, E. M. (1997). Self-enhancing and self-defeating ego orientation: Relations with task and avoidance orientation, achievement, self-perceptions, and anxiety. *Journal of Educational Psychology, 89*, 71–81.

Simon, H. A. (1994). The bottleneck of attention: Connecting thought to motivation. In W. D. Spaulding (Ed.), *Interactive views of motivation, cognition, and emotion. Nebraska Symposium on motivation* (Vol. 41, pp. 1–21). Lincoln, NE: University of Nebraska Press.

Skinner, E. A. (1995). *Perceived control, motivation, & coping.* Thousand Oaks, CA: Sage.

Skinner, E. A. (1996). A guide to constructs of control. *Journal of Personality and Social Psychology, 71*, 549–570.

Spitz, H. H., & Borys, S. V. (1984). Depth of search: How far can the retarded search through an internally represented problem space?

In P. H. Brooks, R. Sperber & C. McCauley (Eds.), *Learning and cognition in the mentally retarded* (pp. 333–358). Hillsdale, NJ: Lawrence Erlbaum Associates.

Spitz, H. H., Minsky, S. K., & Bessellieu, C. L. (1985). Influence of planning time and first-move strategy on Tow of Hanoi problem-solving performance of mentally retarded young adults and nonretarded children. *American Journal of Mental Deficiency, 90,* 46–56.

Sternberg, R. J. (1987). A unified theory of intellectual exceptionality. In J. D. Day & J. G. Borkowski (Eds.), *Intelligence and exceptionality: New directions for theory, assessment, and instructional practices* (pp. 135–172). Norwood, NJ: Ablex.

Switzky, H. N. (1997). Individual differences in personality and motivational systems in persons with mental retardation. In W. E. McLean, Jr. (Ed.), *'Ellis' handbook of mental deficiency, psychological theory, and research* (3rd ed. , pp. 343–377). Mahwah, NJ: Lawrence Erlbaum Associates.

Taylor, S. E., & Pham, L. B. (1996). Mental simulation, motivation, and action. In P. M. Gollwitzer & J. A. Bargh (Eds.), *The psychology of action: Linking cognition and motivation to behavior* (pp. 219–235). New York: Guilford Press.

Tomporowski, P. D., & Tinsley, V. (1997). Attention in mentally retarded persons. In W. E. McLean, Jr.(Ed.), *'Ellis' handbook of mental deficiency, psychological theory, and research* (3rd ed., pp. 219–244). Mahwah, NJ: Lawrence Erlbaum Associates.

Turner, L. A. (1996). Attributional beliefs of persons with mild mental retardation. In M. Lewis & M. W. Sullivan (Eds.), *Emotional development in atypical children* (pp. 149–159). Mahweh, NJ: Lawrence Erlbaum Associates.

Turner, L. A. (1998). Relation of attributional beliefs to memory strategy use in children and adolescents with mental retardation. *American Journal of Mental Retardation 103,* 162–172.

Turner, L. A., Dofny, E. M., & Dutka, S. (1994). Effects of strategy and attribution training on strategy maintenance and transfer. *American Journal on Mental Retardation, 98,* 445–454.

Van Haneghan, J. P., Switzky, H. N., & Baxter, A. (1998). Smith-Magenis Syndrome. In L. Phelps (Ed.), *A 'Practitioner's Handbook of Health Related Disorders in Children* (pp. 603–609). Washington, DC: American Psychological Association.

Vygotsky, L. S. (1978). *Mind in society: The development of higher psychological processes.* Cambridge, MA: Harvard University Press.

Walden, T. A., Knieps, L. J., & Baxter, A. (1991). Contingent provision of social information by parents of normally developing and delayed children. *American Journal on Mental Retardation, 96*, 177–187.

Wehmeyer, M. L. (1994). Perceptions of self-determination and psychological empowerment of adolescents with mental retardation. *Education and Training in Mental Retardation and Developmental Disability. 29*, 9–21.

Wehmeyer, M. L., Kelchner, K., & Richards, S. (1996). Essential characteristics of self-determined behavior of individuals with mental retardation. *American Journal on Mental Retardation, 100*, 632–642.

Wehmeyer, M. L., & Metzler, C. A. (1995). How self-determined are people with mental retardation? The National Consumer Survey. *Mental Retardation, 33*, 111–119.

Weiner, B. (1986). *An attributional theory of motivation and emotion.* New York: Springer-Verlag.

Weisz, J. R. (1979). Perceived control and learned helplessness among mentally retarded and nonretarded children: A developmental analysis. *Developmental Psychology, 15*, 311–319.

White, R.W. (1959). Motivation reconsidered: The concept of competence. *Psychological Review, 66*, 297–333.

Whitman, T. L., 'O'Callaghan, M., & Sommer, K. (1997). Emotion and mental retardation. In W. E. McLean, Jr.(Ed.), *'Ellis' handbook of mental deficiency, psychological theory, and research* (3rded., pp. 77–98). Mahwah, NJ: Lawrence Erlbaum Associates.

Yando, R. & Zigler, E. (1971). Outerdirectedness in the problem-solving of institutionalized and noninstitutionalized normal retarded children. *Developmental Psychology, 4*, 277–288.

Zeigarnik, B. W. (1968). On finished and unfinished tasks (W. D. Ellis, Trans.). In W. S. Sahakian (Ed.), *History of psychology: A source book in systematic psychology* (pp. 441–444). Itasca, IL: F. E. Peacock. (Reprinted from *A source book of gestalt psychology* by W. D. Ellis, Ed., 1938, New York: Harcourt Brace & World)

Zigler, E., & Balla, D. (1982). Rigidity—A resilient concept. In E. Zigler & D. Balla (Eds.), *Mental retardation: The developmental-difference controversy* (pp. 61–82). Hillsdale, NJ: Lawrence Erlbaum Associates.

Zigler, E., Balla, D., & Watson, N. (1972). Developmental and experiential determinants of self-image disparity in institutionalized and non-institutionalized retarded and normal children. *Journal of Personality and Social Psychology, 23*, 81–87.

8

A Sensitivity Theory of End Motivation: Implications for Mental Retardation

Steven Reiss

The Ohio State University Nisonger Center

The sensitivity theory of motivation analyzes complex human behavior into 16 elemental, motivational components. For example, I recently (Reiss, 2000) provided a theoretical analysis of how five meaningful areas of human life (romantic relationships, careers, parenting, sports, and spirituality) can satisfy all or nearly all of the 16 desires . The model also has been related to psychopathology (Reiss & Havercamp, 1996), applied behavior analysis (Reiss & Havercamp, 1997), and rare developmental disorders of genetic origin (Dykens & Rosner, 1999). In other words, the theoretical work has a potentially broad range of application for the underlying concepts. Although it seems unlikely that all or even most of the applications will be proved valid, at this point the theory is interesting for its heuristic value in putting forth new ideas and in stimulating new research. In this chapter, we will review the basic tenets of the model and take a look at three implications for research on mental retardation and developmental disabilities. The implications are self-determination, cooperative living, and dual diagnosis.

STATEMENT OF SENSITIVITY THEORY

Sensitivity theory provides an example of an individual psychology approach to motivation (Allport, 1937). The following is a formal statement of the theory.

Concepts and Definitions

A *motive*, or a *desire*, is a reason to instigate behavior. Motives are divided into *ends* and *means* (Aristotle, 1953). Ends are self-motivating or ultimate goals that people desire for no reason other than that they intrinsically value the goal. Examples of end motives include hunger, status, and power, all of which are sometimes intrinsically desired for no reason other than that is what people want. These goals are called ends because they can serve as the logical end of an explanation of purposeful behavior. Means are aimed at accomplishing intermediate goals that eventually lead to satisfying an end desire—means are not self-motivating and, in fact, are motivational only because they are connected to ends. For example, when a hungry person buys food, the purchase of the food is motivating only because it is an intermediate step toward satiating hunger.

Sensitivity theory is a theory of end motivation. That is, the 16 basic desires are end motives. Although other end motives might be recognized, they explain less behavior than those formally recognized by the theory.

Each end desire forms its own continuum between high and low motivation. *High motivation* implies that the desire in question is strong and is experienced frequently, whereas *low motivation* implies that the desire is weak and is experienced infrequently. For example, a person with high motivation for vengeance seeks out interpersonal competition and enjoys revenge more than most people. In contrast, a person with low motivation for vengeance may actively avoid competition and dislike seeking revenge, unless the provocation is substantial.

A *sensitivity* is a stable individual difference in the strength of an end motive. The most fundamental idea expressed in sensitivity theory is that the strength of universal motives varies from one person to the next. *Anxiety sensitivity*, which falls under the desire for tranquility, is the idea that anxiety is not equally motivating for

TABLE 8.1.
The 16 Fundamental Desires

Social contact	The desire for interaction with other people. Includes the desire for fun/pleasure.
Curiosity	The desire to explore or learn.
Honor	The desire to value one's parents and their heritage, morality, or religion.
Family	The desire to raise one's own children. (Does not include raising other people's children.)
Independence	The desire for self-reliance.
Power	The desire for influence including mastery, leadership, and dominance.
Order	The desire for a predictable environment. Includes the desire for cleanliness and ritual.
Idealism	The desire to improve society.
Status	The desire for social standing. (Includes a desire for attention.)
Vengeance	The desire to get even with others. (Includes the joy of competition.)
Romance	The desire for sex, beauty, and art.
Exercise	The desire to move one's muscles.
Acceptance	The desire for approval from others.
Tranquility	The desire to be free of anxiety, fear, or pain.
Eating	The desire for food (not included in this study.)
Saving	The desire to hoard (including desire to own.)

Note. In Reiss and Havercamp (1998), idealism was called citizenship, acceptance was called sensitivity to rejection, and tranquility was called sensitivity to aversive sensations.

all people (Reiss, Peterson, Gursky, & McNally, 1986). *Acceptance sensitivity* is the idea that individuals are not equally motivated to gain approval from others.

An *individual desire hierarchy* is a summary of a person's priorities among the 16 basic desires. The hierarchy shows which of the 16 basic desires are high (strongly experienced) and which are low (weakly experienced) for a particular person. Generally, the most important basic desires for explaining an individual's behavior are those that are unusually high or unusually low. Those basic desires that are neither high nor low are less important in explaining a person's behavior.

The 16 basic desires are assumed to be universally motivating but individuals differ in how strongly they are motivated by each desire. An *individual desire profile* indicates whether a person is high, average, or low for each of the 16 basic desires for a particular person. Sensitivity theory assumes that each person needs to satisfy his or her desires, or live in accordance with his or her desire profile, in order to have a high quality of life.

Research Identification of 16 Desires

Although many lists of basic desires have been proposed, what is different about the 16 basic desires is that they were developed empirically based on having surveyed large number of people about what is important in their lives. Nearly all other lists of basic motives were based on introspection (Plato, 1966), observations of animals (James, 1950; McDougall, 1926), or psychodynamic research (Murray, 1938).[1]

I began our research by developing a list of every end goal we could think of, consulting psychology textbooks for additional ideas (Reiss & Havercamp, 1998). I also asked colleagues and friends to look at our list and suggest ideas of their own. After about three months of generating a list, I had identified more than 400 possible end goals.

The next step was to pare the list down to 328 basic motives and values. I eliminated the redundancies and those motives that have relatively little psychological significance. For example, I

---

[1]The idea of identifying significant motives by asking people what it is they desire has been opposed by some theorists who have attacked the validity of all self-report measures. Although many self-report measures are problematical, categorical criticisms of these measures is invalid. Self-report measures of end motives, for example, represent a new type of test that appears to have significantly different qualities from traditional personality tests.

eliminated thirst because the desire to drink water does not explain much behavior even though it is essential for survival.

Susan Havercamp and I then asked a group of 401 adolescents and adults from diverse backgrounds to rate the importance of each goal on the list. This generated a large data set in which 401 people rated 328 end goals. These data then were submitted to a series of factor analyses. We found that 15 categories explained well the participants' ratings of the 328 end goals. Subsequently, a 16th category (saving) was added to the list based on theoretical considerations, and the list of 16 desires was demonstrated in a confirmatory factor analysis with an independent sample.

Having identified 16 basic categories of end goals, we interpreted each category psychologically and reviewed the relevant research literatures. Our list was similar to lists of instinctual motives previously published by William James in 1890 (1950) and by William McDougall (1926). Both James and McDougall had argued that these desires have an evolutionary basis and are seen in nearly all people. Much of what people do can be attributed to one or more of these desires.

Havercamp (1998) set out to validate the 16 basic desires, as measured by our self-report instrument, called the Reiss Profile of Fundamental Goals and Motivational Sensitivities. She demonstrated that the instrument has sound psychometric properties, low social desirability, high concurrent validity, and excellent criterion validity. She showed that high scores for certain desires predicted choice of college major or career. For example, philosophers scored very high for curiosity, and soldiers scored very high for power. Havercamp concluded that the Reiss profile has a significant degree of validity.

We also studied the basic desires of people with mental retardation or developmental disabilities. This work showed similar results: People with mental retardation or developmental disabilities are driven by largely the same basic desires seen in the general population (Reiss & Havercamp, 1998). The main differences were as follows. Whereas the desire for attention is expressed by adults as a desire for social status, for people with mental retardation we see the primal desire for attention. Although Havercamp and I had interpreted only one factor for the desire for tranquility, we interpreted three for people with mental retardation or developmental disabilities, including the desires to avoid anxiety (tranquility 1), frustration or task demands (tranquility 2), and pain (tranquility 3). Whereas people without mental retardation or developmental disabilities show a basic desire for parenting, people with mental retardation or developmental disabilities instead showed a desire to help others. Idealism (concern about society) is not an important motive for people with mental retardation. We did not add savings to the list for people with mental retardation or developmental disabilities. Apart from these differences, the basic desires of people with mental retardation or developmental disabilities and those of everybody else are essentially the same.

Because self-report data become increasingly unreliable in people who have difficulty communicating, we developed a ratings instrument to assess the basic desires of people with mental retardation or developmental disabilities. The ratings instrument assesses behavior that either expresses a basic desire directly or is known to be correlated with a basic desire. In 1998, Havercamp and I (Reiss & Havercamp, 1998) showed that the Reiss Profile Mental Retardation or Developmental Disabilities ratings instrument has a 15–factor solution similar to that applicable to the Reiss Profile self-report instrument minus the saving scale. Since the 15 basic desires appear to have a genetic basis (they have evolutionary significance, are seen in nearly all people, and are seen in animals), it is not surprising that Havercamp and I were able to develop similar psychometric instruments for people with and without mental retardation or developmental disabilities. Both I (Reiss, 1999) and Dykens and Rosner (1999) presented validity data showing that the ratings instrument can be used to develop motivational profiles of various groups of people, such as people with autism or Prader-Willi syndrome.

The results of our research showed that people with mental retardation or developmental disabilities, and those without mental retardation or developmental disabilities, want the same things from life. In terms of happiness, they have the same needs all people have. Specifically, they need acceptance, family, stability, friends, mastery, independence, honor, learning, exercise, and attention, and they need to minimize anxiety, frustration, and pain. Social services must provide people with mental retardation or developmental disabilities opportunities and supports to obtain these goals or they may be unable to experience value-based happiness and even may become depressed.

Recently, I (Reiss, 2000b) expanded the sensitivity theory of human motivation into a comprehensive theory of meaningful behavior, including spirituality. My theory holds that all people with mental retardation or developmental disabilities embrace the same 16 basic desires or values (Reiss & Havercamp, 1997). Individuals differ, however, in how they prioritize these values. The theory assumes that these individual differences are much greater than had been assumed by previous psychologists and educators. When it comes to basic desires and values, one size does not fit all.

In (Reiss, 2000a), I assumed that psychological well-being, or *value-based happiness*, requires the general satisfaction of those basic desires that are most valued by a particular individual. For example, a sport-minded person must have a high diet of physical exercise in order to gain value-based happiness. In contrast, a person who places a high value on order must have a neat, clean, and orderly environment. The general idea is that value-based happiness does not require the complete satisfaction of all 16 basic desires and values, only the satisfaction of a person's five or six most important basic desires.

In (Reiss, 2000a), I related the 16 basic desires to religious sentiment in samples of college students, mental retardation service providers, and seminary students. Perhaps the most interesting finding was that religious people do not value self-reliance to the same extent as do nonreligious people; instead, they value interdependence (being able to rely on others to meet their needs). Generally, the results provided additional evidence of the validity of the 16 desires and their link to psychological factors associated with the experience of meaning.

The 16 Basic Desires

The following is the list of basic desires recognized by Reiss' sensitivity theory of motivation. Each of these desires is largely unrelated to all others. Each forms a continuum between high and low motivation. High motivation indicates that the desire is intensely and frequently experienced, whereas low motivation indicates that the desire is weak and infrequently experienced.[2]

Power is the desire to experience influence or what is sometimes called *self-efficacy* or *competence motivation*. This desire is commonly satisfied by achievement, leadership, or domineering behavior. When this desire is satisfied, people feel competent and influential. High power desire is associated with ambition, workaholism, or dominance; low power desire is associated with a lack of ambition or submission.

Independence is the desire for self-reliance or what is sometimes called *autonomy*. This desire is commonly satisfied by doing things on one's own without assistance from others. When this desire is satisfied, people feel free. People with high independence desire dislike needing others, whereas those with low independence desire enjoy being connected to others or a greater reality. Low independence desire is associated with romantic love.

Curiosity is the desire for truth or knowledge. This desire is commonly satisfied by exploration or learning. When the desire is fulfilled, people feel enlightened. High curiosity is associated with exploration, whereas low curiosity is associated with experiencing little interest in learning.

Physical exercise is the desire to move one's muscles. This desire is commonly satisfied by physical activity such as sports or vigorous work. When the desire is fulfilled, people feel fit. High physical exercise is associated with a need for activity, whereas low physical activity is associated with avoidance of physical activity.

Social contact is the desire for interaction with other people. The desire for play or fun falls under this desire because of the primal association between play and social contact. This desire is commonly satisfied by socializing with others through friendships, parties, clubs, or events. When this desire is satisfied, people have a sense of belonging. High social contact is associated with fun-loving behavior, whereas low social contact is associated with a desire for privacy and aloneness.

Vengeance is the desire to get even with others. This desire is commonly satisfied through participation in competitive activi-

---

[2]Strictly speaking, the theory is concerned with the strength of motivation, not with the frequency and strength of feelings.

ties, interpersonal competitiveness, or aggression. When this desire is satisfied, people feel vindicated. High vengeance is associated with aggressive behavior, whereas low vengeance is associated with peacekeeping behavior or kindness.

Honor is the desire to be loyal to one's parents, ethnic group, or heritage. It includes the desire to show character and behave morally, as defined by traditional codes of conduct. This is the desire that connects people to their parents and ancestors. The desire is most commonly satisfied by behaving in accordance with traditional codes of conduct, following ethnic or family tradition. When people behave honorably, they feel loyal and possibly righteous. High honor is associated with moralistic behavior and concern with character. Low honor is associated with unscrupulous behavior and a lack of loyalty.

Family is the desire to raise one's own children. It does not include a general desire for nuturance; it is limited to taking care of one's own. When this desire is satisfied, people experience love. High family desire is commonly satisfied by centering one's activities around one's children. Low family desire is commonly satisfied by not having children.

Order is the desire for a predictable environment. It includes the desire for cleanliness and ritual. It is commonly satisfied by rituals, traditions, cleanliness, and organizing activities. When this desire is satisfied, people feel that their lives are predictable. High order is associated with rule-governed and compulsive behavior, whereas low order is satisfied by preferences for disorganization, flexibility, and ambiguity.

Romance is the desire for sex, including the desire for beauty. It is commonly satisfied by romantic love. When this desire is experienced, people feel lust. High romance is associated with sensualism, whereas low romance is associated with asceticism.

Idealism is the desire to improve society. It is commonly satisfied by becoming involved in social causes. When this desire is satisfied, people feel that the world is just. High idealism is associated with humanitarian activities, whereas low idealism is associated with a lack of interest in societal affairs.

Status is the desire for social standing. (The desire for attention falls under this desire). When this desire is satisfied, people feel worthy and important. Status is most commonly satisfied by seeking wealth or prestige, such as wearing expensive clothes, living in exclusive neighborhoods, or joining exclusive clubs. People with high status are attentive to issues of class, wealth, and prestige. People with low status are inattentive to class, wealth, and prestige.

Acceptance is the desire for approval. When this desire is satisfied, people feel self-confident and happy. When the desire is frustrated, people feel insecure and unhappy. Acceptance is most commonly satisfied when parents accept their children. To a lesser extent, it can be satisfied by close friendships and intimate relationships. It is most commonly frustrated by parental rejection. High acceptance desire leads to concern with issues of criticism and rejection. Low acceptance desire suggests a high capacity to tolerate criticism and rejection.

Tranquility is the desire to be free of anxiety, frustration, or pain. It is associated with feelings of relaxation and calm. People with high tranquility tend to behave fearfully and experience anxiety frequently; those with low tranquility tend to be adventuresome.

Eating is the desire for food. It is commonly satisfied by preparing and consuming meals. People with high eating are attentive to food, whereas those with low eating are much less attentive to food than the average person. Eating is associated with feelings of hunger.

Saving is the desire to collect and own things. A high desire for saving is associated with hoarding, including hoarding money. People with a high desire to save hate wasting anything. A low desire for saving is associated with spendthrift behavior.

Implications for Mental Retardation

Sensitivity theory can help us understand what a person desires most in life. This information can be helpful in promoting self-determination and cooperative living and in diagnosing and treating challenging behavior.

Self-Determination. People with disabilities want greater control over their lives (Braddock, Hemp, Bachelder, & Fujiura, 1998, p. 13; Wehmeyer & Meltzler, 1995). In order to accomplish this goal, which is sometimes called *personal autonomy*, person-centered planners assess needs from the perspective of the individual. The aim is to identify essential lifestyles, or what each individual requires for happiness.

Sensitivity theory may help clarify how researchers should assist people with mental retardation or developmental disabilities in planning their own futures. Under sensitivity theory, personal autonomy is defined as the right to pursue the fundamental goals of one's life, as distinguished from someone else's fundamental goals. The aim of personal futures planning, therefore, should be to identify a person's most important life goals.

Directly asking people questions such as, "What do you want?" and "What goals are important to you?" often does not produce a valid answer. Many people are confused about their goals. Although effective planning must be based on a person's end goals, few people can tell others directly which goals are means and which are ends. For example, if a psychologist asks a person what their end goals are, odds are high they will not understand the question.

Suppose that at a young age—say at time of graduation from high school—you essentially had to develop your life plan. You had to decide where you would live, whom you would live with, what your occupation would be, and what your leisure activities might be. Think how easy it would be to make mistakes. You might think that owning an expensive car would make you happy—and maybe it would—but when you get the car you may become bored with it much faster than you had imagined. You might think that a rich sex life is the key to your happiness—and it may be for some people—but for many sexual interest wanes over the years and relationships based on little else end in bitter divorce. Consider how difficult it is for anyone to know what will make himself or herself happy, and then imagine how much more difficult it might be for a person with mental retardation who may not understand well how choices relate to outcomes.

The risk with personal futures planning is that people lock themselves into choices they later regret. This is a likely outcome in a government-funded system that cannot easily allow for changes in plans. When months or years are required for changes, people can become frustrated and depressed.

Sensitivity theory can help consumers and facilitators make choices likely to lead to enduring happiness. The theory provides a list of the 16 most basic motives that drive human behavior. Facilitators need to assess the five or six most important basic motives for any individual. Sensitivity theory implies that these motives need to be satisfied for a happy lifestyle. The remaining motives are less important to the happiness of the individual.

A three step process is suggested:

Step 1:   *Determine the consumer's two to six most important basic desires.* Administer the Reiss Profile Mental Retardation to parents and caregivers and compute the standardized scores. Interview parents, caregivers, and, if possible, consumers regarding all high or low scores. Look at the case history to get a sense of who this person is. Based on all this information, identify the two to six basic desires that differ most from the Reiss Profile norms or from the individual's peers. These are the most important basic desires for the individual. For example, the most important basic desires for a particular person might be high social contact, low order, and high tranquility. For another, it might be high family, high physical exercise, and high status (attention).

Step 2:   *Teach the consumer to understand how choices relate to the satisfaction of basic needs and desires.* Regarding each choice the consumer needs to make, show the consumer how various options are connected to satisfying the consumer's most important life goals. For example, if social contact is an important goal for a consumer, the facilitator would encourage the consumer to consider how the choice of various residential options or daily schedules might affect opportunities to socialize. If an individual has a strong desire for physical activity, the facilitator can assist the person in understanding this need when choosing a daily schedule.

Step 3.   *Choices are made by educated consumers.* Ask the consumer to make choices based on an understanding of what the consumer desires most (two to six most important end goals) and how various options may or may not satisfy those desires.

This approach encourages consumers to make choices based on their needs, rather than on impulses. Some person-centered planners have misunderstood autonomy as the right to act on any impulse one might experience. This is impulsiveness, not autonomy, and it does not lead to a happy lifestyle. Programs where people with mental retardation or developmental disabilities have been empowered to fire staff arbitrarily, to change their minds every day as to what they want to do, and to behave impulsively grant only the illusion of personal autonomy. True autonomy comes from the pursuit of a person's most important basic desires—of finding friends, jobs, adequate living arrangements, privacy, and so on.

Cooperative Living. Because of financial reasons, adults with mental retardation sometimes must share an apartment or house with others. Sometimes this works out well, but many instances occur in which people do not get along with each other. Thus, there is a need for planners and facilitators to take a closer look at what can be done to increase cooperative living among people sharing a common home, apartment, or room.

Sensitivity theory can help identify people who are likely or unlikely to get along. According to this theory, only compatible people can live together for any length of time. When people are basically compatible, over time their friendship should strengthen. When people are incompatible, however, it is only a matter of time before problems emerge and something has to be done in terms of intervention or reassignment. Thus, sensitivity theory holds that compatibility is the key to cooperative living.

Residential providers usually are given little guidance in assessing compatibility. No theory or conceptual system has been put forth to guide them in this endeavor. Few or no instruments have been developed to provide information for assigning people to cooperative living. Little training is available. It is basically a trial and error process that often works badly, posing significant limitations to the implementation of cooperative living.

Sensitivity theory offers a theoretical rationale and practical methods for assessing compatibility between two people assigned to live together in a small group home, house, or apartment. According to this theory, the principles of bonding and separation relate the 15 basic desires to the assessment of compatibility. These principles are as follows:

- *Principle of Bonding.* People get along best with those whose desire profile is similar to their own. When desire profiles are similar, people can use their relationship to satisfy their desires. For example, all other relevant factors being equal, two ambitious people (indicating high desire for power) are likely to appreciate each other. Similarly, two sociable people are likely to appreciate each other.
- *Principle of Separation.* People grow apart when their desire profiles are dissimilar. When desire profiles are dissimilar, people must go outside the relationship to satisfy their desires. For example, an ambitious person (indicating high power) is unlikely to appreciate a nonambitious person (indicating low power). A sociable person is unlikely to appreciate a private person.

According to sensitivity theory, the following four steps can be followed to assess compatibility of potential housemates:

1. For each consumer, determine the two to six most important basic desires. This can be done by (a) administering the Reiss Profile to parents and caregivers and computing the standardized scores; (b) interviewing parents, caregivers, and, if possible, consumers regarding all high or low scores; and (c) looking at the case history to get a sense of who this person is. Based on all this information, identify those basic desires for which the consumer has high or low motivation. (*High motivation* would be indicated by a standard score at least .7 above the norm, and *low motivation* would be indicated by a standard score .7 below the mean.)
2. Repeat Step 1 for each consumer who is considering the same apartment, house, or small group home.
3. Determine the *compatibility index* for each pair of individuals. Assign the pair a score of +1 for each match regarding important basic desires. A match is indicated either when both individuals are high for the same desire or when both are low for the same desire. For example, if high social contact is an important basic desire for both Susan and Judy, assign the

pair a score of +1. If both Susan and Judy have low order (indi-cating that they dislike structure, organization, and sched-ules), add +1 to the compatibility score. Repeat the process for each match. After you do this, assign a score of -3 to each mis-match. A mismatch is indicated when one person is high for a basic motive and the other is low. For example, if high social contact is one of the important life goals of Susan, but low social contact is one of the important life goals of Judy, they are mismatched on social contact, and a score of -3 is added to the total compatibility index. When assessing mismatches, ignore examples of one person having a high need and the other being average—look only at situations where one per-son is high (more than .7 *SD* above the norm) and the other is low (more than .7 *SD* below the norm) on a basic desire.

4. Using the compatibility index, all available information, what you know about the consumer, and the family's expressed wishes, do the best you can to match the most compatible people.

Dual Diagnosis.   Up to this point, we have seen how sensi-tivity theory can help facilitators with person-centered planning and with matching compatible people in cooperative living arrangements. We now consider a very different application of sensitivity theory, one that is aimed at understanding challenging behavior.

Sensitivity theory recognizes three causes of challenging behavior: aberrant contingencies, aberrant environments, and aberrant motivation (Reiss & Havercamp, 1996, 1997, 1998). The key to identifying the role of each cause in a particular case is the total amount of reinforcement associated with the behavior.

- *Aberrant contingencies* refer to the direct reinforcement of maladaptive behavior and are discussed extensively in the lit-erature on applied behavior analysis. When a problem behav-ior is caused primarily by aberrant contingencies, the individual receives about as much total reinforcement as peers. For example, suppose a teacher pays about as much attention to Tom as to the other children in the class, but for some reason Tom is more likely to be attended primarily when he misbehaves. Under these circumstances, the problem behavior is being directly reinforced by the teacher, so that extinction or reinforcement of incompatible behavior should constitute effective treatment.

- *Aberrant environments*, such as emotionally cold parents or large institutions, do not satisfy ordinary desires and psychological needs. The psychological effects of aberrant environments have been evaluated by developmental researchers (e.g., Zigler, 1971). When a problem behavior is caused primarily by an aberrant environment, the individual receives much less total positive reinforcement than do peers. For example, suppose that an uninvolved parent pays so little attention that a child becomes angry and rebellious. Under these circumstances, the problem behavior is caused by a nonnurturing environment, so that the parents need to change their attitude, or the child needs exposure to other adults, for effective treatment.

- *Aberrant motivation* refers either to a desire for excessive amounts of positive reinforcement or to intolerance of ordinary amounts of anxiety, frustration, or pain (hypersensitivity to aversive stimuli). When a problem behavior is caused primarily by aberrant motivation, the individual receives a very high amount of total reinforcement compared with peers. For example, suppose a teacher both pays attention to Tom when he misbehaves and, as a consequence, pays much more attention to Tom than to nearly all other children in the class. Under these circumstances, the problem behavior may be caused by Tom's seeking unusually high levels of attention. Neither extinction nor the direct reinforcement of incompatible behavior should constitute effective treatment because neither of these approaches can satisfy Tom's need for excessive amounts of attention. Instead, the therapist has to find some way to reduce Tom's desire for excessive amounts of attention. Since it is not clear how this can be done, Havercamp and I (Reiss & Havercamp, 1999) called for innovative approaches and relevant research into this question. Examples of aberrant motivation include children who are addicted to attention, adults who are addicted to sex, and adolescents who are hypersensitive to frustration or anxiety.

Of the three causes of aberrant behavior recognized in sensitivity theory, aberrant motivation is the most novel. People with aberrant motivation do not care about the same things most people care about, at least not to the same extent. Some people dress sloppy because they do not care about order. The behavior is not a result of reinforcement contingencies different from those experienced by neat people. Nor is the behavior a result of sloppy people not paying attention to social conventions or understanding the social value placed on neatness. The problem is that sloppy people do not care about (are not reinforced by) neatness. They do not enjoy neatness, they do not value neatness, and they even may feel uncomfortable when things are too neat or organized.

As recognized by Ellis (1993), disturbances in caring are common in many people with aberrant behavior. For example, some depressed people care so much about a lost loved object they no longer care about anything else. Some people with anxiety disorders care so much about the consequences of experiencing anxiety they no longer want to leave their homes. Some children with developmental disabilities care so much about attention they are willing to become problem children to get it.

Attention (which falls under the desire for status) is a good case in point. Children who care about attention much more than others are said to have a high need for attention. They require large amounts of attention before they satiate. Because these children are the ones that get the most attention, appropriate behavior rarely produces the amount of attention the child desires. In order to satisfy their high need for attention, the children develop conduct problems, because these behaviors offer the best chance the children have for obtaining high amounts of attention.

Applied behavior analysts treat aberrant behavior by modifying response-reinforcement relations. According to sensitivity theory, this may not be enough for an enduing treatment effect. With many aberrant behaviors, the problem is related to how much reinforcement the person desires, not just in what behavior is being reinforced. The individual shows aberrant behavior, not because it is reinforced, but because the person has learned that it leads to a high amount of reinforcement. Because applied behavior analysts do not even try to change the amount of reinforcement people desire, they often produce treatment effects that lack durability.

CONCLUSION

Sensitivity theory puts forth an individual psychology approach to the study of human motivation. Psychologists have primarily assumed that since everybody likes sex and dislikes anxiety, individual differences in the strength of such motives were unimportant for a general theory of human behavior. Indeed, it has taken more than a decade to establish the basic fact of anxiety sensitivity (Reiss et al., 1986; Taylor, 1999) or the idea that anxiety is not equally aversive to all people. Sensitivity theory holds that the key to understanding much of human behavior is individual differences in the most basic pleasures and displeasures of humankind.

Sensitivity theory is concerned with individual differences in 16 specific desires. What is unique about the specific list of desires is that it is based on empirical research with large numbers of people. No other theory of human motivation has put forth a comprehensive set of empirical findings of correlations among the basic desires of humankind. Other theories of motivation are based on speculation, psychodynamic analysis, ethnological research, or laboratory studies in which motives are studied piecemeal. Sensitivity theory represents a rare effort to study basic motivation from a comprehensive, psychometric perspective.

Although everybody is assumed to embrace the 16 basic desires, individuals differ in how they prioritize them. These priorities are called *individual desire hierarchies*. Sensitivity theory assumes that much of human behavior can be understood as an effort to satisfy a person's individual desire hierarchy.

In this chapter, we considered three diverse applications of sensitivity theory to the field of mental retardation or developmental disabilities. Assessment of individual desire hierarchies can help facilitators in person-centered planning identify what each person needs for a high quality of life. It can help facilitators assess compatibility of people being considered for cooperative living arrangements. It leads to a new approach to the study and treatment of dual diagnosis. At this point, readers should understand that these are mostly theoretical applications of the sensitivity approach and that much additional research is needed to test these applications.

REFERENCES

Allport, G. W. (1937). *Personality: A psychological interpretation.* New York: Holt.

Aristotle (1953). *The Nicomachean ethics.* New York: Penguin Books. (Original work published 330 BCE)

Braddock, D., Hemp, R., Bachelder, L., Fujiura, G. (1998). *The state of the states in developmental disabilities.* Washington, D.C.: American Association on Mental Retardation.

Dykens, E. M., & Rosner, B. A. (1999). Refining behavioral phenotypes: Personality—motivation in Williams and Prader-Willi syndromes. *American Journal of Mental Retardation, 114,* 158–169.

Ellis, A. (1993). Fundamentals of rational-emotive therapy for the 1990s. In W. Dryden & L. K. Hill (Eds.), *Innovations in rational-emotive therapy* (pp. 1–32). Newbury Park, CA: Sage.

Havercamp. S. H. (1998). *Reliability and validity of the Reiss profile of Fundamental Goals and Motivational Sensitivities.* Doctoral dissertation, Department of Psychology, The Ohio State University.

James, W. (1950). *The principles of psychology.* (Vol. 2). New York: Dover. (Original work published 1890)

McDougall, W. (1926). *An introduction to social psychology.* Boston: John W. Luce.

Murray, H. A. (1938). *Explorations in personality.* New York: Oxford University Press.

Plato (1966). *The republic* (F. M. Cornford, Trans.). New York: Oxford University Press. (Original work published 375 BCE)

Reiss, S. (1999). The sensitivity theory of aberrant motivation. In S. Taylor (ed)., *Anxiety sensitivity.* New York: Lawrence Erlbaum Associates.

Reiss, S. (2000a). Who am I: The 16 basic desires that motivate our actions and define our personalities. *Beyond pleasure and pain.* New York: Putnam.

Reiss, S. (2000b). Why people turn to religion: A motivational analysis. *Journal for the Scientific Study of Religion.*

Reiss, S., & Havercamp, S. H. (1996). The sensitivity theory of motivation: Implications for psychopathology. *Behavior Research and Therapy, 34,* 621–532.

Reiss, S., & Havercamp, S. H. (1997). The sensitivity theory of motivation: Why functional analysis is not enough. *American Journal of Mental Retardation, 101,* 553–566.

Reiss, S., & Havercamp, S. H. (1998). Toward a comprehensive assessment of functional motivation: Factor structure of the Reiss profiles. *Psychological Assessment, 10,* 97–106.

Reiss, S., & Havercamp. S.M. (1999). Sensitivity theory, functional analysis, and behavior genetics: A response to Freeman et al. *American Journal of Mental Retardation, 104,* 289–293.

Reiss, S., Peterson, R. A., Gursky, D. M., & McNally, R. J. (1986). Anxiety sensitivity, anxiety frequency, and the prediction of fearfulness. *Behaviour Research and Therapy, 26,* 341–345.

Taylor, S. (1999). *Anxiety sensitivity: Theory, research, and treatment.* Mahwah, N.J.: Lawrence Erlbaum Associates.

Wehmeyer, M. L., & Meltzler, C. A., (1995). How self-determined are people with mental retardation? The national consumer survey. *Mental Retardation, 32,* 111–119.

Zigler, E. (1971). The retarded child as a whole person. In H. E. Adams & W. K. Broadman (Eds.), *Advances in experimental clinical psychology* (pp. 47–121). New York: Pergamon Press.

Author Index

Tidman, M., 81
Tinsley, V., 326, 329, 331, 334, 339
Tomassone, J., 59
Tomc, S.A., 303
Tomporowski, P.D., 326, 329, 331, 334, 339
Tonge, B.J., 303
Trabasso, T., 185
Treasure, J., 297
Trent, J.W., Jr., 4
Tsunematsu, N., 268
Tuddenham, R.D., 7
Turner, L.A., 320, 336, 339, 346, 348, 349
Turnure, J.E., 38, 217
Twohig, P.T., 114
Tymchuk, A.J., 223, 224, 233
Tzuriel, D., 59, 77, 85, 87, 88, 94, 107, 111, 112, 113, 114, 117, 118

U

Udwin, O., 261, 302
Upshure, C.C., 268
Urv, T., 199
Utman, C.H., 97

V

Van Acker, R., 293
Van den Berghe, H., 283
Van Haneghan, J.P., 360
Vaughn, S.R., 224
Vaught, S., 85, 87, 88, 94, 107, 113
Verplanken, B., 205
Vida, S., 301
Vietze, P.M., 295, 355
Vinogradov, S., 296
Volkmar, F.R., 271, 289, 295, 301, 302, 306
Von Neumann, J., 205, 220
Vygotsky, L.S., 354

W

Wachs, T.D., 88
Wagner, S., 299, 300
Waite, R., 73, 74
Walden, T.A., 354
Walker, T.G., 182
Walzer, S., 306
Wang, P., 302
Ward, M.J., 155
Wardell, B., 301
Warren, A.C., 300
Warren, B., 171
Watson, M., 296, 301
Watson, N., 60, 64, 73, 349
Weaver, J., 30, 88, 93, 100
Weed, K., 353
Wehmeyer, M.L., 119, 148, 158, 160, 161, 166, 167, 168, 169, 170, 171, 174, 178, 179, 180, 181, 185, 186, 209, 213, 215, 216, 223, 225, 226, 234, 241, 344, 347, 382
Weinberg, R.A., 185
Weiner, B., 59, 60, 68, 69, 70, 333, 346
Weiss, L., 305
Weisz, J.R., 78, 212, 274, 348
Wenig, B., 171
Werlinsky, B., 42, 78
Werner, H., 152, 203
Wessels, K., 81
West, M.D., 171
Wheeler, D., 173
Whidden, E., 293
Whisler, J.S., 59, 70
White, R., 33, 60, 75, 76, 82, 154, 218, 355
Whitman, B.Y., 258, 353, 354
Whitman, T.L., 163
Whitsell, N., 76, 214

Subject Index

For Product Safety Concerns and Information please contact our EU
representative GPSR@taylorandfrancis.com
Taylor & Francis Verlag GmbH, Kaufingerstraße 24, 80331 München, Germany

www.ingramcontent.com/pod-product-compliance
Ingram Content Group UK Ltd.
Pitfield, Milton Keynes, MK11 3LW, UK
UKHW021427080625
459435UK00011B/186